Individualized Therapy of Hypertension

FUNDAMENTAL AND CLINICAL CARDIOLOGY

1. *Drug Treatment of Hyperlipidemia*, edited by Basil M. Rifkind
2. *Cardiotonic Drugs: A Clinical Review, Second Edition, Revised and Expanded*, edited by Carl V. Leier
3. *Complications of Coronary Angioplasty*, edited by Alexander J. R. Black, H. Vernon Anderson, and Stephen G. Ellis
4. *Unstable Angina*, edited by John D. Rutherford
5. *Beta-Blockers and Cardiac Arrhythmias*, edited by Prakash C. Deedwania
6. *Exercise and the Heart in Health and Disease*, edited by Roy J. Shephard and Henry S. Miller, Jr.
7. *Cardiopulmonary Physiology in Critical Care*, edited by Steven M. Scharf
8. *Atherosclerotic Cardiovascular Disease, Hemostasis, and Endothelial Function*, edited by Robert Boyer Francis, Jr.
9. *Coronary Heart Disease Prevention*, edited by Frank G. Yanowitz
10. *Thrombolysis and Adjunctive Therapy for Acute Myocardial Infarction*, edited by Eric R. Bates
11. *Stunned Myocardium: Properties, Mechanisms, and Clinical Manifestations*, edited by Robert A. Kloner and Karin Przyklenk
12. *Prevention of Venous Thromboembolism*, edited by Samuel Z. Goldhaber
13. *Silent Myocardial Ischemia and Infarction: Third Edition*, Peter F. Cohn
14. *Congestive Cardiac Failure: Pathophysiology and Treatment*, edited by David B. Barnett, Hubert Pouleur, and Gary S. Francis
15. *Heart Failure: Basic Science and Clinical Aspects*, edited by Judith K. Gwathmey, G. Maurice Briggs, and Paul D. Allen

16. *Coronary Thrombolysis in Perspective: Principles Underlying Conjunctive and Adjunctive Therapy*, edited by Burton E. Sobel and Désiré Collen
17. *Cardiovascular Disease in the Elderly Patient*, edited by Donald D. Tresch and Wilbert S. Aronow
18. *Systemic Cardiac Embolism*, edited by Michael D. Ezekowitz
19. *Low-Molecular-Weight Heparins in Prophylaxis and Therapy of Thromboembolic Diseases*, edited by Henri Bounameaux
20. *Valvular Heart Disease*, edited by Muayed Al Zaibag and Carlos M. G. Duran
21. *Implantable Cardioverter-Defibrillators: A Comprehensive Textbook*, edited by N. A. Mark Estes III, Antonis S. Manolis, and Paul J. Wang
22. *Individualized Therapy of Hypertension*, edited by Norman M. Kaplan and C. Venkata S. Ram
23. *Atlas of Coronary Balloon Angioplasty*, Bernhard Meier and Vivek K. Mehan

ADDITIONAL VOLUMES IN PREPARATION

Cholesterol Lowering: Clinical and Population Aspects, edited by Basil Rifkind

Individualized Therapy of Hypertension

edited by

Norman M. Kaplan and C. Venkata S. Ram

The University of Texas
Southwestern Medical Center at Dallas
Dallas, Texas

Marcel Dekker, Inc. New York • Basel • Hong Kong

Library of Congress Cataloging-in-Publication Data

Individualized therapy of hypertension / edited by Norman M. Kaplan
and C. Venkata S. Ram.
p. cm. — (Fundamental and clinical cardiology ; 22)
Includes bibliographical references and index.
ISBN 0-8247-9262-9 (alk. paper)
1. Hypertension—Treatment. I. Kaplan, Norman M.
II. Ram, C. Venkata S. III. Series: Fundamental and clinical
cardiology ; v. 22.
[DNLM: 1. Hypertension—therapy. W1 FU538TD v.22 1995 / WG 340
I397 1995]
RC685.H8I44 1995
616.1'3206—dc20
DNLM/DLC
for Library of Congress 94-28741
CIP

The publisher offers discounts on this book when ordered in bulk quantities. For more information, write to Special Sales/Professional Marketing at the address below.

This book is printed on acid-free paper.

MARCEL DEKKER, INC.
270 Madison Avenue, New York, New York 10016

Current printing (last digit):
10 9 8 7 6 5 4 3 2 1

Printed in the United States of America

Series Introduction

Marcel Dekker, Inc., has focused on the development of various series of beautifully produced books in different branches of medicine. These series have facilitated the integration of rapidly advancing information for both the clinical specialist and the researcher.

My goal as editor of the Fundamental and Clinical Cardiology series is to assemble the talents of world-renowned authorities to discuss virtually every area of cardiovascular medicine. In the current monograph, *Individualized Therapy of Hypertension*, Drs. Kaplan and Ram have edited a much needed and timely book. Future contributions to this series will include books on molecular biology, interventional cardiology, and clinical management of such problems as coronary artery disease and ventricular arrhythmias.

SAMUEL Z. GOLDHABER

Preface

At first glance, it may be hard to justify yet another book on the treatment of hypertension. However, this book is unique in that it provides complete coverage of the concept of individualized therapy, the approach that is now being increasingly advocated and practiced. Moreover, it is written by leading authorities in each area that impacts on the individualization of therapy.

Some of these authors have views that are not shared by the editors. But, rather than censor or modify them (in itself a foolhardy and dangerous task), the editors have asked only that each author defend his or her opinion with hard evidence. Therefore, what you have before you is not a cookbook of untested recipes, but a tried and tested set of guidelines that should help in providing the best care for our hypertensive patients.

NORMAN M. KAPLAN and C. VENKATA S. RAM

Contents

Contributors

Michael H. Alderman, M.D. Chairman, Department of Epidemiology and Social Medicine, Albert Einstein College of Medicine, Bronx, New York

Phyllis August, M.D. Associate Professor, Department of Obstetrics and Gynecology, Cornell University Medical College, New York, New York

Henry R. Black, M.D. Chairman, Department of Preventive Medicine, Rush Presbyterian–St. Luke's Medical Center, Chicago, Illinois

Robert J. Cody, M.D. Professor of Medicine and Assistant Division Director, Research Affairs, Department of Internal Medicine, The Ohio State University Medical Center, Columbus, Ohio

John J. Curtis, M.D. Professor of Medicine and Surgery, Department of Medicine, University of Alabama at Birmingham, Birmingham, Alabama

William C. Cushman, M.D., F.A.C.P. Professor, Department of Medicine and Preventive Medicine, University of Tennessee College of Medicine, Memphis, Tennessee

Tomasz Grodzicki, M.D., Ph.D. Department of Gerontology and Family Medicine, Jagiellonian University, Cracow, Poland

R. Brian Haynes, M.D., Ph.D., F.R.C.P.C., F.A.C.P. Professor, Department of Clinical Epidemiology and Medicine, McMaster University, Hamilton, Ontario, Canada

Robert J. Heyka, M.D. Medical Director, West Side Dialysis Center, Department of Hypertension/Nephrology, Cleveland Clinic Foundation, Cleveland, Ohio

Norman M. Kaplan, M.D. Professor of Internal Medicine, and Chief, Hypertension Division, University of Texas Southwestern Medical Center at Dallas, Dallas, Texas

Iris R. Keys, M.D. Assistant Professor, Hypertension Division, Department of Medicine, University of Maryland, Baltimore, Maryland

Marshall D. Lindheimer, M.D. Professor, Departments of Medicine, Obstetrics, Gynecology, and Clinical Pharmacology, University of Chicago, Chicago, Illinois

Franz H. Messerli, M.D. Professor of Medicine, Department of Hypertension, Ochsner Clinic, New Orleans, Louisiana

Olaf B. Paulson, M.D. Professor, Department of Neurology, University Hospital, Rigshospitalet, Copenhagen, Denmark

C. Venkata S. Ram, M.D. Clinical Professor, Hypertension Division, Department of Internal Medicine, University of Texas Southwestern Medical Center at Dallas, Dallas, Texas

Elijah Saunders, M.D. Associate Professor and Head, Hypertension Division, Department of Medicine, University of Maryland, Baltimore, Maryland

Sheldon G. Sheps, M.D. Professor of Medicine and Chair, Mayo Medical School, and Division of Hypertension, Mayo Clinic and Mayo Foundation, Rochester, Minnesota

Svend Strandgaard, M.D. Consultant Physician, Department of Medicine and Nephrology B, Herley Hospital, Herley, Denmark

Donald G. Vidt, M.D. Professor of Medicine, Ohio State University, and Senior Physician, Department of Nephrology and Hypertension, Cleveland Clinic Foundation, Cleveland, Ohio

Myron H. Weinberger, M.D. Director, Hypertension Research Center, and Professor, Department of Medicine, Indiana University School of Medicine, Indianapolis, Indiana

William F. Young, Jr., M.D. Associate Professor of Medicine, Mayo Medical School, and Divisions of Endocrinology, Hypertension, and Internal Medicine, Mayo Clinic and Mayo Foundation, Rochester, Minnesota

1

The Need for a New Approach

NORMAN M. KAPLAN

University of Texas Southwestern Medical Center at Dallas
Dallas, Texas

It has been more than 30 years since the treatment of the nonmalignant forms of hypertension became feasible. During this time, antihypertensive therapy has changed dramatically, in large measure reflecting the availability of a steadily enlarging supply of equally effective but more easily tolerated drugs. For the first decade, the 1960s, all that were available were diuretics, a few adrenergic inhibitors (reserpine, guanethidine, methyldopa), and the direct vasodilator hydralazine. They were often given in a stepwise manner that became stylized as the "diuretic-first, stepped care" approach.

In the 1970s, attempts were made to provide therapy more directly tailored to the individual patient's pathophysiology, in particular, the renin profile. Starting in the mid-1980s with the availability of a rapidly expanding list of drugs (Table 1), the concept of individualized therapy surfaced and has been increasingly advocated. This book is designed to explore the underpinnings of that concept and to provide practical guidelines for the clinical application of individualized therapy.

At the onset, recognition should be given to the continued divergence of opinions by experts in the field. Two examples will serve:

1. The 1993 report of the Joint National Committee (JNC-5), composed of 15 U.S. authorities, stated: "Because diuretics and β-blockers have

Table 1 Antihypertensive Drugs Available in the United States

Volume depleters	Adrenergic inhibitors		Vasodilators
Diuretics	Peripheral	Beta-receptor	Direct
Thiazides	Guanadrel	Acebutolol	Hydralazine
Chlorthalidone	Guanethidine	Atenolol	Minoxidil
Indapamide	Reserpine	Betaxolol	Calcium blockers
Metolazone	Central	Bisoprolol	Amlodipine
Loop diuretics	Clonidine	Carteolol	Diltiazem
Bumetanide	Guanabenz	Metoprolol	Felodipine
Furosemide	Guanfacine	Nadolol	Isradipine
Torasemide	Methyldopa	Penbutolol	Nicardipine
K^+ Savers	Alpha-receptor	Pindolol	Nifedipine
Amiloride	Doxazosin	Propranolol	Verapamil
Spironolactone	Prazosin	Timolol	ACE inhibitors
Triamterene	Terazosin	Combined alpha and beta	Captopril
		Labetalol	Enalapril
			Lisinopril
			Ramipril
			Benzepril
			Fosinopril
			Quinapril

been shown to reduce cardiovascular morbidity and mortality in controlled clinical trials, these two classes of drugs are preferred for initial drug therapy" (1).

2. The 1993 memorandum from a World Health Organization/International Society of Hypertension (WHO/ISH) committee composed of 13 authorities from around the world stated, "The choice of the initial drug therapy of an individual hypertensive patient is a challenge for the physician and should not be restricted, on theoretical or economic grounds, to any one or two of the various classes of drugs that have been tested so far" (2).

I. WHY THE CONTINUED CONTROVERSY

With as many drugs and authorities as are available, uniformity is hardly expected. But two major issues remain unresolved: first, when to start antihypertensive drug treatment; second, which drug to choose for initial and subsequent therapy.

A. When to Start Drug Therapy

Here again, the JNC-5 report (1) and the WHO/ISH memorandum (2) exemplify the issue. JNC-5 states: "If blood pressure remains at or above 140/90 mm Hg during a 3- to 6-month period despite vigorous encouragement of life-style modifications, antihypertensive medications should be started, especially in individuals with target organ damage (TOD) and/or other known risk factors for cardiovascular disease (CVD)."

The 1993 WHO/ISH memorandum is more conservative (Figure 1), advocating drug therapy if the diastolic pressure is 95 mm Hg or above with the proviso that "drug treatment should be considered for such patients [whose diastolic pressure remains between 90 and 95 mm Hg] who are at high risk."

Lest these two recommendations seem to be only a little apart, remember that 40% of the entire population with hypertension, defined by a diastolic pressure of 90 mm Hg or higher, are in the 90 to 95 mm Hg range (3). Therefore, the JNC-5 position recommends drug therapy for millions of patients who likely would not be treated by the WHO/ISH criteria.

In reality, both JNC-5 and the 1993 WHO/ISH memorandum are closer than the previous reports from the two groups published 4 to 5 years before (4,5). Both of the 1993 reports give additional emphasis to go beyond just the level of blood pressure in making the decision, bringing the existence of both target organ damage and other cardiovascular risk factors into the equation.

An even more forceful and structured presentation of the need to consider more than the level of blood pressure has been presented by a group of authorities from New Zealand (6). They start with examples of the need to consider the absolute risk of developing cardiovascular disease based on overall risk status:

> For example, of 100 women aged 60 with mildly raised blood pressure but no other important risk factor for cardiovascular disease, 10 at most are likely to have a major cardiovascular event (stroke, myocardial infarction, or coronary death) in the next 10 years. Thus 90% of the women would remain free of the disease for the 10 years. Most current clinical guidelines for the management of raised blood pressure, however, are based largely on blood pressure while other risk factors affecting absolute risk, although they are considered, are given less emphasis. This means that a 60 year old woman with diastolic blood pressure of 100 mm Hg but no other risk factor—an absolute risk of cardiovascular disease of about 10% in 10 years—may meet the criteria for treatment whereas a 70 year old man with multiple risk factors but a diastolic blood pressure of 95 mm Hg—an absolute risk of about 50% in 10 years—may not.

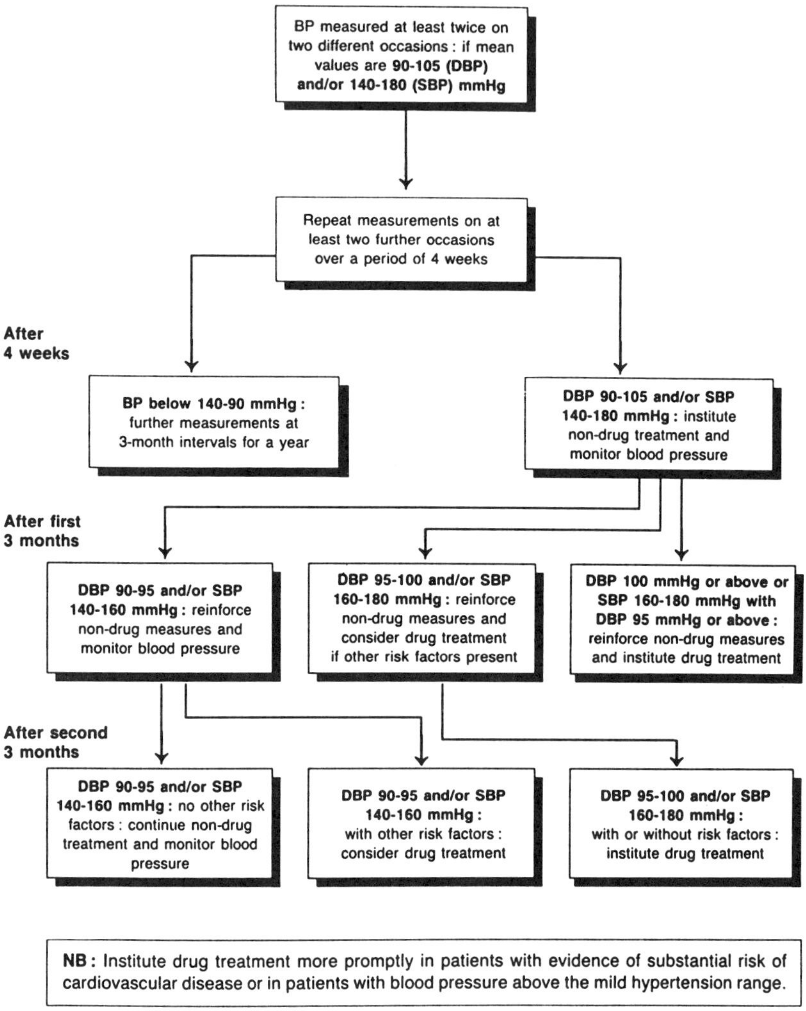

Figure 1 A flow diagram for the definition and management of mild hypertension. DBP, diastolic blood pressure; SBP, systolic blood pressure. (From Ref. 2.)

The New Zealand authors provide a list of the relevant risk factors (Table 2) and then incorporate the number of these risk factors along with various levels of blood pressure in men and women to indicate that "patients with a blood pressure of 150–170 mm Hg systolic or 90–100 mm Hg diastolic, or both, should be given treatment to lower blood pressure if the risk

Table 2 Features Considered in the Decision to Treat

Other risk factors
Cigarette smoking
Total cholesterol/high-density lipoprotein (HDL) cholesterol ratio > 6
Diabetes
Obesity (BMI > 30)
Family history of premature cardiovascular disease (in parent or sibling before age 55)
Symptomatic cardiovascular disease
Angina or silent ischemia
Myocardial infarction
Coronary angioplasty or bypass surgery
Heart failure
Left ventricular hypertrophy by electrocardiogram or echocardiogram
Transient ischemic attacks
Stroke
Peripheral vascular disease
Familial hyperlipidemia
Other target organ damage such as renal disease

Source: Ref. 6.

of a major cardiovascular disease event in 10 years is more than about 20%" (Figure 2).

The concept of determining the need for therapy on the basis of overall risk is developed further in Dr. Alderman's chapter (Chapter 2).

B. Which Drug to Choose

Once having decided upon the need to start drug therapy, the practitioner must choose from among the eight major classes listed in Table 1, usually a single drug as monotherapy for all but a relatively few with such severe hypertension as to require multiple agents from the onset (see Chapter 12).

As noted in JNC-5 (1) and echoed by "official" groups in England (7), Canada (8), and New Zealand (6), a diuretic or a beta-blocker is given preference by most but not all (2). In general, only these two classes are considered for initial therapy along with alpha-blockers, the alpha-beta blocker, calcium blockers, and angiotensin-converting enzyme (ACE) inhibitors. Neither the peripheral nor the central-acting adrenergic inhibitors nor the direct vasodilators are included because of their greater propensity to cause bothersome side effects.

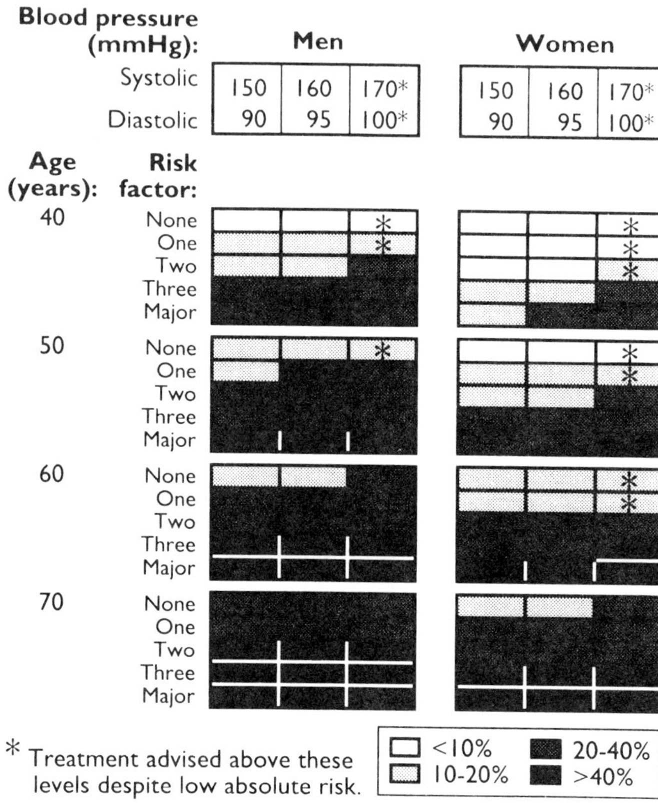

Figure 2 Guidelines for the treatment of hypertension based upon the approximate 10 year risk of a cardiovascular disease event per 100 patients. (From Ref. 6.)

1. Not a Matter of Efficacy

The choice of drug should not be based upon overall efficacy. By the nature of the approval process mandated by the U.S. Food and Drug Administration and most national regulatory agencies, all drugs approved for oral therapy of hypertension must meet the criterion of lowering the blood pressure by about 10% in the majority of patients (9). Therefore, the drugs are formulated to provide equivalent effect overall.

Proof of such equivalency comes from the Treatment of Mild Hypertension Study (TOMHS), which carefully followed a total of 902 patients who were randomly allocated to a placebo or a drug from one of five major classes (10). At the end of 48 months, the average fall in blood pressure with moder-

Table 3 Changes at 48 Months for TOMHS Participants

	Chlorthalidone	Acebutolol	Doxazosin	Enalapril	Amlodipine	Placebo
Systolic BP	−14.6	−13.9	−13.4	−11.3	−14.1	−8.6
Diastolic BP	−11.1	−11.5	−11.2	−9.7	−12.2	−8.6
Echo LV mass (g)	−34	−24	−24	−23	−25	−27
HDL/Total Cholesterol	1.4	1.2	2.6	1.9	1.5	1.2
% remaining on initial Rx	67	78	66	68	82	1.2

Source: Ref. 10.

ate doses of each drug was quite similar for all (Table 3). With all five drugs, similar rates of patient acceptance and side effects were noted. The side effects differed as expected and were not onerous with any drug.

On the other hand, individual patients differ in their responsiveness to different drugs. This differential responsiveness is partly based on demographic factors, as nicely documented in a Veterans Administration Cooperative Study (11). In this study involving over 1200 hypertensive men, about 200 were each randomly assigned to a drug from one of six major classes or a placebo. Although only 41% completed the 1 year trial on the same monotherapy that was initially prescribed, the results document rather impressive differences in the response rate of the patients as characterized by age (younger or older) and race (black or white) (Figure 3). As seen in the fig-

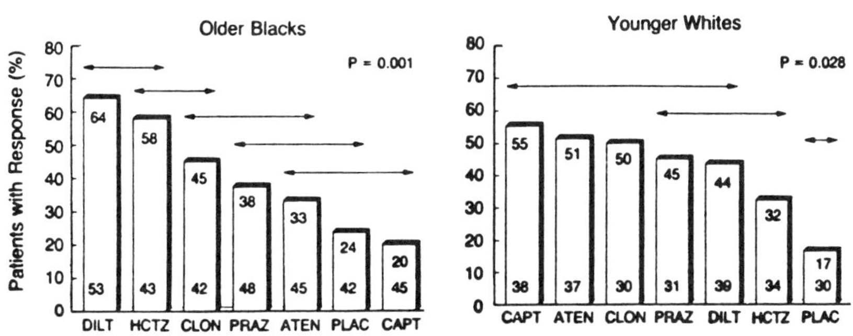

Figure 3 The percentage of good responders in the younger white and older black patients in a Veterans Administration Cooperative Study given a placebo or one of six antihypertensive drugs, each representative of a major class of agents. (From Ref. 11.)

ure, the same drug, captopril, was the *most* effective agent in the younger whites, but the *least* effective drug in the older blacks.

Attempts have been made to use specific features beyond demographic characteristics, in particular the renin profile, to help decide before starting therapy which class of drug would be most efficacious for the individual patient. Although more information about this issue is given in subsequent chapters, I do not believe any features beyond age and race have been proved useful.

2. *Not a Matter of Quality of Life*

In addition to efficacy, drugs must be shown to be safe in order to be approved for use. Beyond overall safety, increasing attention has been given to their effect on various aspects of the quality of life (QOL), as assessed by detailed questionnaires (12). Without considering all of the different results reported by different investigators with the same agents, I believe it is fair to conclude that no one drug or class of drugs is clearly more user-friendly than the others. This conclusion is supported by a meta-analysis of all QOL studies published through 1991, wherein all provided about the same *positive* influence (Figure 4).

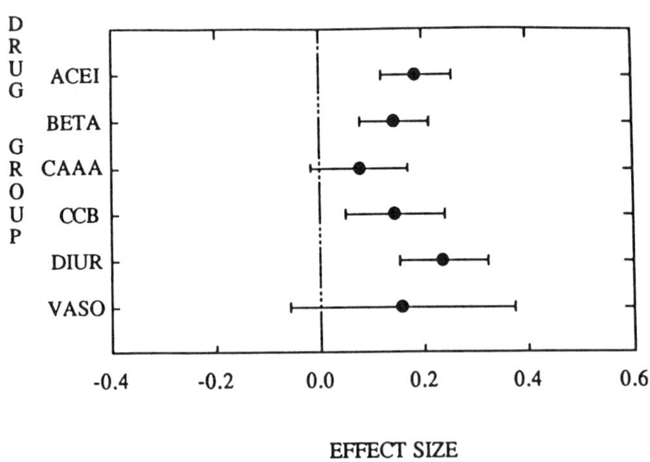

Figure 4 Change in quality of life, portrayed as the effect size with 95% confidence intervals, from a meta-analysis of 9 published trials of 27 groups using 14 drugs from 6 major classes. ACEI, angiotensin-converting enzyme inhibitor; BETA, beta-blocker; CAAA, centrally acting alpha$_2$-agonist; CCB, calcium channel blocker; DIUR, diuretic; VASO, vasodilator. (From Ref. 12.)

3. The Shortfall in Prevention of Coronary Disease

With little reason to make the choice on the basis of either overall efficacy or adverse effects, the issue has been largely focused on the apparent shortfall in protection against coronary events seen in the major clinical trials in which either diuretics or beta-blockers were used as the primary therapy. The evidence is seen in the meta-analysis by Collins et al. of all controlled trials of the treatment of hypertension as of 1990 (13) (Figure 5). This meta-analysis includes four relatively small trials of more severe and complicated hypertension that are not usually included in such reviews. Nonetheless, there is a shortfall in the effects on coronary mortality (an 11% reduction versus the expected 20% to 25% reduction) compared to the full effect on stroke mortality (a 38% reduction versus the expected 40%).

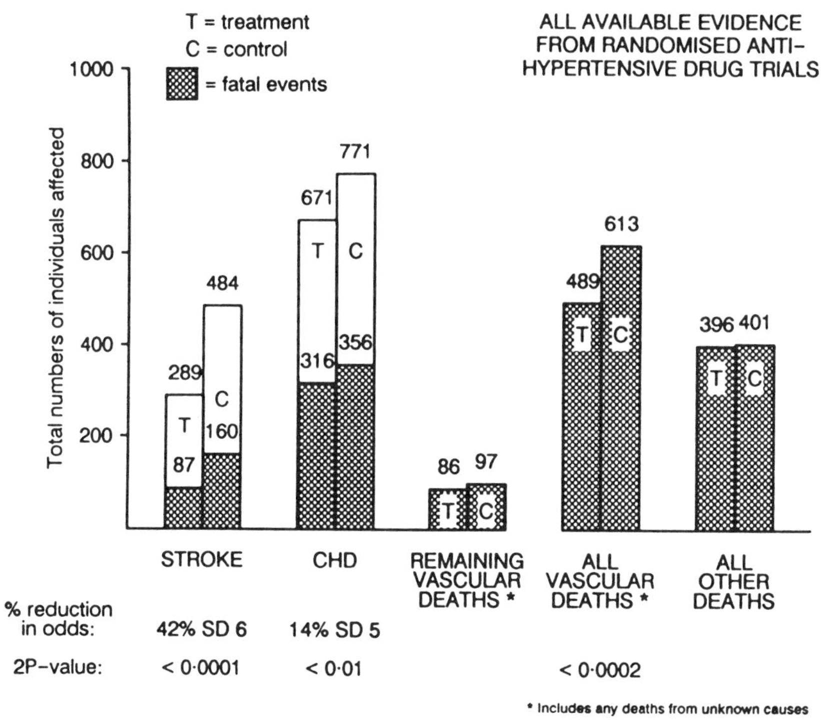

Figure 5 Total mortality and morbidity from various causes in 16 controlled randomized trials of antihypertensive therapy involving 37,000 individuals whose mean diastolic blood pressure at entry was 99 mm Hg. (Mean DBP difference 5–6 mm Hg for 5 years). (From Ref. 13.)

Since the studies shown in Figure 5 were completed, three additional large controlled trials of treatment of the elderly—all using diuretics and/or beta-blockers—have been published (14–16). As shown in Table 4 and explained in more detail in Chapter 4, the protection against all coronary events in these trials in the elderly was more impressive than that seen in the trials involving younger patients (13). However, greater protection was again seen against strokes and no significant reduction in coronary *mortality* was seen.

There are many possible reasons for this shortfall in protection against coronary disease in both younger and older patients (17). Since none of these reasons can be proved or disproved, there seems little purpose in rehashing what has been previously described (17). For now, it is enough to say that biochemical aberrations induced by diuretics and beta-blockers involving electrolytes, lipids, and glucose/insulin may be responsible.

All recognize the biochemical aberrations often induced by diuretics and beta-blockers. Some, however, minimize their impact, claiming that the changes are either slight in degree or short in duration and never shown actually to worsen cardiovascular risk (18). There are data, however, that these changes are significant in degree and persistent for at least 5 years. A recent example comes from a comparison of two groups of 300 hypertensives, similar at onset in all regards, one given a thiazide diuretic, the other treated with various other antihypertensives but no diuretic (19). At the end of 5 years, there was a 19 mg/dl difference in total serum cholesterol level between the two groups of patients, constituting an 8 mg/dl rise in those on diuretics and an 11 mg/dl fall in those not on diuretics. Blood glucose levels were also higher in those who received the diuretic. This study differs from others wherein lesser differences were noted in that it compared only those patients who took the prescribed therapies, thereby avoiding the inclusion

Table 4 Recent Trials of Therapy in Elderly Hypertensive Patients

	SHEP	STOP-HT	MRC
Mean BP at entry	170/77 (100% ISH)	195/102	185/91 (43% ISH)
Events per 1000 patient years (treated versus placebo)/relative risk			
Stroke	.67[a]	.53[a]	.75[a]
Coronary disease	.73[a]	.87[b]	.81[c]
Congestive failure	.45[a]	.49[a]	
All cardiovascular	.68[a]	.60[a]	.83[a]

[a]Statistically significant.
[b]MI only.
[c]Ischemic heart disease.

of patients who were allocated to a regimen but did not take it (i.e., the "intention to treat" approach).

These effects were seen with moderately high doses of diuretics and likely would be minimized with lower doses which have been shown to provide equal antihypertensive efficacy (20). Unfortunately, many patients continue to receive unnecessarily high doses, so the potential for biochemical mischief remains.

Nonetheless, as Dr. Alderman eloquently argues in Chapter 2, diuretics and beta-blockers remain the only drugs that have been tested, and they have been shown to reduce overall mortality, mainly by their impact on strokes. Until currently proceeding controlled trials of alpha-blockers, calcium blockers, and ACE inhibitors are completed, his (and most "official" groups') recommendations to give preference to diuretics and beta-blockers must be heeded.

II. THE RECOGNITION OF VARYING PATIENT NEEDS

Lest the preference for diuretics and beta-blockers be taken as a call for their exclusive use, the special considerations for the initial choice of therapy delineated in JNC-5 (1) should be remembered. These special considerations include the following:

Demography (as noted further in Chapters 4 and 6)
Biochemical changes (as noted further in Chapter 5)
Coexisting conditions (as noted in Chapters 7, 8, and 9, and elsewhere)
Quality of life
Cost

A. Coexisting Conditions

As will be described in many subsequent chapters, a large proportion, by far the majority of hypertensives, have coexisting conditions which may recommend specific choices of initial therapy. Without repeating what is covered by other authors about many of these coexisting conditions in their chapters, I will take the editor's prerogative to provide an overview of the situation (Table 5). My preferences and dislikes are not identical to those of others in the subsequent chapters, but I believe a strong case can be made for the listing in Table 5. Most of the rest of this book looks further into this issue, since it is the overriding indication for individualized therapy.

B. Life-Style Modifications

Although there is no uniformity in the choices of drug therapy, there is universal agreement about the value of nondrug therapies or, as they are called

Table 5 Individualized Choices of Therapy

Coexisting condition	Diuretic	Beta-blocker	Alpha-blocker	Calcium blocker	ACE inhibitor
Older age	+ +	+/−	+	+	+
Black race	+ +	+/−	+	+	+/−
Angina pectoris	+/−	+ +	+	+ +	+
Post myocardial infarction	+	+ +	+	+/−	+ +
Congestive failure	+ +	−	+	−	+ +
Cerebrovascular disease	+	+	+/−	+ +	+
Renal insufficiency	+ +	+/−	+	+ +	+ +
Diabetes	−	−	+ +	+	+ +
Dyslipidemia	−	−	+ +	+	+
Asthma or chronic obstructive pulmonary disease	+	−	+	+	+

$^{++}$Preferred, $^{+}$suitable, $^{+/-}$*usually not preferred*, $^{-}$usually contraindicated.

in JNC-5, life-style modifications (Table 6). Every report strongly recommends their use prior to and parallel with drug therapy.

A vivid portrayal of the value of these life-style modifications is provided in the same TOMHS trial described earlier (10). Recall that all subjects were first begun on a nutritional-hygienic regimen (weight loss, sodium restriction, physical activity, and moderation of alcohol intake). Those assigned to placebo continued to follow this regimen (as did those given one of the five types of antihypertensive drug). As seen in Table 3, those on the nutritional-hygienic regimen plus placebo achieved an average 8.6/8.6 mm Hg fall in blood pressure after 4 years.

This impressive effect is less than that achieved by the addition of a drug. But the greater effect of the drugs obviously incorporates the underlying effect of the life-style modifications, so we can assume that they produced only a 4 to 6 mm Hg additional effect. Moreover, the degree of modifications

Table 6 Life-Style Modifications for Hypertension

1. Stop smoking for overall cardiovascular health.
2. Lose weight, particularly for upper body obesity.
3. Reduce sodium intake to less than 120 mmol/day (2.5 g sodium or 7 g NaCl).
4. Moderate alcohol intake (no more than 2 usual portions per day).
5. Exercise (isotonic) regularly.
6. Maintain adequate potassium, calcium, and magnesium intake.

in life-style over the 4 years was relatively small: weight loss averaged less than 3 kg; sodium restriction averaged only about 15 mmol per day; physical activity and alcohol intake were altered only modestly. The impressive fall in blood pressure then was accomplished by relatively small changes in life-style, changes that should certainly be attainable by most patients given adequate instruction and repeated encouragement. Many of the same techniques described in Chapter 14 to improve compliance with drug therapy can also be utilized to improve compliance with nondrug therapy as well.

III. CONCLUSION

A new approach to the treatment of hypertension is clearly needed and is carefully delineated in the remainder of this book. The term *individualized therapy* may have different connotations for different practitioners. But the guidelines given here and in greater detail subsequently should go far to establish this concept as the best we now have to offer our hypertensive patients to achieve the real goal of therapy: maximal protection against cardiovascular disease with minimal interference with the enjoyment of life.

REFERENCES

1. Joint National Committee on Detection, Evaluation, and Treatment of High Blood Pressure. The fifth report of the joint national committee on detection, evaluation, and treatment of high blood pressure (JNC V). Arch Intern Med 1993; 153: 154–183.
2. The Guidelines Subcommittee of the WHO/ISH Mild Hypertension Liaison Committee. 1993 guidelines for the management of mild hypertension. Hypertension 1993; 22:392–403.
3. Kaplan NM. Hypertension in the population at large. In: Kaplan NM, ed. Clinical Hypertension. 6th ed. Baltimore: Williams & Wilkins, 1994:23–45.
4. Joint National Committee. The 1988 report of the joint national committee on detection, evaluation, and treatment of high blood pressure. Arch Intern Med 1988; 148:1023–1038.
5. Guidelines Subcommittee. 1989 guidelines for the management of mild hypertension: memorandum from a WHO/ISH Meeting. J Hypertens 1989; 7:689–693.
6. Jackson R, Barham P, Bills J, et al. Management of raised blood pressure in New Zealand: a discussion document. Br Med J 1993; 307:107–110.
7. Sever P, Beevers G, Bulpitt C, et al. Management guidelines in essential hypertension: report of the second working party of the British Hypertension Society. Br Med J 1993; 306:983–987.
8. Ogilvie RI, Burgess ED, Cusson JR, et al. Report of the Canadian hypertension society consensus conference: 3. Pharmacologic treatment of essential hypertension. Can Med Assoc J 1993; 149:575–584.
9. Kaplan NM. The appropriate goals of antihypertensive therapy: neither too much nor too little. Ann Intern Med 1992; 116:686–690.

10. Neaton JD, Grimm RH Jr, Prineas RJ, et al. Treatment of mild hypertension study. JAMA 1993; 270:713–724.
11. Materson BJ, Reda DJ, Cushman WC, et al. Single-drug therapy for hypertension in men. N Engl J Med 1993; 328:914–921.
12. Beto JA, Bansal VK. Quality of life in treatment of hypertension. Am J Hypertens 1992; 5:125–133.
13. Collins R, Peto R, MacMahon S, et al. Blood pressure, stroke, and coronary heart disease. Part 2. Short-term reductions in blood pressure: overview of randomised drug trials in their epidemiological context. Lancet 1990; 335:827–838.
14. SHEP Cooperative Research Group. Prevention of stroke by antihypertensive drug treatment in older persons with isolated systolic hypertension. JAMA 1991; 265:3255–3264.
15. Dahlöf B, Lindholm LH, Hansson L, et al. Morbidity and mortality in the Swedish trial in old patients with hypertension (STOP-hypertension). Lancet 1991; 338: 1281–1285.
16. Medical Research Council Working Party. MRC trial of treatment of hypertension in older adults: principal results. Br Med J 1992; 304:405–412.
17. Kaplan NM. Treatment of hypertension: rationale and goals. In: Kaplan NM, ed. Clinical Hypertension. 6th ed. Baltimore: Williams & Wilkins, 1994:145–170.
18. Burris JF, β-Blockers, dyslipidemia, and coronary artery disease. Arch Intern Med 1993; 153:2085–2092.
19. Elliott WJ. Glucose and cholesterol evaluations from diuretic therapy: intention to treat vs. actual on-therapy experience (abstr). Am J Hypertens 1993; 6:9A–10A.
20. Carlsen JE, Køber L, Torp-Pedersen C, Johansen P. Relation between dose of bendrofluazide, antihypertensive effect, and adverse biochemical effects. Br Med J 1990; 300:975–978.

2

The Rationale

MICHAEL H. ALDERMAN

Albert Einstein College of Medicine
Bronx, New York

I. INTRODUCTION

How strange that a chapter be devoted to rationalizing the need for individualized antihypertensive therapy. The very foundation of personal encounter medicine is to care for each patient according to his or her unique circumstances. This discussion is necessary nevertheless, I believe, because of the incongruity between the biology of blood pressure and the characteristics of current practice.

Blood pressure is the physical manifestation of a complicated physiological process. Its measure affords some insight into relative risk for cardiovascular disease. In fact, there is a roughly linear relationship between the height of the pressure and the likelihood of a cardiovascular event. Specifically, large observational studies have shown that there is a constant change in relative risk for a given change in both systolic and diastolic pressures (1). The fixed difference in relative risk associated with a particular difference in pressure persists throughout the usual range of pressures seen in the

---

Much of this material has been previously presented in Alderman, M.H. Blood Pressure Management: Individual Treatment Based on Absolute and the Potential for Benefit. *Annals of Internal Medicine*, 119:329–335, 1993.

community. No arbitrary threshold level of pressure either assures freedom from disease or makes heart attack or stroke inevitable. Thus, no level of pressure is diagnostic of a disease, in the way that detection of the tubercle bacillus in a patient with classic signs and symptoms establishes the diagnosis of tuberculosis. It is simply one of a number of risk factors which together provide an estimate of the actual likelihood of disease in an individual. As will be described in greater detail, blood pressure, by itself, actually defines subgroups composed of individuals of vast prognostic heterogeneity. As a result, the measure of blood pressure, by itself, is a rather poor predictor of outcome for the individual and provides inadequate guidance about the potential for therapy to benefit.

Since blood pressure is continuously related to cardiovascular disease outcomes and since a particular level of pressure tells precious little about prognosis or the potential benefit of intervention, a strategy for decision making that depends exclusively upon the level of pressure seems inappropriate. Nevertheless, clinicians often behave as if it were possible to dichotomize patients into normotensive and hypertensive categories by applying a threshold value.

Why has this happened (2)? Although the search for precision, the need for clinicians to make practical therapeutic decisions, and the advice of authorities have all contributed, perhaps it is the nature of the clinical trial that has done most to determine current practice. After demonstration that reduction of blood pressure could dramatically influence the course of malignant hypertension, the obvious next step was to determine whether similar intervention would influence the outcome of patients with less dramatic presentations. Widespread disagreement about the safety, as well as controversy about the benefit that might be produced by antihypertensive therapy, made clinical trials inevitable. The prolonged and unpredictable course of cardiovascular disease, and the relative rarity of "hard" end-points such as death and/or myocardial infarction and stroke, made a large-scale random study necessary. The most straightforward way to assemble a study population was, and is, to define eligibility by blood pressure. The pattern of admitting patients who met a certain threshold blood pressure (BP) level was established in the initial Veterans Administration (VA) Study (3). Its results were presented in terms of study cohorts that were defined by level of entry blood pressure. Extrapolation, at the most obvious level, suggested that all persons with similar pressures might share the benefit realized in the study. Thus, it is the minimum eligibility criterion of clinical trials that largely determines clinical practice today. Patients with pressures above that magic number are candidates for therapy and those below are not. In short, instead of being the norm, individualized therapy has become the exception for management of blood pressure.

Unfortunately, the simple application of the general conclusions of aggregate studies to an individual, in view of the heterogeneity of patients with the same pressure, may not be the best strategy. The purpose of this volume is to advocate for and indicate the tools needed to pursue another path. Individualization requires that, for the care of each patient, the clinician must address two questions: Should there be treatment? and What should that treatment be? I would contend that these questions can only be answered by a complete evaluation of the patient was well as a detailed knowledge of the results of clinical trials and fundamental research. The task of the physician is to merge these data sources and, with the help of the patient, decide whom to treat and how. On the basis of the totality of available knowledge gleaned from epidemiological, biological, and clinical trial sources, as well as from the examination of the patient, physicians must establish, as precisely as possible, the risk faced by each patient and, therefore, the absolute potential for benefit to be achieved by reduction of that risk by hypotensive therapy.

This chapter examines the first issue, Whom to treat, and makes the case that the decision to treat, just like the form which that treatment should take, must be individualized and cannot be dictated by blood pressure level. The remainder of this volume addresses the second issue, planning specific therapy for different kinds of patients.

II. BLOOD PRESSURE AS A RISK FACTOR

There is a strong, consistent, graded, and independent association between blood pressure and the incidence of stroke and heart attack (1,4,5). Blood pressure is not, however, a disease. It is one of many biological, genetic, and behavioral characteristics whose presence and magnitude affect the relative risk of disease occurrence (6). Neither blood pressure nor other risk factors are invariably present in those who experience a cardiovascular event, nor are they always absent in those who do not. Despite increasing risk, even at the highest end of the blood pressure range, only some will sustain a premature stroke or heart attack. In Framingham, during 15 years of follow-up study, less than one-third of those whose only risk factor was a systolic blood pressure above 195 mm Hg (highest category) had a stroke or heart attack (7). Among the 325,348 MRFIT screenees, those with diastolic pressures of 90 mm Hg or above were about twice as likely to have a heart attack or stroke as were those with diastolic pressures below 90 mm Hg, but only a small percentage suffered an event (8).

Similarly, a lower blood pressure does not confer total protection against a cardiovascular calamity. In fact, more than half (57%) of all heart attacks, and a substantial minority, approaching half of all strokes in some populations studies, occur in persons with normal blood pressure (9,10). In short, blood pressure, like other risk factors, provides quantitative and not qualitative information. Although higher blood pressures are associated with more events, no threshold distinguishes those who will from those who will not experience a cardiovascular disease event.

III. RELATIVE AND ABSOLUTE RISK

Relative and absolute risk are different ways to express the likelihood of events for individuals or groups. The actual quantities are empirically derived from observation of defined populations such as the Framingham study subjects. In practice, by extrapolation, these measures are then used to predict risk for other individuals or groups with characteristics similar to those of the groups studied. *Relative risk* describes the increase (or decrease) in likelihood of an event in one population in comparison to that in some other reference population. It is a ratio which imparts no information about the absolute expected incidence of events. *Absolute risk*, on the other hand, is the expected incidence of events. It is used to estimate the total number of events to be expected by a specific group or, by extension, the actual odds for an individual to have an event.

For blood pressure, relative risk (RR) for heart attack or stroke increases continuously with rising systolic and diastolic blood pressure. Specifically (Figure 1) each 7.5 mm Hg increase in diastolic blood pressure is associated

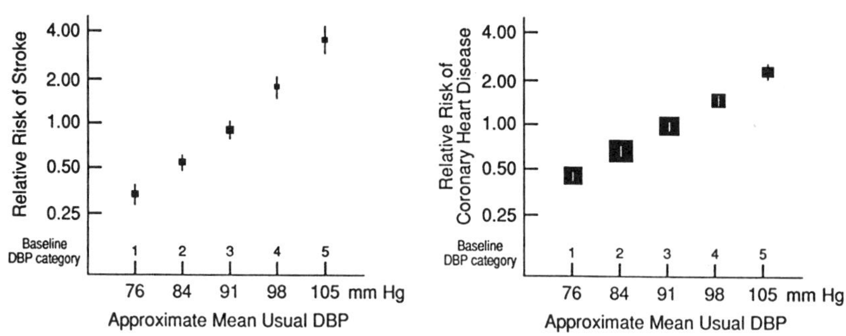

Figure 1 Relative risk of stroke and coronary heart disease by usual diastolic blood pressure. Stroke data were compiled from seven prospective observational studies with 843 events, and coronary heart disease data were compiled from nine prospective observational studies with 4856 events. The five categories of diastolic blood pressure (DBP) are defined by baseline DBP. Estimates of the usual DBP in each category are taken from mean DBP values 4 years post baseline in the Framingham Study. (From Ref. 1.)

with 46% more strokes (RR = 1.46) (1). This figure gives no clue as to the actual number of any particular group who will experience a stroke. Instead, it expresses the relative expectation of an event in two groups that differ only in level of blood pressure. It is noteworthy that the majority of myocardial infarctions occur among patients with "normal" diastolic blood pressure.

This observational association neatly matches experimental experience. In 14 intervention trials a 5 to 6 mm Hg fall in diastolic blood pressure was associated with a 42% drop in cerebrovascular events (11). Moreover, this benefit was about the same whether study subjects had mild, moderate, or severe hypertension. For coronary events, the protection associated with the same blood pressure fall was less than predicted by observational studies. Nevertheless, roughly the same percentage reduction in events occurred for a given blood pressure fall, regardless of initial pressure.

The practical implication of continuously increasing risk associated with rising blood pressure is clear. Reduction of blood pressure should prevent cardiovascular disease regardless of level of initial pressure (11,12). For example, among 50- to 59-year-olds, a 5 mm Hg reduction in diastolic pressure would prevent about 16% of all heart attack deaths (13). By comparison, the alternative approach of treating all the roughly 5% whose diastolic pressures are greater than 100 mm Hg to a diastolic pressure of 85 mm Hg would prevent about 9% of such events. But these two approaches are in no way incompatible. In fact, for that minority of individuals whose cardiovascular disease peril (absolute risk) is great, more substantial blood pressure reduction can and should confer even greater benefit.

In contrast to relative risk, absolute risk quantifies the probability or odds of an event's occurring in a population. In cardiovascular practice, it reflects the summation of an individual's entire constellation of clinical characteristics. It can be estimated with considerable precision by measuring the levels of conventional risk factors and detecting preclinical disease.

The process of defining absolute risk exposes the great prognostic differences among patients, even those with identical blood pressure. For example (Figure 2), a hyperlipidemic, glucose-intolerant 55-year-old male smoker with left ventricular hypertrophy has a distinctly greater risk than does a 55-year-old nonsmoker without cardiac enlargement—at every level of blood pressure. The increasing relative risk associated with increasing blood pressure persists among subjects with higher or lower absolute risk. By contrast, the actual hazard at any given blood pressure level can vary dramatically depending on overall risk. In this example, lower absolute risk subjects, even those with systolic pressures above 195 mm Hg, are only one-tenth as likely to experience an event as are those of the same age and gender, with systolic blood pressures of 105 mm Hg, but at high absolute risk (46/1000 versus 372/1000) (14).

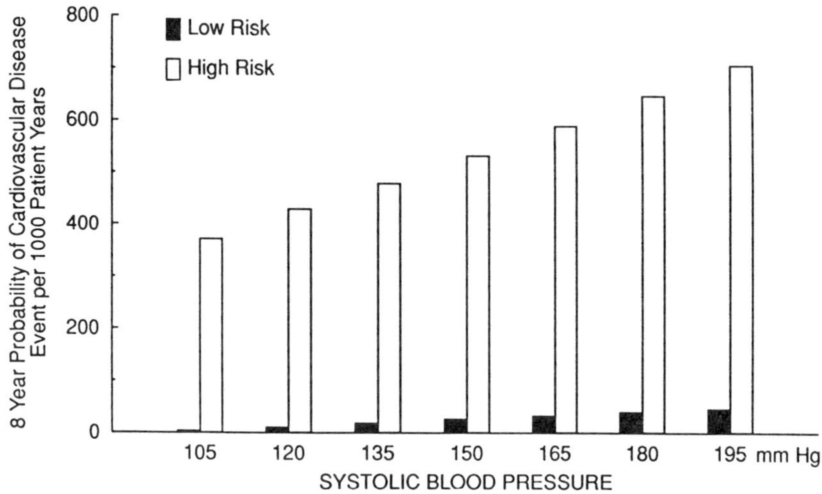

Figure 2 Absolute and relative risk of a cardiovascular disease event in a high- versus a low-risk 55-year-old male by systolic blood pressure. High risk: left ventricular hypertrophy, cigarette smoker, glucose intolerance, cholesterol level = 8.02 mmol/L.

Experimental evidence supports predictions based on these observations. MRC participants, all of whom had the same blood pressure levels, could be divided into high and low risk groups (Table 1). Untreated, the high-risk group experienced 149 events per 1000 patient years; the low-risk group, 3.7 (15). Diuretic based therapy generated equal blood pressure reduction in both groups and produced roughly the same percentage (35% versus 22%) of cardioprotection. However, in the high-risk group, 52 events per 1000 were avoided, while in the low-risk group, the gain was less than 1 per 1000 (16). Thus, it was possible to distinguish within a single blood pressure stratum, in advance and using tools less powerful than those now available, very different levels of risk and potential for benefit.

Table 1 Division into High- and Low-Risk Groups

	High risk	Low risk
Age	65	45
Serum cholesterol level (mmol/L)	8	5
Body mass index	30	27
Myocardial ischemia by ECG	Present	Absent
Cigarettes per day	40	0

IV. CURRENT CLINICAL PRACTICE

Current practice ignores these clinical realities. Many physicians rely on a blood pressure threshold alone to diagnose and guide treatment. By missing the crucial distinction between blood pressure as a quantity (risk factor) versus a quality (disease), many hypertensives, despite little hope of benefit measured by reduction of stroke or myocardial infarction (MI), are subjected to lifelong drug therapy. It is also possible, although unproven, that longer-term trials would reveal the ability of blood pressure reduction to prevent disease progression. At the same time, many high-risk normotensives, among whom occur more than half of all heart attacks, are categorically excluded from the cardioprotective potential of hypotensive therapy.

In the MRC trial, where entry to treatment was based upon a threshold blood pressure, 850 were treated for 1 year, to prevent one stroke (17). The inclusion of many low-risk subjects in the MRC trial undoubtedly contributed to the high treated-to-benefitted ratio, but that is, of course, just the point. Nevertheless, if this modest benefit could be realized at no, or some known small cost, as in childhood vaccination, then the effort might be justified. Unfortunately, treatment carries risk. Every labeled and treated person is exposed to possible adverse consequences (18). Electrolyte and metabolic disturbances are common, and impotence frequent (19). Moreover, it has been postulated, but not proved, that too great a drop in pressure (the J-shaped curve) may actually induce the myocardial infarction that treatment was prescribed to prevent (20,21). All of these proven and postulated consequences of treatment have led some authorities to argue that the equivocal results of antihypertensive trials in regard to MI prevention reflect the net result of heart attacks avoided, minus the others caused by overzealous treatment (22).

But what about the failure to treat those many so-called normotensive persons who are at great absolute risk? Figure 3 shows that a given systolic blood pressure difference predicts roughly similar (30%) cardiovascular protection in three groups with different pressures (23,24). The potential benefit thus varies with absolute risk. Group A (high-risk) men, with seemingly normal systolic pressures (135 mm Hg), have a greater probability of disease than do members of Groups B and C despite their higher starting pressures (165 and 195 mm Hg, respectively). A drop from 135 to 105 could be expected to prevent 103 events in Group A, while the same 30 mm Hg decline would prevent only 45 and 30 events, respectively, in the lower-risk groups, despite their initially higher pressures. Regrettably, no clinical trial has tested this hypothesis. However, since it has been repeatedly shown that the same pressure reduction yields the same benefit in severe, moderate, and mild hypertensives, it is hard to imagine that, at least in the middle range of

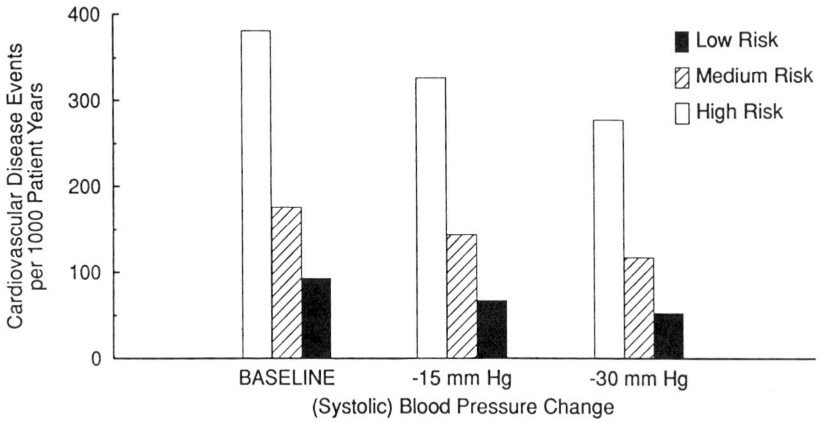

Figure 3 Cardiovascular disease events by systolic blood pressure change for high-, medium-, and low-risk men. High risk: systolic blood pressure = 135 mm Hg, cholesterol level = 8.02 mmol/L, glucose intolerance, left ventricular hypertrophy. Medium risk: systolic blood pressure = 165 mm Hg, cholesterol level = 6.72 mmol/L, glucose intolerance, no left ventricular hypertrophy. Low risk: systolic blood pressure = 195 mm Hg, cholesterol level = 4.78 mmol/L, no glucose intolerance, no left ventricular hypertrophy.

blood pressure (80 to 100 mm Hg), benefit would disappear simply because some arbitrary threshold had been breached.

As noted, treatment does carry risk. The notion of treating "normotensive" subjects is, at first glance, threatening. However, as noted, the risk of disease determines the absolute potential for benefit and since the hazard of treatment remains relatively stable, concentrating treatment on high-risk patients (even with less than 90 mm Hg diastolic blood pressure) seems the most prudent way to maximize the benefit to cost ratio. In fact, results from the recently reported SOLVD study are reassuring in that regard (25). There, blood pressure reduction in high-risk normotensive subjects reduced the incidence of myocardial infarction. In SOLVD, although involving a very special group of patients from whom wide extrapolation is unjustified, a treatment induced fall in diastolic pressure from 76 to 72 mm Hg, compared with no change in the control group, was associated with a 28% reduction in heart attacks. Consistent with that experience is the recently completed Trial of Treatment for Isolated Systolic Hypertension in the Elderly (SHEP), in which reduction of normal diastolic blood pressure was associated with a decline in cardiovascular morbidity and mortality (26). All SHEP patients did have elevated systolic pressure, which was also reduced. The point is that reduction of both, or either, systolic and diastolic pressures appears useful, and this seems to be true on both sides of the imaginary threshold conventionally used to separate normal from abnormal.

V. AN ALTERNATIVE CLINICAL STRATEGY

Provision of hypotensive drugs should depend on absolute risk and potential for benefit rather than blood pressure level alone. As noted, a variety of tools are available—and more soon will be—to measure absolute risk in individual patients. The known risk factors themselves provide a good start. They tend to cluster, probably because of their common metabolic influences, and this multiplies liability (27). Smokers with an unfavorable family history and high cholesterol and fasting blood sugar levels are at considerable risk of a cardiovascular disaster—even when diastolic blood pressure is 85 mm Hg! Other factors, such as plasma renin (28) and insulin levels (29), promise to increase the list of factors that can together provide a closer approximation of absolute risk. Detection of vascular disease in its preclinical state improves identification of high-risk patients. It is now possible to detect traces of urinary albumin (30), and early narrowing of peripheral vessels (31) and, by echocardiography, to describe cardiac size precisely (32). Together, risk factors and preclinical disease form the basis for identifying persons whose potential for benefit justifies blood pressure reduction, even when the pressure is normal. Indeed, formal strategies to quantify total risks are being developed and applied (33,34).

The American Heart Association, for example, has produced a scheme which uses the Framingham study experience as the basis for assigning specific numeric values to various demographic characteristics, as well as to the presence and extent of risk factors (35–37). The sum of these numbers (Figure 4) can be used to provide an index of absolute probability of an event for each individual. In the examples presented in Figure 4, it can be seen that different 55-year-old white males can have either clearly normal (B) or clearly hypertensive (C) levels of systolic pressure and the same absolute risk. By the same token, at either pressure (136 and 170 mm Hg), the probability of events can be lower or higher than average for all persons of that age and gender. Since a given reduction in blood pressure can be expected to produce a roughly equivalent percentage decline in risk of events, it is likely that with the same degree of blood pressure reduction, more subjects at greater absolute risk, like A and D, would benefit than those like B and C. For every patient, quantification of risk, albeit imperfect, can provide useful clues to the baseline risk and the potential for benefit that therapy could yield (see Figure 2, Chapter 1). This approach is readily amenable to computer analysis. Thus, the implications of different therapeutic options could be readily explored.

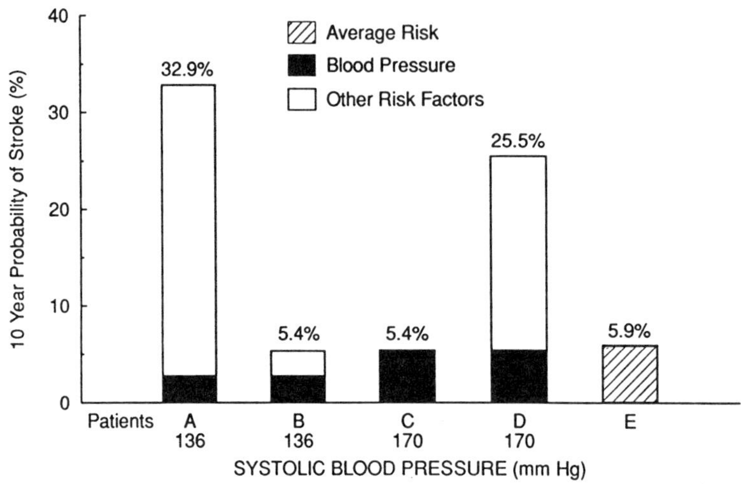

Figure 4 Ten year probability of stroke by systolic blood pressure for four 55-year-old white males with different risk factors. Patient A = previously treated, history of cardiovascular disease and diabetes, cigarette smoker, left ventricular hypertrophy; Patient B = cigarette smoker; Patient C = no other risk factors; Patient D = history of diabetes, cigarette smoker, and left ventricular hypertrophy; Patient E = average risk.

Replacement of an antihypertensive treatment policy dictated by threshold with one driven by a risk/benefit analysis will certainly complicate the lives of physicians and patients. Absent simple guidelines, it is likely those relatively few patients with the highest levels of blood pressure (diastolic BP greater than 104 mm Hg) will continue to receive antihypertensive drug therapy regardless of the constellation of other factors. Similarly, those at the lowest levels (diastolic BP less than 80 mm Hg), regardless of absolute risk, should probably not have drug treatment.

In practice, important changes in thinking are needed for that vast majority of persons whose pressures are at or near—on both sides—the current arbitrary threshold. At this juncture, it is worth emphasizing the imprecision with which pressure is measured. Even with the most laborious and time consuming approaches, the assignment of a specific blood pressure value to an individual patient is an inexact science. The middle zone (80 to 104 mm Hg diastolic or 140 to 180 mm Hg systolic) includes about 70% of all adults (38). Within this range, I believe that the decision to apply drugs for each individual should be based on absolute risk.

Clearly, present knowledge cannot guarantee that all those at high risk will be identified. However, existing tools can better discriminate between those who might benefit and those whose risk is so slight that treatment offers little promise of help than does an arbitrary blood pressure cut point. Comprehensive patient assessment will identify some in the ranges previously described as normotensive who, by virtue of family history, glucose intolerance, minimal renal dysfunction, peripheral vascular disease, left ventricular hypertrophy, and/or a high serum cholesterol level, are at increased cardiovascular risk. Blood pressure reduction should produce real benefit for these patients. The other modifiable risk factors should, of course, also be pursued with vigor. In fact, it may sometimes be possible, by eliminating or reducing other risk factors, to convert a high-risk subject into a low-risk subject and thus reduce the call for antihypertensive drugs. Studies to quantify the precision and test the validity of this approach ought to be high on the research agenda of preventive cardiology.

There will be other patients with diastolic pressures in the neighborhood of 100 mm Hg, who do not smoke and have low cholesterol and fasting blood sugar levels, a low Renin Profile, a normal echocardiogram result, and no evidence of renal dysfunction, who should be spared drug therapy. The experience of control subjects in the Australian National Trial of Antihypertensive Treatment provides reassurance about the safety of withholding drug therapy (39). Fully 78% of untreated subjects whose initial diastolic pressure was 100 to 104 mm Hg had pressures at some time during the study of less than 100 mm Hg (40). Most importantly, that majority whose pressure tended to fall spontaneously had event rates indistinguishable from those of individuals who were treated to reach the same pressure. Excess morbidity was limited to the 22% of control subjects whose pressure remained the same or rose during the study. Presumably, in mild hypertensives without other risk factors or evidence of preclinical disease, a rise in blood pressure would precede any adverse pressure-related cardiovascular outcome. Thus, regular patient monitoring could provide the appropriate signal for timely intervention.

This new paradigm must be effectively communicated to patients. Options will have to be presented so that absolute risk, and the potential for benefit, are clearly spelled out. Then, each patient's unique way of weighing risk and benefit, informed by these quantitative clues, can lead to rational decision making. Since personal values and preferences differ, individual therapeutic decisions in the same circumstances can legitimately be expected to vary.

VI. SUMMARY

The issue is not whether blood pressure is a risk factor for cardiovascular disease, or whether its reduction saves lives. That has been convincingly demonstrated. What is at issue is how best to apply that knowledge. Logic argues for displacing the whole community's pressure distribution downward. If it were possible to safely and easily lower everyone's BP even slightly, the result would be more disease prevention than any conceivable clinical strategy. Regrettably, knowledge about what is needed to achieve this goal and how to do it leave much to be desired. Investment in fundamental and applied research to improve dietary and behavioral approaches to attaining these goals is much needed.

But physicians do have powerful and varied tools to dramatically lower blood pressure in individual patients. Knowing how and when to use those tools wisely is the challenge. Blood pressure must be seen as what it is—a reflection of relative risk, a risk factor, and only one of the multiplicity of factors that together determine absolute risk. Blood pressure reduction does not cure (because high blood pressure is not a disease), but rather lowers the odds of developing real disease (heart attack, stroke, and renal failure). The need for hypotensive therapy should therefore be determined by the absolute likelihood of a stroke or heart attack, and the associated opportunity for their prevention, and not by any particular blood pressure level. There must be some proportionality between potential for benefit and burden of intervention. The demanding task of clinical medicine is to define those parameters, to assist the patient in assessing their implications, and, in implementing the therapeutic choice that follows, to provide the best possible care.

The relation of blood pressure to cardiovascular disease is continuous and, therefore, reliance on a threshold value to determine therapeutic behavior is inappropriate. Instead, effective and efficient clinical management should be based upon quantitative assessment of each individual's absolute risk and potential for benefit.

REFERENCES

1. MacMahon S, Peto R, Cutler J, et al. Blood pressure, stroke, and coronary heart disease. Part 1. Prolonged differences in blood pressure: prospective observational studies corrected for the regression, dilution bias. Lancet 1990; 335:765–774.
2. Pickering GW. Normotension and hypertension: the mysterious viability of the false. Am J Med 1978; 65:561–563.
3. Veterans Administration trial: effects of treatment on morbidity in hypertension. JAMA 1970; 213(7):1143–1152.
4. Kannel WB, Sorlie P. Hypertension in Framingham. In: Paul O, ed. Epidemiology Control of Hypertension. Miami: Symposium Specialists, 1975:553–592.
5. Kannel WB. Hypertension and the risk of cardiovascular disease. In: Laragh JH, Brenner WM, eds. Hypertension: Pathophysiology, Diagnosis, and Management. New York: Raven Press, 1990:101–125.

6. Stokes J III, Kannel WB, Wolf PA, et al. The relative importance of selected risk factors for various manifestations of cardiovascular disease among men and women from 35 to 64 years old: 30 years of follow-up in the Framingham Study. Circulation 1987; 75(suppl V):V-64–V-73.
7. Madhavan S, Alderman MH. The potential effect of blood pressure reduction on cardiovascular disease: a cautionary note. Arch Intern Med 1981; 141:1583-1588.
8. Kannel Wb, Neaton JD, Wentworth D, et al. Overall and coronary heart disease mortality rates in relation to major risk factors in 325,348 men screened for MRFIT. Am Heart J 1986; 112:825–836.
9. Kannel WB. Some lessons in cardiovascular epidemiology from Framingham. Am J Cardiol 1976; 37:269–281.
10. Kannel WB, Wolf PA, Verter J, McNamara PM. Epidemiological assessment of the role of blood pressure in stroke: The Framingham Study. JAMA 1970; 214:301–310.
11. Collins R, Peto R, MacMahon S, et al. Blood pressure, stroke and coronary heart disease II: short term reductions in blood pressure: overview of randomized drug trials in their epidemiological context. Lancet 1990; 335:827–838.
12. Kottke TE, Gatewood LC, Wu SC, Park HA. Preventing heart disease: is treating the high risk sufficient? J Clin Epidemiol 1988; 4:1083–1093.
13. Law MR, Frost CD, Wild NJ III. Analysis of data from trials of salt reduction. Br Med J 1991; 302:819–824.
14. Kannel WB, McGee Dl, Gordon T. A general cardiovascular risk profile: The Framingham Study. Am J Cardiol 1976; 38:46–51.
15. Medical Research Council Working Party. Stroke and coronary heart disease in mild hypertension: risk factors and the value of treatment. Br Med J 1988; 296:1565–1570.
16. Marmot MG. Epidemiology and the art of the soluble. Lancet 1986; 1:897–900.
17. Medical Research Council Working Party. MRC trial of treatment of mild hypertension: principal results. Br Med J 1985; 291:97–104.
18. Alderman MH, Lamport B. Labelling of hypertensives: a review of the data. J Clin Epidemiol 1990; 43:195–200.
19. Raftery EB. The metabolic effects of diuretics and other antihypertensive drugs: a perspective as of 1989. Int J Cardiol 1990; 28:143–150.
20. Alderman MH, Ooi WL, Madhavan S, Cohen H. Treatment induced blood pressure reduction and the risk of myocardial infarction. JAMA 1989; 262(7): 920–924.
21. Farnett L, Mulroy CP, Linn Wh. The J-curve phenomenon and the treatment of hypertension. JAMA 1991; 265:489–495.
22. Oliver MF. Risks of correcting the risks of coronary disease and stroke with drugs. N Engl J Med 1982; 306:297–298.
23. Alderman MH, Madhavan S. Management of the hypertensive patient: a continuing dilemma. Hypertension 1981; 3:192–197.
24. Gordon T, Kannel WB, ed. Framingham Study: An Epidemiological Investigation of Cardiovascular Disease, Bethesda, Maryland: Section 27, U.S. Department of Health, Education and Welfare, National Institutes of Health, 1971.

25. The SOLVD Investigators. Effect of enalapril on survival in patients with reduced left ventricular ejection fractions and congestive heart failure. N Engl J Med 1991; 325:293-302.
26. SHEP Cooperative Research Group. Prevention of stroke by antihypertensive drug treatment in older persons with isolated systolic hypertension: final results of the systolic hypertension in the elderly program (SHEP). JAMA 1991; 265: 3255–3264.
27. Kannel WB, Neaton JD, Wentworth P, et al. Overall and coronary health disease mortality rates in relation to major risk factors in 325,348 men screened for MRFIT. Am Heart J 1986; 112:825–836.
28. Alderman MH, Madhavan S, Ooi WL, et al. Association of the remin-sodium profile with the risk of myocardial infarction in patients with hypertension. N Engl J Med 1991; 32416):1098–1104.
29. Ducimetiere P, Eschwege E, Papoz L, et al. Relationship of plasma insulin levels to the incidence of coronary heart disease mortality and myocardial infarction in a middle-aged population. Diabetologia 1980; 19:205–210.
30. Yudkin JS, Forrest RD, Jackson CA. Microalbuminuria as predictor of vascular disease in non-diabetic subjects. Lancet 1988; 2:530–533.
31. Piguoli P, Tremoli E, Poli A, et al. Intimal plus medial thickness of the arterial wall: a direct measurement with ultrasound imaging. Circulation 1986; 74:1399–1406.
32. Koren MJ, Devereux RB, Casale PN, et al. Relation of left ventricular mass and geometry to morbidity and mortality in uncomplicated essential hypertension. Ann Intern Med 1991; 114:345–352.
33. Tunstall-Pedoe H. The Dundee Coronary Risk-Disk for management of change in risk factors. Br Med J 1991; 303:744–748.
34. Randall T, Muir J, Mant D. Choosing the preventive workload in general practice: practice application of the Coronary Prevention Group Guidelines and Dundee Coronary Risk-Disk. Br Med J 1992; 305:227–231.
35. Anderson KM, Wilson PWF, Odell PW, Kannel WB. An updated coronary risk profile: a statement for health professionals. Circulation 1991; 83:356–362.
36. Wolf PA, D'Agostino RB, Belanger AJ, Kannel WB. Probability of stroke: a risk profile from the Framingham Study. Stroke 1991; 22:312–318.
37. Kannel WB. Pulling it all together: the cardiovascular outlook. Am Heart J 1992; 123:264–266.
38. Horan MJ. Implications for research and policy in the treatment of hypertension: medical considerations. Hypertension 1989; 13(suppl 1):1-164–1-166.
39. The Management Committee. The Australian therapeutic trial in mild hypertension. Lancet 1980; 1:1261–1267.
40. Alderman MH. The indications for treatment with antihypertensive drugs. In: Sleight P, Freis E, eds. Cardiology. Vol. 1. Hypertension. London: Butterworth Scientific, 1982.

3

Uncomplicated Hypertension

WILLIAM C. CUSHMAN

University of Tennessee College of Medicine
Memphis, Tennessee

HENRY R. BLACK

Rush Presbyterian–St. Luke's Medical Center
Chicago, Illinois

The risk of cardiovascular events and death increases progressively in acculturated populations with increases in both systolic and diastolic blood pressure throughout the range of pressures (1). This risk is further progressively increased in individuals with other cardiovascular risk factors, such as elevated cholesterol level or cigarette smoking, but is also considerably higher once complications such as myocardial infarction or stroke have occurred, or when end organ damage, such as left ventricular hypertrophy, is present. This chapter will primarily address the rationale and methods of intervention for the prevention and treatment of hypertension in the individual without complications or target organ damage ascertained by routine studies. Since everyone possesses demographic characteristics such as age or race, however, there will of necessity be some overlap with other chapters in this book. In addition, as we become increasingly more sophisticated in identifying cardiovascular risk factors and discovering subclinical evidence of target organ damage, we may discover that all patients with high blood pressure have complications and that the "uncomplicated" hypertensive patient does not exist.

I. CLASSIFICATION OF BLOOD PRESSURE

Since the risk of cardiovascular events and death increases progressively throughout the distribution of blood pressure in a population, why must we classify patients by blood pressure levels at all? The first and most obvious reason is that we as clinicians must frequently make *categorical* decisions as to what, when, and to what intensity life-style changes or antihypertensive medications should be recommended or prescribed to an individual "patient." A classification system based at least in part on blood pressure ranges/categories allows an estimation of risk that can be remembered and applied in the practical decision-making process that occurs during everyday practice.

The second reason for a classification system is that decisions about when to initiate drug therapy for hypertension have primarily been based on the entry blood pressure criteria of the cohorts who benefited from treatment in prospective randomized clinical trials which demonstrated a reduction in cardiovascular events with antihypertensive medications. Without this type of clinical trial evidence, we can have little confidence that drug treatment based on blood pressure level or range will result in more benefit than harm. We must always bear in mind that the objective of treating hypertension is to reduce the associated morbidity and mortality and not simply to lower blood pressure. These trials have generally shown that the higher the risk, the greater the absolute benefit with treatment, so it is reasonable that we categorize patients carefully so we can be as confident as possible that our therapy will serve our patients well.

It has been argued that since in the outcome trials an average achieved difference in treated blood pressure between the intervention and control groups of about 5 mm Hg diastolic or 10 mm Hg systolic reduced events by an average of 33%, regardless of the entry blood pressure, the decision to treat hypertension should be based on the absolute estimated cardiovascular risk for an individual and whether a one-third reduction in risk is meaningful for that person (2). The risk estimate for a certain level of blood pressure is highly variable, depending on concomitant conditions and risk factors. Clearly, the higher the predicted absolute risk, the greater the reduction of risk in absolute terms by this one-third relative risk reduction. In the examples used by Jackson et al., a 70-year-old man with multiple risk factors, but a diastolic blood pressure of 95 mm Hg, has a 50% absolute risk for development of cardiovascular disease in 10 years, while a 60-year-old woman with a diastolic blood pressure of 100 mm Hg as her only risk factor has an absolute risk of 10% in 10 years. A one-third reduction in relative risk for each would reduce absolute risk by 17% versus 3%, respectively.

However, the practice of most clinicians and the recommendations of the U.S. Joint National Committee (JNC V) on Detection, Evaluation, and

Treatment of Hypertension (3), as well as most other national and international consensus committees in hypertension (4), have been primarily to consider the entry criteria or other experience from randomized outcome trials in recommending the blood pressure levels at which drug treatment should be initiated. The stages or severity classifications of hypertension have been based on both outcome trials and prospective epidemiological data. The 1993 Fifth U.S. Joint National Committee has based a new classification system (Table 1) for blood pressure and hypertension predominantly on epidemiological risk (3). The recommendations for initiation of treatment based on *diastolic* blood pressure still rely on clinical trial experience from studies which measure clinical endpoints (death, coronary heart disease, stroke, and congestive heart failure), but systolic recommendations rely both on epidemiological data and the remarkable benefits of treatment demonstrated in the systolic hypertension trials which have been reported in the 1990s.

The new JNC V Report defines "normal" blood pressure as below 130/85 mm Hg ("optimal" is 120/80 mm Hg), "high normal" as 130 to 139 mm Hg systolic and/or 85 to 89 mm Hg diastolic, and "hypertension" as 140 mm Hg systolic or 90 mm Hg diastolic, or above, on the basis of at least two readings at each of two or more visits, assuming reasonably proper technique. The high normal category identifies individuals who deserve closer follow-up observation because they are at higher risk for cardiovascular events and the ultimate development of definite hypertension (5). They are definitely strong candidates for life-style interventions or treatment of other risk factors for the prevention of hypertension and cardiovascular disease.

Table 1 Classification and Management of Confirmed Blood Pressure

Category	Systolic (mm Hg)	Diastolic (mm Hg)	Management
Normal	<130	<85	Recheck in 1–2 years.
High normal	130–139	85–89	Recheck in $\leqslant 1$ year; life-style modifications.
Stage 1	140–159	90–99	Life-style modifications 3–6 months; consider drug therapy if $\geqslant 95$ mm Hg diastolic, $\geqslant 150$ mm Hg systolic, or high risk.
Stage 2	160–179	100–109	Life-style modifications and drug therapy.
Stage 3	180–209	110–119	Same as stage 2, but a second drug may be added sooner or simultaneously.
Stage 4	$\geqslant 210$	$\geqslant 120$	

II. STAGING OF HYPERTENSION AND GUIDELINES FOR INITIATING THERAPY

The new U.S. (JNC V) staging system of hypertension (Table 1) emphasizes that all levels of hypertension, both systolic and diastolic, are associated with increased risk for fatal and nonfatal cardiovascular events and warrant effective long-term therapy with life-style changes with or without the addition of antihypertensive medications (3).

All the national and international guidelines reported in 1993 acknowledge a persistent level of blood pressure above which drug treatment should be initiated, even for the low-risk or uncomplicated patient, either immediately or after a trial of life-style (nonpharmacological) intervention (4). For systolic blood pressure, 160 mm Hg or greater was cited by all except the United States (greater than or equal to 150 mm Hg) and New Zealand (greater than or equal to 170 mm Hg) guidelines. For diastolic blood pressure, 95 or 100 mm Hg or above was equally cited as the level above which drug treatment should eventually be initiated for the uncomplicated individual. (By comparison, the morbidity outcome trials generally used entry blood pressure criteria of 90 or 95 mm Hg diastolic or above or 160 to 180 mm Hg systolic or greater.) However, in one way or another each consensus report recognized that there were levels of blood pressure in which higher-risk patients should be treated with drugs and lower-risk patients might be effectively managed with life-style interventions alone. In the U.S. guidelines (JNC V) this range was 140 to 150 mm Hg systolic and 90 to 95 mm Hg diastolic, but included 140 to 170 mm Hg systolic and 90 to 100 mm Hg diastolic in the various other guidelines. The JNC V "stage 1 hypertension" is most consistent with this range within which "individualization" in the decision to initiate drug treatment is recommended: 140 to 159 mm Hg systolic and 90 to 99 mm Hg diastolic. We agree, however, with JNC V that the "uncomplicated" patient with persistent blood pressure elevations above 150 mm Hg systolic or 95 mm Hg diastolic after 3 to 6 months of encouragement of life-style modifications should be started on antihypertensive medication. Although the prospective trials did not specifically address the 150 to 159 mm Hg systolic blood pressure range, this level confers a long-term risk similar to a diastolic blood pressure of 100 to 105 mm Hg and was the observed level of systolic blood pressure during follow-up observation for the placebo group in the Systolic Hypertension in the Elderly Program (SHEP) trial (6).

III. BLOOD PRESSURE GOALS OF THERAPY

All but one of the 1993 national and international guideline committees give specific absolute blood pressure level goals for drug therapy (4). The Canadian,

United Kingdom, United States, and The World Health Organization/International Society of Hypertension (WHO/ISH) (in elderly) guidelines all recommend reducing diastolic blood pressure below 90 mm Hg. For a systolic goal, either below 160 mm Hg (U.K.), below 140 mm Hg (U.S., WHO/ISH in elderly), 140 to 160 mm Hg (U.S. in isolated systolic hypertension), or 120 to 130 mm Hg (WHO/ISH in young) is given. The New Zealand guidelines focus on reducing absolute risk and assume reductions of 10/5 mm Hg as a (minimum) goal. We agree with a general goal of below 140/90 mm Hg, but below 160 mm Hg systolic may be more than adequate for those with markedly elevated systolic pressures (above 180 mm Hg).

The "J curve" concept, that the risk of coronary events is increased if diastolic blood pressure is lowered too far with antihypertensive therapy (7), is considered an unproven hypothesis and should not affect therapeutic decisions. The ongoing Hypertension Optimal Treatment (HOT) international trial may answer this question definitively, but both SHEP and the Treatment of Mild Hypertension Study (TOMHS) are consistent with lower cardiovascular event rates with diastolic blood pressures averaging below 80 mm Hg (6,8).

IV. BLOOD PRESSURE MEASUREMENT

Care should be taken to follow standardized methods of measuring blood pressure in order to prevent misclassification of blood pressure levels (9, 10). A mercury sphygmomanometer is preferred and the cuff size should be appropriate for midupper arm circumference: greater than 32 cm requires at least a "large" adult cuff. The patient should be sitting quietly in a chair (with back supported) in a quiet room without having smoked within several hours. Although the bell of the stethoscope is recommended, the diaphragm is easier to use and provides similar readings to the bell. The mercury column should be lowered at 2 mm Hg per beat or second; the first Korotkoff sound which is followed by several consecutive Korotkoff sounds is systolic blood pressure, and the level at which there is a consistent disappearance of sounds or at which the last beat is heard is diastolic blood pressure.

"Pseudohypertension," a higher blood pressure reading by sphygomomanometer than by an arterial catheter, may occur in older individuals. It is caused by calcification of the brachial artery and is suspected if hypotensive symptoms develop in the absence of hypotension readings by indirect measurement. It may be screened for by "Osler's" maneuver: a "positive" test is a persistently palpable radial artery when the cuff is inflated above the systolic pressure level. Diastolic determinations appear to be affected more than systolic. Unfortunately, several groups have demonstrated that the classification of patients as Osler maneuver positive or negative has an unacceptable intra-

and interobserver variation (11,12). However, pseudohypertension is rare and individuals with this condition have not been excluded from epidemiological or interventional hypertension studies demonstrating risks or benefits of treatment. Therefore patients with pseudohypertension may be assumed to benefit from treatment.

V. LIFE-STYLE MODIFICATIONS (NONPHARMACOLOGICAL TREATMENT)

Many life-style interventions have been examined or recommended to prevent or treat hypertension, but the strength of supportive data for each intervention varies (13). There are four modalities that have sufficient evidence from prospective intervention trials to be recommended by JNC V and other consensus committees on the management of hypertension (Table 2): weight, salt, and alcohol reduction, and increased physical activity (3,4).

A. Weight Reduction

Weight loss has produced the most consistent and largest reductions in blood pressure, primarily in upper normal and stage 1 and 2 hypertension (13–15). The average blood pressure reduction observed in hypertensive patients is usually 1 to 2 mm Hg per kg weight loss. The response varies among patients, but there is almost always a response. In the Trials of Hypertension Prevention (TOHP), weight loss by diet and increased physical activity was more effective in lowering blood pressure and preventing the onset of hypertension than any other modality tested, although neither exercise nor alcohol reduction was studied (16). As with other studies, the more weight loss the greater the reduction in blood pressure (17). But it is crucial to bear in mind that patients do not have to achieve ideal body weight to obtain a

Table 2 Life-Style Modifications for Prevention or Treatment of Hypertension

Weight reduction	Reduction of 1–2 mm Hg per kg weight loss, if overweight
Dynamic exercise	⩾20 minutes, ⩾3 times a week (>30 min if walking) of low to moderate intensity dynamic exercise
Alcohol moderation	⩽2 drinks[a] per day average, if drinking more
Sodium restriction	70–100 mmol per day intake as trial for sodium sensitivity/responsiveness

[a]1 drink = 12 oz beer, 5 oz wine, or 1.5 oz 80 proof liquor.

substantial reduction in blood pressure. A 4–5 kg weight loss may be very helpful and achievable over time.

In addition to its effect on blood pressure, weight loss has other potential benefits, such as improving lipid levels, insulin sensitivity, left ventricular mass, and sense of well-being.

B. Exercise

A number of cross-sectional and prospective observational studies have shown that either regular vigorous physical exercise, leisure time physical activity, or physical fitness is associated with lower blood pressure levels and a lower prevalence of hypertension (18).

The great majority of randomized controlled studies over the past decade or so demonstrate a convincing antihypertensive effect for both systolic and diastolic blood pressure. Reviews including studies up to 1989 have concluded that regular physical exercise lowers blood pressure in patients with hypertension from 5 to 15 mm Hg systolic and 5 to 10 mm Hg diastolic compared to that of a control condition or group (18,19). The results of a recent carefully designed and conducted randomized, parallel study (20) of 27 mildly hypertensive men with an average age of 44 years and blood pressure of 138/95 mm Hg is consistent with that conclusion: the net effect on blood pressure of 10 weeks of a dynamic exercise regimen was −7/−10 mm Hg. The exercise regimen consisted of walking, jogging, and/or stationary bicycling for 30 minutes, four times a week for 10 weeks, at 65% to 80% of maximal achieved heart rate on a baseline exercise test. The control regimen consisted of slow calisthenics and stretching for the same duration and frequency, but while always maintaining less than 60% maximal heart rate.

Regular dynamic exercise may be as effective in lowering blood pressure as weight reduction and also confers other benefits, such as facilitating weight loss and improving lipid levels and insulin sensitivity. The exercise prescription should be for low to moderate intensity (e.g., 50% to 70% maximum heart rate) dynamic exercise of at least 20 to 30 minutes duration, at least three times a week. It is rarely necessary to order a formal stress test before recommending an exercise program, although it may be prudent if the patient appears to have a moderate or high probability of having coronary artery disease. Certainly, the patient with known coronary disease or symptoms should receive appropriate testing.

C. Salt Reduction

Populations with little access to salt are essentially free of hypertension, and dietary sodium is directly associated with blood pressure in observational studies (21).

The majority of reported trials and meta-analyses report that moderate sodium restriction significantly reduces systolic and diastolic blood pressure (22), but to a lesser degree than what has been achieved by a reduction in weight or alcohol intake or increased physical activity. In one meta-analysis, for example, the average change in blood pressure in hypertensive patients with a reduction of sodium of about 70 mmol/day was $-4.9/-2.6$ mm Hg (23). Blacks, the elderly, the obese, diabetics, and hypertensive patients appear to be more sensitive to changes in dietary salt intake over several days than others, but there are few long-term data to confirm that salt reduction has a more persistent antihypertensive effect in these "salt-sensitive" groups.

It is recommended by all the hypertension consensus committees to consider reduction in dietary sodium from the 150 to 200 mmol/day typical average intake to below 100 mmol/day in all hypertensive patients (4). This degree of sodium reduction can usually be achieved by not adding salt while cooking or at the table and by avoiding heavily salted food, especially snacks. However, long-term compliance has been difficult to achieve and other modalities may be more effective in lowering blood pressure, so priorities and patient choices may lead to a different emphasis. Individualization is generally encouraged. If a patient selects salt reduction as a life-style modification, compliance may be enhanced with regular feedback concerning urinary sodium excretion, by either timed collections or semiquantitative dipstick estimates of urinary chloride concentration (24).

D. Alcohol Reduction

Alcohol intake of three or more drinks per day is associated with higher average blood pressures in many epidemiological studies (25,26). While heavy drinking declines somewhat with age, the effect of alcohol on blood pressure is greater with increasing age (27).

There have been 10 randomized controlled trials reporting the effect of alcohol reduction on blood pressure. The average net reductions in blood pressure observed were up to 8 mm Hg for systolic pressure and up to 6 mm Hg for diastolic pressure, for differences in alcohol intake of one to six drinks* per day. For example, the first well-controlled randomized trial in hypertensive patients demonstrated a reduction in blood pressure of 5/3 mm Hg ($p < 0.001$ for both systolic and diastolic) with an average reduction of four drinks per day maintained for 6 weeks in moderate to heavy drinkers (28). Although more clinical trial evidence is needed, especially to confirm that an antihypertensive effect is sustained long-term (29), it is prudent to recom-

*A standard drink is defined as approximately 14 grams of ethanol and is contained in 12 oz of beer, 5 oz of table wine, or 1.5 oz of distilled spirits.

mend a limitation of alcohol intake to no more than two drinks a day in normotensive and hypertensive individuals, both for prevention or treatment of hypertension and for prevention of the other significant risks of heavy drinking (3). Hypertensives who drink an average of one to two drinks of alcoholic beverages per day may continue that amount so long as there are no other reasons to reduce or stop drinking (30).

E. Life-Style Recommendations

A combination of several life-style modalities may be very effective in reducing blood pressure (15), but asking an individual to change too many habits at once can lead to poor compliance. For those drinking an average of more than two drinks of alcohol per day, initial emphasis should be on at least moderating alcohol intake. Smoking cessation should also carry a very high priority, not because it will lower blood pressure, but because it is an independent risk factor for cardiovascular disease as well as a host of other diseases. Otherwise, the combination of dietary changes to reduce weight and increased physical activity is the most prudent regimen for the sedentary overweight individual with upper normal blood pressure or stage 1 hypertension.

VI. CONSIDERATIONS IN THE SELECTION OF ANTIHYPERTENSIVE DRUGS

Many drugs are available that lower blood pressure effectively in hypertension either as single-drug or combination therapy (3). On the basis of the evidence currently available, we recommend considering all of the following factors when selecting an initial drug for treatment of hypertension (Table 3): (1) Has the drug been successful in reducing morbidity and mortality in trials of antihypertensive therapy? (2) Are there important concomitant conditions which specifically indicate or contraindicate a certain class or classes of drugs? (3) Do patient characteristics, such as age or race, predict the antihypertensive response to a drug? (4) Can the patient afford the drug?

Table 3 Considerations in the Selection of Antihypertensive Drug Therapy

1. Hypertension morbidity and mortality trial experience
2. Important concomitant conditions: indications or contraindications
3. Patient characteristics (e.g., age and race)
4. Economic considerations
5. Quality of life and symptomatic adverse effects

and (5) Will it affect his/her quality of life? Other considerations, such as presumed effects on left ventricular mass or a patient's renin profile, have not yet been proved to be important differentiating factors in making a drug selection. There are situations when the first factor should be the only consideration, and there are other situations when one or several of the others will take precedence.

A. Morbidity/Mortality Trial Experience

All five consensus hypertension committees who made recommendations in 1993 acknowledge that only therapeutic regimens that include a base of a diuretic or a beta-blocker have demonstrated a reduction of events in morbidity and mortality trials (Table 4) (4,31). Four of the five, Canada, New Zealand, the United Kingdom, and the United States, recommend diuretics and beta-blockers as the preferred initial classes of drugs for treatment of hypertension because of this experience in outcome trials (2,3,4,32). The WHO/ISH guidelines, however, list the classes in order of proven benefit in outcome trials: (1) diuretics, (2) beta-blockers, and (3) angiotension-converting enzyme (ACE) inhibitors, calcium antagonists, and alpha$_1$-receptor blockers (33). However, they go on to say that "no evidence is so far available that benefits are due to any particular class of antihypertensive agents

Table 4 Recommendations for Preferred Drugs for Initial Therapy of Uncomplicated Hypertension by 1993–94 Hypertension Guidelines Committees

Canada	Monotherapy with either low-dose thiazide diuretic or beta-blocker
New Zealand	Low-dose diuretics and low-dose β-blockers should be considered as first-line treatment
United Kingdom	Two classes of drugs have been adequately and extensively tested in outcome trials: diuretics (thiazides) and beta-blockers
United States	Because diuretics and beta-blockers have been shown to reduce morbidity and mortality, these two classes are preferred for initial drug therapy
WHO/ISH	Several classes can be recommended as first-line treatment.[a] They are, in order of proven benefit based on morbidity and mortality studies, (1) diuretics, (2) beta-blockers, and (3) ACE inhibitors, calcium antagonists, and alpha$_1$-receptor blockers

[a]ACE, angiotensin-converting enzyme; WHO/ISH, World Health Organization/International Society of Hypertension.

rather than to the lowering of blood pressure per se"; therefore, the clinician may choose among the available classes on the basis of a variety of factors, not just the experience of outcome trials in hypertension. Although all the other reports clearly give preference to considering diuretics and beta-blockers first, some members of the U.K. and U.S. committees were in more agreement with the WHO/ISH position (4).

The other classes of drugs recommended as alternatives to diuretics and β-blockers in the various guidelines include ACE inhibitors, calcium antagonists, alpha$_1$-receptor blockers, and (in the U.S. guidelines) alpha-beta-blockers. Except in the WHO/ISH guidelines, the concern about these classes was that they had not yet been demonstrated to be effective in morbidity and mortality trials. There is agreement that they lower blood pressure as well as diuretics or beta-blockers in many patients, and therefore should be at least as beneficial. However, as has been demonstrated in the treatment of other diseases (e.g., congestive heart failure and ventricular arrhythmias), unexpected adverse morbid or mortal effects of drugs that offset their beneficial effects may only become apparent in prospective outcome trials. All the committees acknowledged that other classes may be selected if diuretics and beta-blockers were contraindicated, ineffective, or not tolerated, or if another class of drug was indicated for a concomitant condition.

We agree that diuretics, especially in hypertensive patients over age 60 years, and beta-blockers in addition for those less than 60 years, should be considered first in the treatment of uncomplicated essential hypertension. Diuretics should be given special preference in patients with isolated systolic or systolic-preominant hypertension. If the preferred agent is contraindicated, ineffective, or not tolerated, or if another class of drug is clearly indicated for a concomitant condition, then an alternative should be selected.

It seems likely that the newer classes of antihypertensive agents would reduce morbidity and mortality at least as well as diuretics and β-blockers. Trials testing this question are ongoing or being planned. For example, the U.S. National Heart, Lung and Blood Institute has initiated a randomized, double-blind clinical trial comparing a diuretic, a calcium antagonist, an alpha$_1$-receptor blocker, and an ACE inhibitor in the treatment of high-risk hypertensive patients. The primary endpoints compared will be fatal and nonfatal coronary events, although other endpoints, such as strokes, heart failure, and total mortality, will also be examined.

B. Concomitant Conditions

Other chapters will discuss how to individualize therapy on the basis of concomitant conditions in the complicated hypertensive patient. As a general principle, however, an antihypertensive drug or class should be given preference that is likely to reduce the risk of events or mortality more by treating the concomitant condition than a diuretic or beta-blocker would in the treatment of the hypertension alone. The use of an ACE inhibitor in a hypertensive patient with congestive heart failure is the most obvious example. Where the benefit is not as clear as this, the clinician is faced with a decision made difficult because of insufficient evidence from outcome trial experience.

C. Predictors of Antihypertensive Efficacy

Quite often the selection of an antihypertensive drug is based on a prediction of what is most likely to control blood pressure. This is especially true if an initial agent selected is ineffective or not tolerated. All classes of antihypertensive agents recommended for potential single-drug therapy will lower blood pressure to normal levels in about 50% of stage 1 and 2 hypertensive patients. However, there is considerable interindividual diversity in response. In recent years there have been attempts to identify patient characteristics that predict better or worse antihypertensive responses to certain classes of drugs in order to prevent unsuccessful therapy. The most consistent patient characteristics that have been helpful in predicting responses are age and race.

In 1993, a VA cooperative study (34) comparing six different classes of antihypertensive drugs and placebo as single agents examined their ability to control blood pressure and be tolerated ("success") over 1 year in younger (age below 60 years) and older (age 60 years or above) white and black men with average untreated diastolic blood pressure of 99 mm Hg (Figure 1) (34). The active drugs were a diuretic (hydrochlorothiazide), a beta-blocker (atenolol), an ACE inhibitor (captopril), a central agonist (clonidine), a calcium antagonist (diltiazem), and an alpha$_1$-receptor blocker (prazosin). Clonidine and prazosin had significantly worse adverse effects and intolerance rates than the other drugs. The 1 year success rates in younger whites were greater for captopril (55%), atenolol (51%), and clonidine (50%) than for hydrochlorothiazide (32%). In older whites, atenolol (68%) and diltiazem (64%) were more successful than prazosin (48%), but all were reasonably effective. Diltiazem (64%) was superior to all the other classes in younger African-Americans. However, in older blacks the calcium antagonist (64%) and the diuretic (58%) were very effective, but all of the rest were successful less than 50% of the time. In fact, as monotherapy the beta-blocker (33%) and the ACE inhibitor (20%) were no more effective than placebo (24%) in this group. These data demonstrate important differences in response rates for single-drug therapy in these four age–race groups that can assist in the choice of drugs when efficacy is the determining factor.

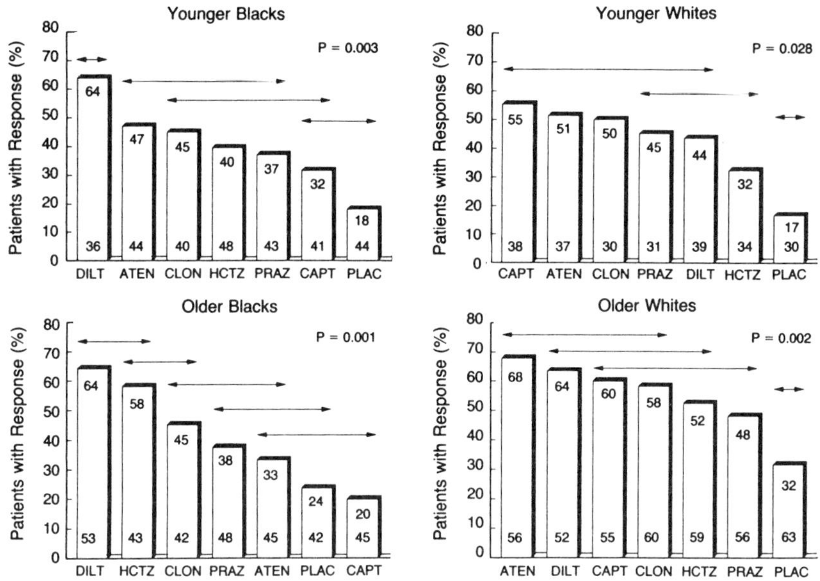

Figure 1 Single-drug therapy success rates (percentage of randomized patients with diastolic blood pressure <90 mm Hg during titration and <95 mm Hg at 1 year) for younger (age <60 years) and older (age ≥60 years) blacks and whites. The arrows group the drugs whose effects do not differ from each other by >15%. The numbers at the top of the bars indicate success rate (%); the numbers at the bottom indicate the number of patients in each group. P values were derived by a chi-square test comparing treatments. HCTZ, hydrochlorothiazide; ATEN, atenolol; CAPT, captopril; CLON, clonidine; DILT, diltiazem; PRAZ, prazosin; PLAC, placebo. (From Ref. 34. Reprinted, by permission of the New England Journal of Medicine.)

Another recently completed trial of antihypertensive therapy, the Treatment of Mild Hypertension Study (TOMHS), compared representative drugs from all the same classes as the VA study, except for a central agonist (8). This study began with milder hypertensives than the VA trial and included aggressive life-style interventions with weight and sodium reduction and increased physical activity in all patients: blood pressure was reduced from an average of 141.1/90.5 mm Hg by 9.1/8.6 mm Hg with nondrug interventions alone (in the placebo group). Therefore, it is not surprising that differences in efficacy were not observed among the active drugs. There were also not enough African-Americans (20%) to analyze separately. However, this trial importantly demonstrates that any of the classes recommended as first-line agents are very effective in uncomplicated mildly hypertensive patients if combined with significant changes in life-style.

Combining antihypertensive drugs with different mechanisms of action so that they have at least additive effects will control blood pressure in almost all stage 1 and 2 uncomplicated hypertensive patients and, especially if a diuretic is included, obliterate any age-race differences in response rates (35).

D. Economic Considerations

While antihypertensive therapy is not as expensive as treatment for some other chronic diseases, cost is often a barrier to successful management, since hypertension is usually an asymptomatic condition and some patients may choose to avoid the expense of drugs. Some patients are simply unable to afford expensive antihypertensive regimens. Fortunately, the medications that have been used in outcome trials, such as diuretics, propranolol, and reserpine, are now very inexpensive. Moreover, most classes of antihypertensive agents have relatively inexpensive representatives. There are other costs to therapy, such as laboratory tests, office visits (including time away from work), and management of any complications of drug therapy, but there is little evidence that these costs should differ significantly between drugs on the basis of the experience in blinded trials (6,8,34).

E. Quality of Life

There are reports of differences in cognitive-behavioral or other quality of life effects between antihypertensive drugs, but the clinical or long-term effects of these differences have not been made clear. However, central agonists do seem to cause symptomatic adverse effects more than the other classes of commonly used antihypertensive medications, including reserpine (34, 36). When symptoms do appear to be caused by an otherwise preferred medication, a trial of a lower dose or a drug free period may allow subsequent continuation of the medication. A serious adverse effect believed to be caused by a medication should certainly lead to its discontinuation.

VII. STEPDOWN OF DRUG THERAPY

Decreasing or withdrawing therapy in uncomplicated patients whose blood pressure is well controlled should be considered if there is uncertainty about the initial diagnosis, if the disease process may have changed (e.g., because of life-style changes), or in order to minimize unnecessary therapy. However, it must be remembered that many hypertensive individuals are currently not on medications or are prescribed insufficient doses, especially if ACE inhibitors or calcium antagonists are being used (3,34).

VIII. CONCLUSIONS

Uncomplicated stage 1 and 2 hypertension should be managed initially with life-style modifications, including weight, sodium or alcohol intake reduction, and/or physical exercise, for 3 to 6 months. Drug therapy should then be added if systolic blood pressure is 150 mm Hg or above and/or diastolic is 95 mm Hg or above. In some patients drug treatment should be initiated if blood pressure is 140 to 150 mm Hg systolic and/or 90 to 95 mm Hg diastolic. The goal of drug therapy is blood pressure below 140/90 mm Hg for most patients. There are many classes of medications from which to choose, but those used in successful morbidity and mortality trials should be considered first, especially low-dose diuretics in hypertensive patients over age 60 years. However, in many patients other factors, such as concomitant conditions or antihypertensive effectiveness, will indicate a trial of another class of drug.

REFERENCES

1. National High Blood Pressure Education Program Working Group. National High Blood Pressure Education Program Working Group Report on Primary Prevention of Hypertension. Arch Intern Med 1993; 153:186–208.
2. Jackson R, Barham P, Bills J, et al. The management of raised blood pressure in New Zealand. Br Med J 1993; 307:107–110.
3. Joint National Committee on Detection, Evaluation, and Treatment of High Blood Pressure. The Fifth Report on Detection, Evaluation, and Treatment of High Blood Pressure (JNC V). Arch Intern Med 1993; 153:154–183.
4. Alderman MH, Cushman WC, Hill MN, Krakoff LR. International roundtable discussion of national guidelines for the detection, evaluation, and treatment of hypertension. Am J Hypertens 1993; 6:974–981.
5. Sagie A, Larson MG, Levy D. The natural history of borderline isolated systolic hypertension. N Engl J Med 1993; 329:1912–1917.
6. SHEP Cooperative Research Group. Prevention of stroke by antihypertensive drug treatment in older persons with isolated systolic hypertension: final results of the Systolic Hypertension in the Elderly Program (SHEP). JAMA 1991; 265: 3255–3264.
7. Cruickshank JM, Thorp JM, Zacharias FJ. Benefits and potential harm of lowering blood pressure. Lancet 1987; 1:581–584.
8. Neaton JD, Grimm RH, Prineas RJ, et al. Treatment of Mild Hypertension Study: final results. JAMA 1993; 270:713–724.
9. Perloff DP, Grim C, Flack J, et al. Human blood pressure determination by sphygmomanometry. Circulation 1993; 88(5, Part 1):2460–2470.

10. Cushman WC, Cooper KM, Horne RA, Meydrech EF. Effect of back support and stethoscope head on seated blood pressure determinations. Am J Hypertens 1990; 3:240–241.
11. Tsapatsaris NP, Napolitana GT, Rothchild J. Osler's maneuver in an outpatient clinic setting. Arch Intern Med 1991; 151:2209–2211.
12. Hla KM, Samsa GP, Stoneking HT, Feussner JR. Observer variability of Osler's maneuver in detection of pseudohypertension. J Clin Epidemiol 1991; 44:513–518.
13. Horan MJ, Blausyein MP, Dunber JB, et al. NIH Report on Research Challenges in Nutrition and Hypertension. Hypertension 1985; 7:818–823.
14. Langford HG, Davis BR, Blaufox MD, et al. Effect of drug and diet treatment of mild hypertension on diastolic blood pressure. Hypertension 1991; 17:210–217.
15. Applegate WB, Miller ST, Elam J, et al. Nonpharmacologic intervention to reduce blood pressure in older patients with mild hypertension. Arch Intern Med 1992; 152:1162–1166.
16. Trials of Hypertension Prevention Collaborative Research Group. The effects of nonpharmacologic interventions on blood pressure of persons with high normal levels: results of the Trials of Hypertension Prevention (phase I). JAMA 1992; 267:1213–1220.
17. Stevens VJ, Corrigan SA, Obarzanek E, et al. Weight loss intervention in phase I of the Trials of Hypertension Prevention. Arch Intern Med 1993; 153:849–858.
18. Cushman WC. Physical activity, fitness, and blood pressure. In: Izzo JL, Black HR, Taubert KA, eds. Hypertension Primer. Council on High Blood Pressure Research (American Heart Association), 1993:161–163.
19. Arroll B, Beaglehole R. Does physical activity lower blood pressure: a critical review of the clinical trials. J Clin Epidemiol 1992; 45:439–437.
20. Martin JE, Dubbert PM, Cushman WC. Controlled trial of aerobic exercise in hypertension. Circulation 1990; 81:1560–1567.
21. Intersalt Cooperative Research Group. Intersalt: an international study of electrolyte excretion and blood pressure: results for 24 hour urinary sodium and potassium excretion. Br Med J 1988; 297:319–328.
22. Kaplan NM. Salt and blood pressure. In: Izzo JL, Black HR, Taubert KA, eds. Hypertension Primer. Council on High Blood Pressure Research (American Heart Association), 1993:167–169.
23. Cutler JA, Follmann D, Elliott P, Suh I. An overview of randomized trials of sodium reduction and blood pressure. Hypertension 1991; 17(Suppl 1):I-27–I-33.
24. Dubbert PM, Cushman WC. Adherence to sodium restriction in the treatment of hypertension (abstr). Am J Hypertens 1990; 3:110A.
25. Klatsky AL, Friedman GD, Siegelaub AB, Gerard. Alcohol consumption and blood pressure: Kaiser-Permanente multiphasic health examination data. N Engl J Med 1977; 296:1194–1200.
26. MacMahon S. Alcohol consumption and hypertension. Hypertension 1987; 9: 111–121.
27. Criqui MH, Wallace RB, Mishkel M, et al. Alcohol consumption and blood pressure: the LRC prevalence study. Hypertension 1981; 3:557–565.

28. Puddey IB, Beilin LJ, Vandongen R. Regular alcohol use raises blood pressure in treated hypertensive subjects: a randomized controlled trial. Lancet 1987; 1:647–651.
29. Cushman WC, Bingham SF, Cutler JA, et al. Prevention and Treatment of Hypertension STudy (PATHS): effect of alcohol reduction on blood pressure: design and baseline characteristics (abstr). Am J Hypertens 1991; 4:109A.
30. Friedman GD, Klatsky AL. Is alcohol good for your health? N Engl J Med 1993; 329:1882–1883.
31. Collins R, Peto R, MacMahon S, et al. Drug treatment of hypertension: an overview of the unconfounded randomized trials in the context of observational epidemiology. Lancet 1990; 335:827–838.
32. Seever P, Beevers G, Bulpitt C, et al. Management guidelines in essential hypertension: report of the Second Working Party of the British Hypertension Society. Br Med J 1993; 306:983–987.
33. The Guidelines Committee of the WHO/ISH Mild Hypertension Liaison Committee. 1993 guidelines for the management of mild hypertension. Hypertension 1993; 22:392–403.
34. Materson BJ, Reda DJ, Cushman WC, et al. Single-drug therapy for hypertension in men: a comparison of six antihypertensive agents with placebo. N Engl J Med 1993; 328:914–921.
35. VA Cooperative Study Group on Antihypertensive Agents. Low-dose captopril for the treatment of mild to moderate hypertension. I. Results of a 14-week trial. Arch Intern Med 1984; 144:1947–1953.
36. Materson BJ, Cushman WC, Goldstein G, et al. Treatment of hypertension in the elderly. I. Blood pressure and clinical changes: results of a Department of Veterans Affairs cooperative study. Hypertension 1990; 15:348–360.

4

The Elderly Hypertensive

TOMASZ GRODZICKI

Jagiellonian University
Cracow, Poland

FRANZ H. MESSERLI

Ochsner Clinic
New Orleans, Louisiana

I. INTRODUCTION

Despite several recent reviews (1–8), there is still widespread confusion regarding the definition, treatment, and prognosis of essential hypertension in patients older than age 65. Some of the following misconceptions, which unfortunately are still commonly believed by practicing physicians, may contribute to this disarray:

1. Arterial pressure increases with age, and therefore an elevated blood pressure is believed to be a normal finding in the elderly population.
2. Function and perfusion of vital organs diminish with age, and elevated pressure is regarded as a physiological compensatory process serving to maintain or enhance blood flow through restricted vascular beds.
3. Elderly patients have predominantly systolic hypertension, and many physicians believe that only diastolic hypertension is a harbinger of heart attack, stroke, or death.
4. High blood pressure does not carry the increased cardiovascular risk for older patients that it does for younger patients.

Although arterial pressure increases with age in Westernized populations and the prevalence of hypertension may reach 50% in patients older than age 65 (9,10), there is nothing benign about hypertension in the elderly. The Veterans Administration Cooperative Study has shown that 63% of those over age 60 with untreated hypertension will suffer a cerebral vascular accident, congestive heart failure, myocardial infarction (MI), or dissecting aneurysm within 5 years. Further studies from the United States (11,12), Belgium (13), and Scandinavia (14) confirm these findings. Even patients with purely systolic hypertension have a much higher mortality rate from all cardiovascular and renal diseases than patients without hypertension.

In an elderly patient with established essential hypertension, two distinctly different pathogenetic processes have been taking place. On one hand, progressive aging per se affects the cardiovascular system and can result in age-specific changes; on the other hand, the cardiovascular system of an elderly hypertensive patient has been exposed to long-standing hypertension that, by itself, damages various target organs. Distinguishing the two pathogenetic factors—age and hypertension—becomes increasingly difficult in the elderly hypertensive patient.

II. PATHOPHYSIOLOGY

Arterial hypertension in the elderly is characterized by a low cardiac output (1) secondary to a low stroke volume and relative bradycardia (15). At the same time, elderly hypertensive patients have higher systolic and diastolic pressures (15–17), elevated left ventricular stroke work, and a distinctly increased total peripheral resistance than younger patients (15,17). Lund-Johanson (18) documented a distinct fall in cardiac output in mildly hypertensive patients followed for 17 years. This fall was caused by reduction of both stroke volume and heart rate and an increase in total peripheral resistance, both during rest and after treadmill exercise.

Even in healthy, normotensive individuals, left ventricular mass progressively increases throughout life, reaching its greatest magnitude in senescence (19). Moreover, echocardiographic criteria of left ventricular hypertrophy (LVH) are reached considerably earlier in life when arterial hypertension is present. LVH by echocardiographic criteria can be found in up to 50% of elderly patients with hypertension (15,20). It is considered an adaptive process of the myocardium that compensates for increased afterload. However, data from the Framingham cohort (21,22) and Cornell indicate that patients with LVH are at greater risk for sudden death (and other cardiovascular morbidity and mortality) than subjects who have a normal heart. At any given level of arterial pressure, these subjects have a far more serious prognosis than those without LVH.

Arterial compliance decreases with age as a result of progressive atherosclerosis and medial hypertrophy, and therefore systolic hypertension becomes common in the elderly population (23).

Advancing age is associated also with a decline in renal blood flow in normal subjects, a phenomenon that is aggravated in patients with arterial hypertension (24). Renal vascular resistance remains distinctly elevated in elderly hypertensive patients, reflecting diffuse nephrosclerosis from long-standing essential hypertension. As a consequence, more patients experience albuminuria, a marker of renal involvement and future renal failure.

In normotensive subjects, intravascular volume changes little with progressing age (25). However, our study performed in hypertensive subjects revealed a significantly lower intravascular volume in elderly patients than in younger patients with similar blood pressure (17). Elderly patients with decreased intravascular volume and diminished reactivity of the baroreceptor reflex are particularly vulnerable to postural and postprandial hypotension.

Neuroendocrine factors also change throughout life. Plasma renin activity decreases with advancing age (26). In contrast, norepinephrine levels increase progressively with age more in normotensive than in hypertensive patients (27), an increase which probably reflects a mechanism that compensates for progressive down regulation of beta-receptors.

III. THERAPEUTIC APPROACH

A. General Guidelines

The optimal choice of antihypertensive strategy should be based on the results of the long-term controlled therapeutic trials. Unfortunately, all major multicenter trials—EWPHE (28), SHEP (29), STOP (30), and MRC (31)—included patients without concomitant disorders, such as recent stroke and myocardial infarction; overt heart failure; or dementia, and their results cannot be directly extrapolated to most of the patients being seen by a physician. The results obtained in apparently healthy (apart from hypertension) subjects may be used as a guide but should not be widely extrapolated. Therefore, we still are not able to draw firm conclusions about whether and how the patient with cardiovascular complications or multiple coexisting diseases should be treated. However, we recommend considering the results of studies that also evaluate soft and surrogate endpoints in choosing the optimal antihypertensive drug. Ideally, this choice should be based on the following criteria:

History and clinical findings
Hemodynamic profile of hypertension
Target organ damage (heart, kidneys, and brain)
Coexisting risk factors and diseases
Concomitant therapies
The patient's mental, psychological, social, and economic condition, especially in the elderly

B. Life-Style Modifications

Nonpharmacological measures such as salt restriction, weight loss, and perhaps mild exercise should be encouraged in the overweight, inactive elderly patient. Excess adipose tissue expands intravascular volume and additionally burdens the left ventricle by enhancing preload (32). This may further impair left ventricular function and thereby accelerate the decline of its performance. The Framingham Study (33) has indicated that obese hypertensive patients are at particularly high risk for congestive heart failure. Similarly, elderly patients are more susceptible to the effects of fluid and salt overload: an excessive salt load (particularly when combined with alcohol, as often happens after birthday parties, etc.) may temporarily overload the extracellular fluid volume space by more than 2000 ml and thereby give rise to congestive heart failure and acute pulmonary edema. Such a dismal course of events is particularly likely to occur in an elderly patient whose heart already has a poorly compensated contractile function.

However, there are several reasons why the elderly patient's compliance with dietary measures may be notoriously poor: first, the elderly tend to have a very established, rigid daily schedule and life-style and may be reluctant to consider any changes; second, it is cumbersome, time-consuming, and expensive to prepare fresh (unprocessed and therefore low-salt) meals three times a day, whereas canned food and TV dinners (high in salt) are much more convenient to prepare; third, because the taste buds of elderly persons lack sensitivity, they tend to use more salt to overcome lack of taste; and fourth, dietary salt restriction in the elderly may have little antihypertensive effect (and thus impress neither patient nor physician), although this restriction prevents diuretic-induced hypokalemia. In addition, the elderly may be unable to follow a daily exercise program because of concomitant problems, such as osteoarthrosis, peripheral vascular disease, Parkinson's disease, dementia, lack of appropriate facilities, or even fear of assault.

Although it is often difficult to motivate elderly patients to change their life-style and diet habits and to encourage them to participate in a regular physical fitness program, the benefits of such nonspecific measures often outweigh the frustration created by the hindrances.

C. Selection of Antihypertensive Agents

As outlined previously, the elderly hypertensive patient is characterized by a distinct hemodynamic, renal, endocrine, and fluid-volume profile that gradually evolves with advancing age. On the basis of this profile, one can compose a "wish list" that enumerates all the desirable properties of an ideal hypertensive drug in this age group (Table 1). Despite equal antihypertensive potency, some agents are preferable to others under certain clinical condi-

Table 1 "Ideal" Antihypertensive Agent in the Elderly Should

Not further depress cardiac performance or systemic blood flow
Lower systemic and renal vascular resistance
Improve cardiac and vascular compliance
Reduce or prevent left ventricular hypertrophy
Not further contract intravascular volume or impede sodium and water handling by the kidney
Not adversely affect other cardiovascular risk factors
Have a smooth onset of action and a receptor half-life of more than 12 hours, allowing once-daily dosage
Not be contraindicated because of concomitant disorders or medications
Be inexpensive

tions, although no single drug available at present would completely fulfill all requirements.

D. Diuretics

Diuretics are efficacious antihypertensive agents in elderly patients with essential hypertension. In most studies in which diuretics were used as first-line therapy, a marked reduction of total and nonfatal strokes has been reported. In the British Medical Research Council study (34), patients receiving diuretics had an even lower stroke rate than those with similar blood pressures who received a placebo. Thus, diuretics may well have a "cerebroprotective" effect. In contrast, the effects of diuretics on the prevention of coronary artery disease and acute MI have been less impressive. Findings from the European Working Party on High Blood Pressure in the Elderly (28) show a significant reduction in total cardiac mortality but not in the occurrence of acute MI. Recently, the STOP trial (30) has shown a significant reduction of primary endpoints (94 versus 58; $p = 0.0031$) and stroke morbidity and mortality (53 versus 29; $p = 0.0081$). This placebo-controlled, double-blinded study has documented a distinct reduction in cardiovascular morbidity in patients who were treated with hydrochlorothiazide plus amiloride, alone or in combination with atenolol, metoprolol, and pindolol, when compared with the placebo group. However, as in many previous studies, no significant reduction in endpoints of coronary artery disease was achieved. Most recently published results of the MRC Trial in the Elderly (31) performed in 4396 subjects aged 65 to 74 years and followed for 5 years showed that the treatment group (HCTZ + amiloride or atenolol) experienced fewer strokes (25%, $p = 0.04$), coronary events (19%, $p = 0.08$), and all cardiovascular events (17%, $p = 0.03$). This protective effect occurred only in the diuretic group (31% fewer strokes, p = 0.04; 44% reduction in coronary events, p = 0.0009; and a 35% reduction in all coronary events, p = 0.0005) but not in patients on atenolol. Moreover, the number of withdrawals was consistently higher in the beta-blocker-treated group than among those receiving a diuretic (respectively, 333 versus 160 patients). The recent SHEP study also documented that diuretics reduce coronary morbidity in a very selective population with isolated systolic hypotension (29).

Since hypertension may be linked with another age-dependent disease—osteoporosis—it should be noted that long-term therapy with thiazide diuretics has been reported to reduce osteoporosis and consequently the incidence of hip fractures (35,36).

Conversely, diuretics are known to cause some metabolic disturbances, partially overriding the beneficial blood-pressure-lowering effect on cardiac mortality. The most important metabolic disturbances are hypokalemia, altered metabolism of glucose and lipids, hyperreninemia, and increased adrenergic stimulation (37). In patients with hypertension and diabetes, diuretics have been shown to be associated with an accelerated decline in renal function and very high mortality (38). This effect may be associated with the minimal effect of diuretic therapy on albuminuria, an established predictor of diabetic and hypertensive renal disease that may lead to renal failure. Their effect of increasing uric acid generally contraindicates diuretics in the presence of gout.

Also in patients with left ventricular hypertrophy and ventricular ectopy, diuretics, through hypokalemia and hypomagnesemia, may aggravate electrophysiological instability and cause more serious arrhythmias. Moreover, their influence on LVH reduction is unpredictable and seems to depend mainly on a decrease of left ventricular interior diameters (39). The influence of diuretics on vascular changes also appears to be less beneficial in comparison with that of newer agents. Dahlof and colleagues, by evaluating retinal vascular changes after 26 weeks of double-blind treatment with hydrochlorothiazide and enalapril, reported that only the angiotensin-converting enzyme (ACE) inhibitor decreased the reflection of the retinal wall and reduced the narrowing of arteries (40). In contrast, hydrochlorothiazide did not have any effects, although blood pressure was lowered to the same degree.

In conclusion, diuretics in low doses are good antihypertensive agents that have been shown to reduce morbidity and mortality from strokes. We also consider diuretics (in low doses) to be excellent step-two agents in combination therapy in patients receiving ACE inhibitors or other agents. Furthermore, in elderly patients with congestive heart failure secondary to left ventricular systolic dysfunction as well as in patients with states involving fluid volume overload, loop diuretics remain a cornerstone of management.

E. Beta-Blockers

Most beta-blockers lower arterial pressure by decreasing cardiac output secondary to a fall in heart rate without affecting or even increasing total peripheral resistance. The high prevalence of heart failure, sick-sinus syndrome, and other concomitant diseases, such as glucose intolerance and diabetes, peripheral artery disease, and chronic obstructive pulmonary disease, clearly makes beta-blockers a poor choice for treatment of elderly hypertensive patients. Beta-blockers should also be avoided in elderly patients with isolated systolic hypertension, since the negative chronotropic effect of these agents in patients with rigid big arteries tends to elevate systolic pressure and lower diastolic pressure (18). It must be emphasized, however, that the hemodynamic effects of beta-blockers are not all alike.

Labetalol (an alpha-beta-blocker), pindolol, bopindolol (a beta-blocker with high sympathomimetic activity), and celiprolol have been shown to maintain cardiac output and dilate peripheral vasculature (41–43). Celiprolol, by exerting its antihypertensive effect at least to some extent through beta$_2$-stimulation (which produces vasodilatation), appears to have an attractive hemodynamic profile for treatment of the hypertensive elderly patient.

Apart from these considerations, beta-blockers remain an excellent choice for patients concomitantly suffering from a hyperkinetic heart syndrome. Beta-blockers have also been clearly documented to reduce reinfarction and mortality rates in post–myocardial infarction (post-MI) hypertensive patients and therefore remain a good choice in this clinical situation (44). They are also useful when combined with dihydropyridine calcium antagonists in hypertensive patients with angina pectoris without left ventricular failure or other contraindications.

F. Centrally Acting Antiadrenergic Drugs

Low doses of centrally acting antiadrenergic agents (methyldopa, clonidine, guanabenz, etc.) have been used in the past to treat hypertension in the elderly. However, with the advent of more modern antihypertensive drugs with a cleaner side-effect profile, these drugs have been largely abandoned. Centrally acting antiadrenergic drugs should be used in combination therapy only as third- and fourth-step agents.

G. Alpha-Blockers

Alpha-blockers exert their antihypertensive effect by reducing total peripheral resistance while maintaining or increasing cardiac output. Since they also dilate capacitance vessels, orthostatic hypotension has been shown to occur and to be a meaningful risk in elderly patients with rigid arteries and reduced baroreceptor activity. In the past, this has been a particular problem with the first dose of prazosin and after inappropriate escalation of the dose. Pretreatment with a diuretic made patients much more susceptible to this first-dose effect. However, orthostatic hypotension is very uncommon with the more modern agents, such as terazosin and doxazosin. The postsynaptic alpha-blockers have been shown to affect dyslipoproteinemia favorably; they lower total cholesterol and increase high-density lipoprotein cholesterol. Although the long-term benefits of these lipid effects remain to be determined (particularly in the elderly), postsynaptic alpha-blockers should be considered first-line agents in hypertensive patients with dyslipoproteinemias. The other important indication for these drugs is prostatic hypertrophy, wherein the alpha-blockers have been shown to diminish partially the symptoms of dysuria and urinary retention.

H. Calcium Antagonists

Calcium antagonists inhibit calcium entry into vascular smooth muscle and therefore lower arterial pressure by reducing total peripheral resistance (45). Their effect on the capacitance vessels is minimal, and orthostatic hypotension is therefore an uncommon adverse effect of calcium-channel blockade. Apart from their common property of inhibiting calcium entry into cells, calcium antagonists exhibit varying pharmacological effects.

For practical purposes, it is useful to divide them into the dihydropyridine and nondihydropyridine derivatives.

1. Dihydropyridine Calcium Antagonists (Nifedipine, Nitrendipine, Nicardipine, Isradpine, Felodipine, and Amlodipine)

When given in acute conditions, all dihydropyridine calcium antagonists produce a reflexive increase in heart rate and cardiac output and a marked reduction in total peripheral resistance. With chronic administration, this cardioacceleration diminishes somewhat and seems to disappear completely with the new agents (isradipine, felodipine, and amlodipine). Dihydropyridine calcium antagonists seem to decrease left ventricular mass to a lesser extent than the nondihydropyridine derivatives. In general, an increase in renal blood flow and glomerular filtration rate can be observed. Dihydropyridine calcium antagonists are excellent antihypertensive agents in elderly hypertensive patients with concomitant bradycardia. However, acute release formulations, such as liquid nifedipine, should be strictly avoided in elderly patients, since they may precipitate an inappropriate reduction in arterial pressure with profound cardioacceleration leading to myocardial ischemia and even acute MI. This sequence of events has not been documented with the sustained release formulation (Procardia XLR or Adalat SR). The newer calcium antagonists (isradipine, felodipine, and amlodipine) appear to have little if any negative inotropic or chronotropic effect. Thus, they do not slow sinus-node activity and atrioventricular (A-V) conduction or diminish left ventricular contractility. Of note, these agents do not stimulate the activity of the sympathetic nervous system or the renin-angiotensin-aldosterone system. In contrast to other calcium antagonists, the newer calcium antagonists have been shown to have a favorable effect on systemic and regional hemodynamics in patients with congestive heart failure. Isradipine, felodipine, and amlodipine can therefore be considered agents of choice in hypertensive elderly patients with coronary artery disease and systolic dysfunction.

2. Nondihydropyridine Calcium Antagonists (Verapamil, Diltiazem, and Gallopamil)

As with the dihydropyridine calcium antagonists, the acute administration of verapamil, diltiazem, or gallopamil results in cardioacceleration. With prolonged administration, however, heart rate falls below pretreatment levels. All three of these agents have negative chronotropic and inotropic effects; that is, they slow sinus-node activity and A-V node conduction. Their use therefore should be avoided in patients with second-degree heart block or congestive failure from systolic dysfunction. In contrast, nondihydropyridine calcium antagonists, particularly verapamil, are excellent agents in patients with congestive heart failure secondary to impaired filling or diastolic dysfunction, a common sequela of long-standing hypertension and LVH.

A recent study has documented that verapamil given 1 week after acute MI diminishes reinfarction rate and increases survival (46). The decrease in reinfarction rate induced by verapamil was similar to that documented with beta-blockers. In patients with non-Q-wave infarction, diltiazem has been documented to reduce reinfarction rates (47).

Although beta-blockers remain the agents of choice in the management of post-MI patients, calcium antagonists that slow heart rate should be considered when beta-blockers are contraindicated or when patients cannot tolerate them (48).

The nondihydropyridine calcium antagonists have been shown to reduce LVH markedly. Concomitantly, these agents improve left ventricular filling, reduce ventricular ectopy associated with LVH, improve myocardial ischemia, and preserve contractile function. Given that LVH has been identified as one of the most powerful cardiovascular risk factors, this effect can hardly be ignored. However, whether or not reduction of LVH, as induced by calcium antagonists, will diminish the morbidity and mortality of a given patient remains to be determined.

3. Antiatheromatous Effects

Calcium antagonists have been shown to exert antiatheromatous effects in certain experimental models (49) and in some clinical studies have inhibited the development of new atheromatous lesions in the coronary circulation. Calcium antagonists, besides lowering blood pressure, may interfere with endothelial and platelet mechanisms, prevent calcium overload of the cells, inhibit smooth muscle proliferation or bind lipoproteins and esters of hydrolysis of cholesterol in liposomes, and decrease arterial wall matrix synthesis (50). No effect on existing atheromatous plaque was observed. These recent findings make calcium antagonists a very attractive choice in elderly hypertensive patients at risk of or suffering from atherosclerosis.

In summary, the evidence in favor of using calcium antagonists in elderly patients with hypertension is based on the beneficial effects of these agents over and above the reduction in blood pressure. The desirable effects in patients with angina pectoris (both groups of calcium antagonists); secondary prevention after MI and reduction of LVH (verapamil and diltiazem); decrease of albuminuria (verapamil, diltiazem); lack of undesirable effects on glucose, lipid, and uric acid metabolism; and promising antiatheromatous effect establish them as first-line antihypertensive drugs in elderly patients.

I. Angiotensin-Converting Inhibitors

Angiotensin-converting enzyme (ACE) inhibitors lower arterial pressure by decreasing total peripheral resistance while maintaining or enhancing systemic and regional blood flow (51). Since ACE inhibitors affect capacitance vessels, thereby diminishing preload to the left ventricle, they have the potential to produce orthostatic hypotension. Despite the fact that plasma renin activity is often low and unresponsive in elderly hypertensive patients, ACE inhibitors have been shown to lower blood pressure effectively and safely in the geriatric population. This clearly demonstrates that the antihypertensive effect of ACE inhibition is not solely dependent on circulating plasma renin activity. Since ACE inhibitors lower both preload and afterload to the left ventricle, they are the agents of choice in hypertensive patients with congestive heart failure from systolic dysfunction. ACE inhibitors are the only agents that have been shown to prolong life in patients with severe congestive heart failure (class III and IV, New York Heart Association). ACE inhibitors also reduce LVH to a greater extent than any other antihypertensive agent and do not cause deterioration in left ventricular function (39). Their beneficial effects on renal hemodynamics include an increase in renal blood flow with concomitant reduction in microalbuminuria.

ACE inhibitors should be used with caution, if at all, in elderly patients with significant renal impairment and hyperkalemia. In this situation, high doses of ACE inhibitors have been shown to worsen renal function and lead to life-threatening hyperkalemia. Milder degrees of hyperkalemia are not uncommonly seen with ACE inhibition, since in elderly patients the mechanism of potassium excretion is often disturbed as a result of hyporenimic hypoaldosteronism, renal failure, or both.

ACE inhibitors, when given after acute MI, have been shown to prevent progressive dilatation of the left chamber (remodeling). The multicenter study Survival and Ventricular Enlargement Trial (SAVE) in post-MI patients with left ventricular dysfunction (EF $< 40\%$) showed significant reduction in risk of total (19%), as well as cardiovascular mortality (21%) ($p = 0.019$, and $p = 0.014$, respectively), lower risk of reinfarction (25%) ($p = 0.015$), and other cardiovascular endpoints in patients treated with captopril when compared with the placebo group (52). Conceivably, the lower incidence of new myocardial infarctions in SOLVD and SAVE trials might be attributable to an ACE inhibitor mediated decrease in coronary tone, or the improved subendocardial perfusion, or slower thickening of the vascular wall (53).

Much ink describing differences in efficacy and safety among various ACE inhibitors has been wasted. From a practical standpoint, blood-pressure-lowering properties are rather similar for all ACE inhibitors, provided that an adequate dose is given. Clearly, in unstable hemodynamic situations, short-acting agents are preferable to long-acting ACE inhibitors. With prolonged administration, and in stable hemodynamic situations, the once-a-day formulations (lisinopril, ramipril, benazepril, fosinopril, monopril, and trandolapril) are more convenient than the twice-daily (b.i.d.) or thrice-daily (t.i.d.) ACE inhibitors.

J. Combination Therapy

The combination of an ACE inhibitor with a calcium antagonist has been particularly useful in our hands. Hypertensive heart disease in the elderly is commonly associated with both systolic and diastolic dysfunction (54). Combining an ACE inhibitor with a calcium antagonist exerts a favorable effect on both pathogenetic components. Such a combination has also been shown to reduce proteinuria and albuminuria to the greater extent than a calcium antagonist or ACE inhibitor separately (55). A nondihydropyridine calcium antagonist should be chosen in patients with predominantly diastolic dysfunction, whereas a dihydropyridine derivative, such as isradipine, felodipine, or amlodipine, is the combination agent of choice in patients with predominantly systolic dysfunction. In all patients with congestive heart failure, a loop or thiazide diuretic is most often needed to prevent fluid accumulation.

The combination of an ACE inhibitor with low doses of a thiazide diuretic will enhance antihypertensive efficacy. This combination is usually well tolerated in the elderly, although occasionally orthostatic hypotension is observed. Potassium-sparing diuretics should not be combined with ACE inhibitors in the geriatric population because of the danger of hyperkalemia. In the post-MI patient with or without hypertension, it is tempting to combine two "cardioprotective" strategies—for example, a beta-blocker and a calcium antagonist that slows heart rate. No study has shown that this combination is more efficacious than either drug alone. Since both drugs have negative inotropic and chronotropic effects, their combination may result in exacerbation of congestive failure or heart block.

K. Hypertension and Concomitant Diseases

Concomitant risk factors in diseases are common in the elderly hypertensive patient. Table 2 provides information regarding the drugs of choice in special clinical situations. In patients with distinct metabolic abnormalities, such as impaired glucose tolerance, dyslipoproteinemia, either an ACE inhibitor, a calcium antagonist, or a postsynaptic alpha-blocker may be the

Table 2 Selection of Drug of Choice Therapy and Usually Contraindicated Agents Based on Coexisting Condition or Medication

Concomitant disease	Drug of choice	Usually contraindicated
Diabetes	Calcium antagonist	Beta-blocker
	ACE inhibitor	Diuretic[a]
Dyslipidemia	Alpha-blocker	Beta-blocker
	Calcium antagonist	Diuretic[a]
	ACE inhibitor	
Coronary artery disease	Beta-blocker	
	Calcium antagonist	
Left ventricular hypertrophy	ACE inhibitor	Diuretic
	Calcium antagonist	Alpha-blocker
Congestive heart failure	ACE inhibitor	Beta-blocker
	Diuretic	Nondihydropyridine calcium antagonist
Renal failure	ACE inhibitor[b]	Beta-blocker
	Calcium antagonist	
	Diuretic	
Chronic obstructive pulmonary disease (COPD)	Calcium antagonist	Beta-blocker
Prostatic hypertrophy	Alpha-blocker	
Arthritis—nonsteroidal anti-inflammatory drugs (NSAIDs)	Calcium antagonist	

[a]In doses exceeding 25 mg/day.
[b]Caution of excessive increase of potassium and creatinine levels.

drug of choice. In a recent study from Finland in which 892 patients were followed for 3.5 years, the incidence of diabetes mellitus was 4.3 in normotensive subjects, 12.9 in hypertensive patients treated with either a beta-blocker or a diuretic, and 6.3 in hypertensive patients treated by other drugs (56). This study clearly attests to the deleterious influence of diuretics and beta-blockers on metabolic abnormalities associated with hypertension. In patients with coronary disease, either cardioselective beta-blockers or calcium antagonists should be considered as first-line therapy. Patients with left ventricular failure are candidates for either ACE inhibitors or certain calcium antagonists depending on the pathogenetic cause of congestive heart failure. Patients who suffer from chronic obstructive pulmonary disease are clearly not good candidates for beta-blockers and should probably be treated with a calcium antagonist. An ACE inhibitor is usually well tolerated in this situation, although particular attention has to be paid to cough, which is a common side effect of this class of drugs. Patients who suffer from prostatic hypertrophy will profit from a postsynaptic alpha-blocker as a first-line antihypertensive drug. Nonsteroidal anti-inflammatory drugs are commonly given to elderly patients and may interfere with the effect of various antihypertensive agents, with the possible exception of calcium antagonists.

L. Hypertensive Urgencies and Emergencies

Hypertension-associated emergencies in elderly patients require special caution because of often coexisting disseminated atherosclerosis which may result in coronary insufficiency, renal artery stenosis, cerebrovascular disease, or poor baroreflex reactivity. An inappropriate abrupt decrease in blood pressure may lead to a dangerous decrease in organ blood flow and ischemic episodes may ensue (57). In such a case, we advise very careful evaluation of the hypertensive patient's recent medication history to prevent hazardous maneuvers (58). When high blood pressure is associated with life threatening disorders, such as myocardial infarction, pulmonary edema, or cerebral edema, we suggest using short-acting agents given intravenously—nitroglycerin and nitroprusside sodium—and monitoring the patient very carefully (see Chapter 13). The sublingually or orally administered agents, such as nifedipine or labetalol, should be used with great caution as the magnitude of blood pressure decrease and time of action can hardly be predicted and side effects may be more dangerous than the high blood pressure itself (59).

IV. SUMMARY

Hypertension in the elderly is usually an asymptomatic disease and should remain so when treated. Although it clearly puts the patient at a higher risk of stroke, sudden death, congestive heart failure, and acute MI, the benefits of antihypertensive treatment still remain disputable in the overall geriatric population. The hemodynamics, renal function, fluid volume, and endocrine mechanisms of blood pressure elevation in elderly patients are very different from these mechanisms in young people with similar blood pressure elevations. Individualized treatment should aim not only to lower arterial pressure but at the same time to reduce target organ damage, such as nephrosclerosis, coronary artery and cerebrovascular disease, and left ventricular hypertrophy, leading to a longer and better life. The marked increase in availability of newer antihypertensive agents makes the decision about which drug to prescribe much more difficult. Although the last Joint National Committee (60) recommended beta-blockers and thiazides as the preferred drugs, the 1993 Guidelines of WHO and ISH for the Management of Mild Hypertension (61) and the Second Working Party of the British Hypertension Society (62) recommended calcium antagonists, ACE inhibitors, and alpha-adrenergic blockers on an equal basis. While waiting for the results of ongoing SYST-EUR and Chinese trials, we suggest individualizing the drug choice according to the stage of hypertension (target organ damage), concomitant diseases, other medications, and mental and economic condition of the elderly hypertensive patient.

REFERENCES

1. Messerli FH, ed. Cardiovascular Disease in the Elderly, 3d ed. Norwell, MA: Kluwer Academic, 1993.
2. Gavras H, Gavras I, eds. Hypertension in the Elderly. Boston: John Wright, 1983.
3. Mann SJ. Systolic hypertension in the elderly: pathophysiology and management. Arch Intern Med 1992; 152:1977–1984.
4. Psaty BM, Furberg CD, Kuller LH, et al. Isolated systolic hypertension and subclinical cardiovascular disease in the elderly: initial findings from the Cardiovascular Health Study. JAMA 1992; 268:1287–1291.
5. Lakatta EG, Cohen JD, Fleg JL, et al. Hypertension in the elderly: age- and disease-related complications and therapeutic implications. Cardiovasc Drugs Ther 1993; 7:643–653.
6. Cushman WC, Rutan GH. Isolated systolic hypertension in the elderly. Cardiovasc Risk Factors 1992; 2:133–139.
7. Fletcher AE, Bulpitt CJ. Epidemiological aspects of cardiovascular disease in the elderly. J Hypertens 1992; 10:551–558.
8. Applegate WB. Hypertension in elderly patients. Ann Intern Med 1989; 110: 901–915.
9. National Health Survey. Vital and Health Statistics USA: Blood Pressure of Adults by Age and Sex, Washington, D.C.: U.S. Government Printing Office, 1964:9.

10. National Health Survey. Vital and Health Statistics. Series 11, No. 150. Blood Pressure of Persons 18 to 74 years, United States, 1971–72. Bethesda, MD: U.S. Department of Health, Education and Welfare, 1975.
11. Kannel WB, Gordon T. Evaluation of cardiovascular risk in the elderly: the Framingham study. Bull NY Acad Med 1978; 54:573–591.
12. Shekelle RB, Ostfeld AM, Klawans HL Jr. Hypertension and risk of stroke in an elderly population. Stroke 1974; 5:71–75.
13. Forette F, Henry JF, Forette B, et al. Hypertension arterielle du sujet age prevalence en milieu long sejour. Nouv Presse Med 1975; 4:2991–2998.
14. Svärdsudd K, Tibblin G. Mortality and morbidity during 13.5 years' follow up in relation to blood pressure: the study of men born in 1913. Acta Med Scand 1979; 205:483–492.
15. Messerli FH, Ventura HO, Glade LB, et al. Essential hypertension in the elderly: hemodynamics, intravascular volume, plasma renin activity, and circulating catecholamine levels. Lancet 1983; 2:983–986.
16. Teresawa F, Kuramoto K. The study on the hemodynamics in old hypertensive subjects. Jpn Circ J 1973; 37:723–729.
17. Messerli FH. Essential hypertension in the elderly. Triangle 1985; 24:35–47.
18. Lund-Johansen P. Heart pump function and total peripheral resistance in mild essential hypertension: a 17-year follow-up study. In: Folkow B, Nordlander M, Strauer BE, et al. eds. Hypertension: Pathophysiology and Clinical Implications of Early Structural Changes. Molndal, Sweden: Hassle, 1985:392–407.
19. Messerli FH. Clinical determinants and consequences of left ventricular hypertrophy. Proceedings of a symposium: Left Ventricular Hypertrophy in Essential Hypertension: Mechanisms and Therapy. Am J Med 1983; 75 (suppl 3A): 51–63.
20. Messerli FH. Individualization of antihypertensive therapy: an approach based on hemodynamics and age. J Clin Pharmacol 1981; 21:517–528.
21. Kannel WB. Prevalence and natural history of electrocardiographic left ventricular hypertrophy. Am J Med 1983; 75(suppl 3A):4–11.
22. Kannel WB, Gordon T, Offutt D. Left ventricular hypertrophy by electrocardiogram: prevalence, incidence and mortality in the Framingham study. Ann Intern Med 1969; 71:89–105.
23. Colandrea MA, Friedman GD, Nichaman MD, et al. Systolic hypertension in the elderly: an epidemiologic assessment. Circulation 1970; 41:239–245.
24. Hollenberg NK, Epstein M, Basch RI, et al. "No man's land" of the renal vasculature: an arteriographic and hemodynamic assessment of the interlobar and arcuate arteries in essential and accelerated hypertension. Am J Med 1969; 47: 845–854.
25. Chien S, Usami S, Simmons RL, et al. Blood volume and age: repeated measurements on normal men after 17 years. J Appl Physiol 1966; 21:583–588.
26. Weidmann P, de Myttenaere-Bursztein S, Maxwell MH, et al. Effect of aging on plasma renin and aldosterone in normal man. Kidney Int 1975; 8:325–333.
27. Goldstein DS. Plasma catecholamines and essential hypertension: an analytical review. Hypertension 1983; 5:86–99.

28. Amery A, Birkenhäger W, Brixko P, et al. Mortality and morbidity results from the European Working Party on High Blood Pressure in the Elderly trial. Lancet 1985; 1:1349–1354.
29. SHEP Cooperative Research Group. Prevention of stroke by antihypertensive drug treatment in older persons with isolated systolic hypertension: final results of the Systolic Hypertension in the Elderly Program (SHEP). JAMA 1991; 265: 3255–3264.
30. Dahlöf B, Lidholm LH, Hansson L, et al. Morbidity and mortality in the Swedish Trials in Old Patients with Hypertension (STOP-Hypertension). Lancet 1991; 338:1281–1285.
31. Medical Research Council Working Party. MRC trial of treatment of hypertension in older adults: principal results. Br Med J 1992; 304:405–412.
32. Messerli FH. Cardiovascular effects of obesity and hypertension. Lancet 1982; 1:1165–1168.
33. Hubert HB, Feinleib M, Menamacre PM, et al. Obesity as an independent risk factor for cardiovascular disease: a 26-year follow-up of participants in the Framingham Heart Study. Circulation 1983; 67:968–977.
34. Medical Research Council Working Party. MRC trial of treatment of mild hypertension: principal results. Br Med J 1985; 291:97–104.
35. Wasnich RD, Banfante RJ, Yano K, et al. Thiazide effect on the mineral content of bone. N Engl J Med 1983; 309:344–347.
36. Ray WA, Griffin MR, Downey W, et al. Long-term use of thiazide diuretics and risk of hip fracture. Lancet 1989; 1:687–690.
37. Gilfford RW Jr. 1990. Diuretics in hypertension. In: Messerli FH, ed. Cardiovascular Drug Therapy. Philadelphia: WB Saunders, 1990:298–309.
38. Warram JH, Laffel LM, Valsania P, et al. Excess mortality associated with diuretic therapy in diabetes mellitus. Arch Intern Med 1991; 151:1350–13536.
39. Dahlof B, Pennert K, Hansson L. Reversal of left ventricular hypertrophy in hypertensive patients: a meta-analysis of 109 treatment studies. Am J Hypertens 1992; 5:95–110.
40. Dahlof B, Stenkula S, Hansson L. Hypertensive retinal vascular changes: relationship to left ventricular hypertrophy and arteriolar changes before and after treatment. Blood Pressure 1992; 1:35–44.
41. Flamenbaum W, Dubrow A. Labetalol. In: Messerli FH, ed. Cardiovascular Drug Therapy. Philadelphia: WB Saunders, 1990:573–591.
42. Reid JL. Celiprolol. In: Messerli FH, ed. Cardiovascular Drug Therapy. Philadelphia: WB Saunders, 1990:554–560.
43. Man in't Veld AJ, Schalekamp MADH. How intrinsic sympathomimetic activity modulates the haemodynamic responses to beta-adrenoreceptor antagonists: a clue to the nature of their antihypertensive mechanism. Br J Clin Pharmacol 1982; 13(suppl 2):245S–248S.
44. Wikstrand J, Kendall M. The role of beta receptor blockade in preventing sudden death. Eur Heart J 1992; 13 (suppl D):111–120.
45. Bühler FR, Hulthen L. Calcium channel blockers: a pathophysiologically based antihypertensive treatment concept for the future. Eur J Clin Invest 1982; 12:1–3.

46. The Danish Study Group on Verapamil in Myocardial Infarction. Effect of verapamil on mortality and major events after acute myocardial infarction (The Danish Verapamil Infarction Trial II—Davit II). Am J Cardiol 1990; 66:779–785.
47. The Multicenter Diltiazem Postinfarction Trial Research Group. The effect of diltiazem on mortality and reinfarction after myocardial infarction. N Engl J Med 1988; 319:385–392.
48. Bühler FR, Hulthén UL, Kiowski W, et al. Beta blockers and calcium antagonists: cornerstones of antihypertensive therapy in the 1980's. Drugs 1984; (suppl 6):9888–9894.
49. Henry PD. Ahterosclerosis, calcium and calcium antagonists. Circulation 1985; 72:456–459.
50. Parmley WW. Vascular protection from atherosclerosis: potential of calcium antagonists. Am J Cardiol 1990; 66:16I–22I.
51. Dunn FG, Oigman W, Ventura HO, et al. Enalapril improves systemic and renal hemodynamics and allows regression of left ventricular mass in essential hypertension. Am J Cardiol 1984; 53:105–108.
52. Pfeffer MA, Braunwald E, Moye LA, et al. Effect of captopril on mortality and morbidity in patients with left ventricular dysfunction after myocardial infarction: results of the survival and ventricular enlargement trial: the SAVE investigators. N Engl J Med 1992; 327:669–677.
53. Cohn JN. The prevention of heart failure—a new agenda (editorial). N Engl J Med 1992; 327:725–727.
54. Grodzicki T, Messerli FH, McLoughlin M, Soria F. Systolic and diastolic dysfunction in 24 elderly hypertensive patients (abstr). J Hypertens 1992;
55. Bakris GL, Barnhill BW, Sadler R. Treatment of arterial hypertension in diabetic humans: importance of therapeutic selection. Kidney Int 1992; 41:912–919.
56. Mykkanen M, Haffner SM, Kuusisto J, et al. Hypertensives with beta-blockers or diuretic therapy have an increased risk for type 2 diabetes.
57. Wachter RM. Symptomatic hypotension induced by nifedipine in the acute treatment of severe hypertension. Arch Intern Med 1987; 147:556–558.
58. Messerli FH, Kowey P, Grodzicki T. Sublingual nifedipine for hypertensive emergencies (letter). Lancet 1991; 338:881.
59. Dubiel JP, Kawecka-Jaszcz K, Kocemba J, et al. Acute and long-term treatment of hypertension with nifedipine in the elderly. J Hum Hypertens 1990; 4: 410–414.
60. Joint National Committee on the Detection, Evaluation, and Treatment of Blood Pressure. The 1992 Report of the Joint National Committee on the Detection, Evaluation, and Treatment of Blood Pressure (JNC-V). Arch Intern Med 1993; 153:154–183.
61. 1993 Guidelines for the Management of Mild Hypertension. Memorandum from a WHO/ISH Meeting. J Hypertens 1993.
62. Sever P, Beevers G, Bulpitt C, et al. Management guidelines in essential hypertension: report of the second working party of the British Hypertension Society. Br Med J 1993; 306:983–987.

5

The Obese, Dyslipidemic, and/or Diabetic Hypertensive

MYRON H. WEINBERGER
Indiana University School of Medicine
Indianapolis, Indiana

I. INTRODUCTION

The risk of a cardiovascular event's occurrence in a hypertensive patient is enhanced by the presence of other risk factors, many of which are more frequently observed in hypertensives than in those with normal blood pressure levels. The initial observations of the long-term Framingham Study identified cigarette smoking, hypercholesterolemia, diabetes, and left ventricular hypertrophy on electrocardiogram as important cardiovascular risk factors which act to amplify the risk presented by high blood pressure alone (1). Additional risk factors include sedentary life-style and obesity, dyslipidemia manifested by elevated triglyceride and low high-density lipoprotein levels, insulin resistance, impaired carbohydrate tolerance, and male gender. Furthermore, the concurrence of several of these factors, particularly obesity, dyslipidemia, and insulin resistance, with elevated blood pressure has led to the description of a clinical syndrome incorporating these abnormalities (2), with preliminary evidence of a familial distribution of these factors, suggesting a genetic basis for them (3). This chapter will review the epidemiological evidence in support of these associations, the possible mechanisms involved, and the implications of the presence of these factors for the treatment of hypertension as well as the impact of specific antihypertensive agents upon them.

II. OBESITY

While the association between body weight and blood pressure has long been recognized, only recently have we understood the possible causes of this relationship and its implications. One of the limitations of the indirect sphygmomanometric technique typically used for blood pressure measurement is its dependence on an idealized relationship between arm circumference and cuff bladder size. Thus when a standard-size adult cuff is used on the arm of an obese individual with increased arm circumference, an artifactual elevation of blood pressure due to the suboptimal distribution of force against the brachial artery often results. This can be remedied by the use of larger cuffs for such individuals (4). The standard adult cuff provides accurate readings in individuals with an arm circumference of less than 35 cm, typically those having a body mass index (BMI) less than 34, and weighing less than 95 kg (4). The use of a large adult cuff or a cuff designed for blood pressure measurement in the thigh provides accurate blood pressure readings in individuals with increased arm circumference but does not influence the accuracy of readings in those with normal arm dimensions (4).

While a large number of cross-sectional studies have demonstrated a relationship between body weight and blood pressure (5,6), relatively few longitudinal studies have confirmed this relationship (7). Moreover, the distribution of body mass may also be important since a closer correlation with blood pressure has been observed for upper body fat than for total body mass (8,9).

A. The Physiological Features of Obesity Hypertension

The features associated with weight-related blood pressure changes are identified, but the mechanisms responsible for them are not yet clear. Most investigators have observed an increase in cardiac output and extracellular fluid volume in association with obesity (6,10,11). In normotensive obese subjects peripheral resistance is decreased, whereas in hypertensives it is increased (6). While some studies have shown an increase in extracellular fluid volume (11), obesity hypertension is generally not considered to be a salt- and volume-dependent phenomenon (12,13). Central obesity has also been found to be associated with an increased vasoconstrictor response to stress (10). Despite these hemodynamic alterations associated with obesity, some epidemiological observations suggest that nonobese hypertensives have higher mortality rates than obese hypertensives (14), suggesting that the combination of obesity and hypertension is somehow protective. This appears paradoxical in view of the known adverse effects of obesity and particularly in view of the recent recognition of the constellation of cardiovascular disease risk factors in individuals with coexistent hypertension, insulin resistance, dyslipidemia, and obesity.

Obesity per se independent of changes in blood pressure is associated with increases in cardiac output and total blood volume, thus indicating that, at the same mean arterial pressure, obese individuals have lower total peripheral resistance than do lean individuals. However, the increased cardiac output is associated with increased preload and left ventricular dilatation, which then lead to an increase in afterload (15). Despite the increased cardiac output and blood volume, vascular resistance in the renal and systemic circulation is reduced and blood flow is increased in obese hypertensives when compared to their lean counterparts (16,17). This could contribute to the decreased morbidity and mortality among obese hypertensives previously cited (14).

B. Mechanisms for Obesity Hypertension

The mechanism for these differences in blood flow and resistance in obese subjects may be related to alterations in adrenergic activity or to the vascular responses to adrenergic stimuli. Egan and colleagues demonstrated that obese men had increased forearm blood flow under basal measurements when compared to nonobese subjects and obese subjects demonstrated a comparatively greater rise in blood flow in response to administration of an alpha-adrenergic blocking agent, phentolamine (18). These observations were interpreted as evidence of increased alpha-adrenergic tone in the vasculature of obese men. Many prior studies had implicated the sympathetic nervous system in the relationship between obesity and blood pressure. Obese borderline hypertensives were found to have higher levels of plasma norepinephrine and epinephrine than nonobese subjects along with increased levels of plasma renin activity (19). When the obese individuals lost weight, the reduction in blood pressure was correlated with decreases in plasma norepinephrine levels, suggesting a causal relationship (19). Additional studies confirming these interactions have recently been reviewed by Tuck, who has speculated about their potential relevance to the pharmacological treatment of obese hypertensives (20).

In rats, increased sensitivity to the thermic effects of norepinephrine during overfeeding has been demonstrated, but such an effect has not been observed in obese humans (21). However, in that study a difference in the disappearance rate of norepinephrine from plasma after infusion of exogenous norepinephrine was observed in obese Pima Indians compared to lean controls (21). These findings led the authors to propose that differences in the metabolic clearance rate of catecholamines may be important in some forms of obesity.

Several studies have attempted to clarify the relationships among body weight, blood pressure, catecholamine or sympathetic nervous system activity, and insulin and glucose responses. In a study of older men, body mass index and total caloric intake were found to be correlated with urinary norepinephrine excretion (22). Furthermore, individuals with elevated levels of blood glucose and/or insulin had higher norepinephrine excretion. No comment was made concerning the relationship of these findings to blood pressure. In a recent review of factors associated with obesity-related hypertension (23) the authors cited studies reporting higher, normal, or lower levels of catecholamines in obese hypertensives. These investigators also reported that the blood pressure was more closely correlated with upper body fat than with adiposity per se. They observed an increase in plasma volume and cardiac output in obese subjects, both of which declined with weight loss. They also observed a decrease in plasma insulin levels with weight loss in their subjects but found no correlation between the insulin changes and the changes in blood pressure (23). However, in a group of obese adolescents in whom increases in both insulin levels and blood pressure were observed, both decreased with weight loss (24).

Not all studies confirm this finding of fasting hyperinsulinemia in hypertensives. In a large study of obese and nonobese normotensive and hypertensive subjects no relationship was seen between fasting insulin levels and blood pressure (25). However, significant correlations were observed between postglucose-administration insulin levels and blood pressure in nonobese subjects but not in obese individuals (25). Hall has recently reviewed the experimental evidence linking insulin and blood pressure (26). He concludes that species differences exist since in the dog, chronic infusion of insulin has no effects on sodium and water balance or on blood pressure, but blood pressure rises with insulin administration in rats (26). He further suggests that the inconsistent observations in humans may reflect heterogeneity in the response of our species (26).

Studies in a Japanese population demonstrated reduced fractional excretion of sodium in obese hypertensives and greater blood pressure response to salt restriction or to the natriuretic effects of infused dopamine than in nonobese subjects (27). These observations suggest that the dopaminergic system, one which favors sodium and water excretion, in addition to the noradrenergic system, which favors salt retention, may also be important in this form of hypertension. In fact, over a decade ago we proposed that the relationship between urinary excretion of dopamine and its metabolites and that of norepinephrine, which we dubbed the "natriuretic index," reflected the sum of these opposing effects on the renal excretion of sodium and might thus be involved in salt-dependent forms of hypertension (28).

The kidney has been implicated in the pathophysiology of hypertension in obesity in other ways. Renal biopsy of 17 massively obese subjects with significant proteinuria but no other evidence of systemic disease revealed focal glomerulosclerosis in 9 subjects and diabetic nephropathy in 5 (29).

Although the authors did not report blood pressure observations in their subjects, they speculated that the renal lesions may result from the glomerular hyperfiltration known to occur in obesity (29). Since none of the subjects found to have diabetic nephropathy on biopsy had clinical evidence of diabetes mellitus, they concluded that occult diabetic nephropathy may also be common in obese individuals and may antedate the clinical presentation of diabetes mellitus.

C. Effects of Weight Loss

In a study of over 300 obese subjects, weight loss was associated with a significant decrease in blood pressure although not all of the subjects had hypertension (30). As with most blood pressure interventions, the magnitude of blood pressure reduction was proportional to the initial blood pressure level. For the entire population studied an average of 1 kg change in weight (increase or decrease) was associated with a corresponding change in blood pressure of 1 mm Hg systolic and diastolic (30). The decline in blood pressure was more rapid early in the weight loss period than later. This nonlinear relationship between weight loss and blood pressure decline has been described as a "floor effect" by other investigators (31). Indeed, in most reviews of the relationship between weight loss and blood pressure this observation has been cited as well as the fact that not all obese hypertensives demonstrate a fall in blood pressure with weight loss (6). It should be emphasized that most but not all studies have shown that weight reduction is associated with a fall in blood pressure. In one well-controlled, carefully performed study, despite an average weight loss of 4.1 kg over a 6 month period, there was no significant decrease in blood pressure (32). This study, involving mild hypertensives, may not have had adequate sensitivity to detect a significant change in blood pressure with such small changes in weight in a heterogeneous group of patients without marked blood pressure elevation.

Weight reduction in hypertensives is associated with a variety of hemodynamic and humoral changes. These include reduction in intravascular volume and cardiac output in concert with a decrease in sympathetic nervous system activity (15). Other investigators have confirmed the decrease in norepinephrine level and the response of mean arterial pressure to upright posture after weight loss in obese hypertensives (19). Among obese borderline hypertensive subjects, weight loss was associated with a decrease in both blood pressure and sympathetic nervous system activity as measured by direct recording from peroneal nerve fibers (33). However, some have found a decrease in blood pressure, plasma volume, and cardiac output with weight loss without a change in body fat content or norepinephrine level (23).

The role of sodium balance in the decrease in blood pressure with weight loss is controversial. In a study of obese hypertensive men, blood pressure decreased only when weight loss was accompanied by restriction of dietary sodium intake but not with equivalent weight loss without reduction in sodium (34). However, another study of the effects of rapid weight loss found that the reduction of blood pressure in obese hypertensives was independent of sodium intake (35). Using a different experimental design, Rissanen and colleagues concluded that salt intake had little effect on the reduction of blood pressure seen with weight loss in obese hypertensives (36).

Beilin has recently reviewed the evidence connecting body weight and blood pressure from the perspective of epidemiological evidence as well as from interventional studies (37). Although the wide variety of study designs does not permit the use of traditional meta-analytical statistics to compare the findings, Beilin concludes that the majority of well-controlled intervention trials indicate a significant reduction in blood pressure associated with weight loss in obese hypertensives (37). His conclusions regarding the role of dietary sodium intake in these findings are more guarded and equivocal: An effect is deemed likely but not certain (37).

Several recent studies have attempted to compare the effects of several nonpharmacological (life-style) interventions on blood pressure in different hypertensive or prehypertensive populations. In the Primary Prevention of Hypertension trial some 200 subjects with high-normal blood pressure (diastolic pressure 85 to 89 mm Hg or 80 to 84 mm Hg and 10% to 50% above ideal body weight) were followed for 5 years after being randomized to a multiple intervention, consisting of weight loss for the obese, reduction in dietary salt intake and reduction in alcohol consumption for those who drank, or to a control group (38). Net weight loss averaged 2.7 kg, sodium intake was reduced by 25%, and reported alcohol intake by 30% in the intervention group. The incidence of subsequent development of frank hypertension was reduced by over half in the intervention group. It appeared that weight loss was the most effective of the interventions in preventing the development of hypertension (38). However, the multifactorial nature of the study design made it difficult to identify a single responsible component. In a larger study of over 800 subjects with diastolic pressures of 78 to 89 mm Hg the effects of various dietary interventions, including caloric reduction, sodium reduction, reduced caloric and sodium intake, and reduced sodium and increased potassium intake, were compared to those of a control group over a 3 year period (39). At the end of this period average weight reduction was 4%, sodium reduction 10%, and no change in potassium intake was seen (39). All four intervention groups had lower mean blood pressure at the end of the study than did the control group. The weight loss group had the greatest blood pressure decrease (39).

Among 2182 subjects with diastolic pressures between 80 and 89 mm Hg who were randomly assigned to one of seven intervention groups including life-style modifications (weight reduction, sodium reduction, stress management) or controls who were assigned to placebo or one of four nutritional supplements (calcium, magnesium, potassium, or fish oil) over an 18 month period, a clearer picture of the value of individual interventions in influencing blood pressure emerged (40). The weight loss group had an average of 3.9 kg reduction associated with the greatest decrease in blood pressure. Sodium reduction that averaged 44 mmol/day was associated with a smaller, but statistically significant ($p = 0.05$) decrease in blood pressure. Despite evidence of good compliance, none of the other groups utilizing stress management or supplementation with calcium, magnesium, potassium, or fish oil demonstrated a significant change in blood pressure (40). In this study also, weight reduction was associated with a frequency of development of hypertension that was half that of the corresponding control group over the 18 month period of study. Sodium reduction had a smaller but discernible effect on the prevention of hypertension (40).

In the Trial of Antihypertensive Interventions and Management (TAIM) 593 mild hypertensives (diastolic pressure 90 to 100 mm Hg) were randomly assigned to usual, weight loss, or low sodium–high potassium diets and then randomly assigned to receive placebo, chlorthalidone, or atenolol (41). Weight loss was associated with a greater decrease in blood pressure among those with the highest pretreatment renin levels and had an additive antihypertensive effect with both drug treatments. A low sodium–high potassium diet had less effect than weight loss in combination with pharmacological therapy but still produced an additive reduction in blood pressure (41). In a study of 64 obese, hypertensive men the effects of a weight and sodium reduction diet were compared to those of a beta-blocker-based, stepped-care pharmacological regimen (42). Despite a decrease in weight in the diet group and an increase in the drug treatment group, blood pressure reduction was significantly better in the drug treated than in the nonpharmacological group. The diet treatment was more effective in lowering plasma insulin and triglyceride levels than was drug therapy (42). Another aspect of the TAIM study examined the effect of two specific antihypertensive agents on weight loss in mild hypertension (43). They found that atenolol treatment was associated with less weight loss than that of the placebo group, while chlorthalidone treatment enhanced weight loss when compared to placebo (43).

D. Conclusions Regarding Obesity

In general, it is clear that obesity is associated with an increased risk of hypertension and that it is often associated with the presence of other factors such as insulin resistance, carbohydrate intolerance, dyslipidemia, and left ventricular hypertrophy (44), all of which amplify the risk of cardiovascular disease and death. The mechanisms involved in obesity related hypertension include increased extracellular fluid volume, cardiac output, and sympathetic nervous system activity. Weight reduction is associated with reduction of blood pressure in the obese, whether hypertensive or normotensive, and may reduce the risk of development of hypertension in the latter. Maintaining weight loss is a difficult task and requires much motivation and support. Not all obese hypertensives have a fall in blood pressure following weight loss, nor is it always adequate even in those whose blood pressure does respond to normalize elevated levels. However, as adjunctive therapy with antihypertensive agents, an additive effect has generally been seen. In addition, weight loss often improves the abnormal lipid profile and carbohydrate intolerance of the obese hypertensive.

III. DYSLIPIDEMIA

The initial Framingham Heart Study report identified hypercholesterolemia as an important independent risk factor for coronary artery disease (45). Moreover, the Multiple Risk Factor Intervention Trial (MRFIT), although confined to males, demonstrated a continuous risk of coronary artery disease and cholesterol levels above 180 mg/dl (4.68 mmol/L) with a doubling of risk at levels above 220 mg/dl (46). In a 30 year follow-up evaluation of Framingham study subjects it was found that the cardiovascular disease death rate increased 1% for every 1% increase (milligrams per deciliter [mg/dl]) of serum cholesterol. Moreover, no threshold effect was observed from 180 mg/dl upward (47), confirming the continuous relationship observed in the MRFIT population (46).

A. High-Density Lipoprotein Cholesterol

In 1977 further information from the Framingham study cohort identified the high-density lipoprotein (HDL) fraction as a better predictor of coronary artery disease risk in both men and women than total cholesterol during a 4 year period (48). Levels of low-density lipoprotein (LDL) were weaker predictors of heart attacks, and triglycerides were found to be related to coronary events only in females (48). This observation was confirmed in 12 year follow-up evaluation of the same cohort, demonstrating the important predictive value of HDL in both men and women (49). In addition, this study quantified the impact of varying levels of total cholesterol at different HDL levels on coronary risk, further demonstrating the relatively greater importance of HDL in predicting coronary artery disease risk (49). A more recent report from the Framingham study has provided additional quantitative information (50). Over a 6 year period a 1% increase in total cholesterol was related to a 2% increase in coronary artery disease risk while a 1% decrease in HDL was associated with a 4% increase in risk (50). Moreover these relationships held even for total cholesterol levels less than 200 mg/dl and were valid in both men and women. In this analysis of the Framingham data triglycerides were found to be related to coronary risk in both men and women, but the significance of this association was lost when adjusted for HDL levels in men but not in women. This report also identified factors associated with reduced levels of HDL such as lack of estrogen treatment in postmenopausal females, obesity, abstinence from ethanol, sedentary lifestyle and lack of exercise, tobacco smoking, and treatment with beta-adrenergic blocking drugs. This information has provided new insights into some of the factors regulating or modifying lipoprotein levels and has enhanced our understanding of treatment.

B. Interventional Studies

While Framingham and other epidemiological observations have provided important information regarding the relationship between various lipid and lipoprotein components and the risk for vascular disease, interventional studies have provided confirmation of these associations by proving the benefit of intervention in reducing these risks. A review of the voluminous literature reporting the effects of a variety of interventions in individuals with dyslipidemia and even with normal lipid profiles is beyond the scope of this chapter. Suffice it to say that the evidence is overwhelming and compelling to indicate the benefit of improvement of the lipid profile for virtually all individuals. Gordon and Rivkind reviewed the observational studies conducted in Framingham, Honolulu, Tromso, Minnesota, and the nationwide MRFIT studies (51). They comment that the evidence from interventional studies indicates that the greatest benefit in reducing the risk of coronary artery disease results from raising HDL levels (51). In general, they report that treatment with niacin and gemfibrozil raises HDL levels about 10% to 15% while treatment with cholestyramine, colestipol, HMG coenzyme A reductase inhibitors, and clofibrate have lesser effects. Probucol lowers both HDL and total cholesterol levels and thus may not be an ideal choice for the individual whose primary abnormality is reduced HDL level. Estrogens and diphenylhydantoin raise HDL levels; androgens, most progestins, and beta-blockers reduce them (51).

C. Triglycerides

Many observational studies have reported a relationship between triglyceride levels and coronary artery disease risk, but this association has been considered to be controversial because of the common association of increased levels of low-density lipoproteins and reduced levels of high-density lipoproteins in individuals with elevated triglyceride levels (52). The connection between triglyceride levels and coronary artery disease is further obscured by the fact that triglyceride levels are the most variable of all lipid components, being influenced by many factors which are less likely to affect the measurements of other lipids or lipoproteins (52). Nonetheless, triglycerides have recently emerged as an important independent risk factor for cardiovascular disease (52).

D. Lipoprotein (a)

Recent evidence has implicated yet another lipoprotein as the most powerful predictor of coronary risk yet identified. This is the fraction identified as lipoprotein (a) (Lp [a]), which has structural homology with plasminogen, providing a link between atherogenic and thrombotic plasma components (53). This lipoprotein and its associated apolipoprotein (a) appear to be genetically determined and thus to be the most important lipid abnormalities in familial dyslipidemia (53). A genetic component of cardiovascular disease has been strengthened by recent observations which have linked the familial occurrence of hypertension with that of dyslipidemias and premature coronary artery disease (54).

E. Familial Dyslipidemic Hypertension

The association of familial hypertension with dyslipidemia was initially described among sibships in which two or more individuals with hypertension were recognized before age 60, and in which 48% demonstrated an abnormality of plasma lipid concentrations (54). These abnormalities included elevated triglyceride level in 30%, elevated low-density lipoprotein level in 19%, and reduced HDL level in 39%. Obviously many subjects had more than one lipid abnormality. This association was named familial dyslipidemic hypertension (FDH) (54) and was followed by a report linking it to coronary artery disease (55). In the latter study families with two or more siblings with coronary artery disease before the age of 55 were evaluated and 75% of those affected were found to have dyslipidemia, most frequently of the pattern defined in FDH and most often consisting of increased triglyceride and/or reduced HDL level (55).

Despite the convincing epidemiological and interventional data linking various lipid and lipoprotein factors to cardiovascular disease, it is quite clear that there is marked heterogeneity in their clinical manifestations. Clues to the existence of differences in the metabolism of these substances and in the response of the vascular endothelium to them have recently emerged and provide new insights into vascular disease (56). Differences in receptors for low-density lipoprotein have been demonstrated among humans and a genetic basis for these differences has been identified (57). It has also been shown that oxidation of low-density lipoproteins markedly increases their uptake by endothelial cells and thus their atherogenicity (56). Moreover, this process can be inhibited by antioxidants such as vitamin E or inhibitors of phospholipase A2 (56). Lipoproteins can also be glycated, a possible mechanism to explain the increased atherogenicity of lipoproteins in patients with diabetes mellitus (56).

F. Therapeutic Implications

While it has long been recognized that the presence of elevated blood pressure augments the cardiovascular consequences of hypercholesterolemia (1), more recent data have confirmed and extended these observations (58). Experimental aninmal models such as the hyperlipidemic Watanabe rabbit have shown a marked increase in atherogenesis when blood pressure is elevated in the presence of hypercholesterolemia (59). Moreover, the use of antihypertensive agents to lower blood pressure does not consistently reduce the risk of cardiovascular morbidity if cholesterol levels rise (60). Indeed in this intervention trial the response of serum cholesterol level to treatment appeared to be a more important determinant of cardiovascular events than did the change in blood pressure (60).

In the Watanabe hypercholesterolemic rabbit, administration of the angiotensin-converting enzyme inhibitor captopril was associated with a reduction in atherosclerosis despite higher levels of circulating cholesterol (61), suggesting that antihypertensive agents may modulate the atherogenic process. For these reasons it is important to be aware of the effects of antihypertensive drugs on factors such as circulating lipids and lipoproteins and on insulin sensitivity and carbohydrate tolerance since it is reasonable to anticipate that such agents may modify or modulate human atherogenesis as well.

In general, diuretics have been shown to induce increases in triglycerides and total cholesterol levels but to have no consistent effects on HDL (62). These effects are dose-dependent and can be minimized by using lower doses of diuretics, or by choosing indapamide, which appears to have less adverse lipid effects than are seen with hydrochlorothiazide at comparable antihypertensive doses. Beta-adrenergic blocking agents, both cardioselective and nonselective, consistently raise triglyceride and lower HDL levels (62). These lipid changes are not seen with beta-blockers having intrinsic sympathomimetic activity (ISA) or with combination alpha- and beta-adrenergic blocking drugs (e.g., labetalol). The centrally acting antisympathetic agents, the angiotensin converting enzyme inhibitors, and the calcium channel entry blockers appear to have no effects on the lipid profile, whereas the alpha-adrenergic blockers are unique among antihypertensive drugs because of their favorable actions to reduce atherogenic lipid levels and to increase HDL levels (62). Little information regarding the effects of direct-acting vasodilators such as hydralazine and minoxidil on lipid and lipoprotein components is available.

Since some studies of the effects of antihypertensive drugs on lipids were short in duration or associated with longer-term changes that were not different from baseline levels, it has been assumed that the drug-induced lipid alterations are transitory. However, most well-controlled trials including a placebo group or those which have examined lipid values after drug withdrawal indicate that the observed changes persist as long as the drugs are taken.

The adverse effect of beta-adrenergic blocking drugs on the lipid profile appears to be offset by beneficial effects of these agents in reducing the risk of sudden death after acute myocardial infarction. A recent analysis of the BHAT trial demonstrated that propranolol raised triglyceride levels by an average of 17% and lowered HDL levels by 6%, despite dietary modifications, weight loss, or smoking cessation in these post–myocardial infarction patients (63). The authors calculated that the adverse effects of propranolol on lipids could have increased the all-cause mortality by about 2% but did not negate the 20% reduction in mortality and morbidity seen in the propranolol-treated subjects (63).

IV. INSULIN RESISTANCE, DYSLIPIDEMIA, AND HYPERTENSION

Despite myriad earlier reports of the frequent concurrence of carbohydrate intolerance with hypertension, Modan and colleagues were the first to document that this association was linked by hyperinsulinemia, which they observed in a high proportion of their study subjects who manifested obesity, carbohydrate intolerance, and elevated blood pressure (64). These observations, made in a population of Israelis, were confirmed in a different population by Ferrannini and colleagues (65). Although the latter study utilized nonobese study subjects, the syndrome has been expanded to include obesity and dyslipidemia, the latter typically reflected by elevated low-density lipoprotein and triglyceride levels and reduced HDL concentrations (2,66). Current scientific evidence suggests that insulin resistance at the tissue level can be directly responsible for many of these abnormalities.

The link between insulin resistance and obesity has been long recognized, but the mechanisms responsible are still being elucidated. This constellation of abnormalities is being identified in increasing numbers of hypertensive patients now that clinicians are more aware of its presence and have a greater understanding of the factors which may contribute to the syndrome. The marked increase in risk for morbidity and mortality conferred by the presence of these multiple abnormalities has mandated more comprehensive evaluation of susceptible individuals and a thoughtful approach to treatment of each of the components in such a way as to minimize increasing the risk for cardiovascular disease. This consideration is most necessary in choosing antihypertensive therapy since the large number of agents available and their vastly differing effects on insulin sensitivity and on lipid and lipoprotein components require careful thought. Table 1 outlines the known effects of the varying classes of antihypertensive drugs on insulin sensitivity and on components of the lipid profile. Among all of the different drug groups only the alpha$_1$-adrenergic blocking agents have been shown to have a consistently beneficial effect on insulin sensitivity and on both the atherogenic and antiatherogenic (HDL) lipid components. Angiotensin-converting enzyme inhibitors have been shown to improve insulin sensitivity and to be neutral in their effects on lipids and lipoproteins. The antisympathetic agents, calcium channel entry blockers, and direct vasodilators (hydralazine, minoxidil) have not been shown to have any effect on insulin sensitivity or lipids. Beta-adrenergic blocking agents, except those with intrinsic sympathomimetic activity and the combined alpha-beta-blockers (labetalol, bucindolol), are known consistently to worsen insulin sensitivity, to raise triglyceride levels (and less consistently cholesterol levels), and to lower HDL levels consistently. Diuretics worsen insulin sensitivity and raise triglyceride levels. The diuretic effects appear to be dose-dependent and perhaps less likely to occur with indapamide than with other diuretics. In the future, agents which improve insulin sensitivity such as metformin (67) and ciglitazone (68) may be available to ameliorate all of the components of the insulin resistance syndrome including hypertension and dyslipidemia.

Table 1 Effect of Antihypertensive Agents on Insulin and Lipid Levels

	Improve	Neutral	Worsen
Insulin sensitivity	A, ACE	AS, C, V	B[a], D
Total cholesterol level	A	ACE, AS, C, V	
Triglyceride level	A	ACE, AS, C, V	B[a], D
LDL level	A	ACE, AS, C, V	
HDL level	A	ACE, AS, C, D, V	B[a]

[a]Except those with ISA and alpha-beta blocking agents. A, alpha$_1$-adrenergic blocking agents; ACE, angiotensin-converting enzyme inhibitors; AS, antisympathetic agents; B, beta-adrenergic blocking agents; C, calcium channel blocking agents; D, diuretics; V, direct vasodilators.

V. SUMMARY

Obesity, insulin resistance, dyslipidemia, and hypertension are independent and powerful risk factors for cardiovascular disease. When they are present in combination, their risk is additive. Moreover, the concurrence of these disorders is more frequent than would be expected on a random basis and is almost certainly linked mechanistically. The treatment of individual components of these syndromes must consider the impact of intervention on the other factors and the potential effect on cardiovascular disease risk. This is particularly important in the selection of antihypertensive therapy since the effects of these drugs on factors beyond blood pressure alone must be considered.

Although both diuretics and beta-blockers may be useful for the control of hypertension and other cardiac problems in patients with obesity, dyslipidemia, or diabetes, their multiple adverse effects support the preference for agents which are either metabolically neutral (ACE inhibitors and calcium channel entry blockers) or beneficial (alpha-blockers) in such patients.

REFERENCES

1. Anderson KM, Odell PM, Wilson PWF, Kannel WB. Cardiovascular disease risk profiles. Am Heart H 1991; 121:293–298.
2. Kaplan NM. The deadly quartet. Arch Intern Med 1989; 149:1514–1520.
3. Williams RR, Hunt SC, Hopkins PN, et al. Familial dyslipidemic hypertension. JAMA 1988; 259:3579–3568.
4. Linfors EW, Feussner JR, Blessing CL, et al. Spurious hypertension in the obese patient. Arch Intern Med 1984; 144:1482–1485.
5. Stamler R, Stamler J, Riedinger WF, et al. Weight and blood pressure: findings in hypertension screening of one million Americans. JAMA 1978; 240:1607–1610.
6. Dustan HP. Obesity and hypertension. Ann Intern Med 1985; 103 (6 pt 2):1047–1049.
7. Witteman JCM, Wilett WC, Stampfer MJ, et al. A prospective study of nutritional factors and hypertension among US women. Circulation 1989; 80:1320–1327.
8. Weinsier RL, Norris DJ, Birch R, et al. The relative contribution of body fat and fat pattern to blood pressure level. Hypertension 1985; 7:578–585.
9. Kanai H, Matsuzawa Y, Kotani K, et al. Close correlation of intra-abdominal fat accumulation to hypertension in obese women. Hypertension 1990; 16:484–490.
10. Jern S, Bergbrant A, Bjorntorp P, Hansson L. Relation of central hemodynamics to obesity and body fat distribution. Hypertension 1992; 19:520–527.
11. Raison J, Achimatos A, Asmar R, et al. Extracellular and interstitial fluid volume in obesity with and without associated systemic hypertension. Am J Cardiol 1986; 57:223–226.

12. Reisin E, Abel R, Modan M, et al. Effect of weight loss without salt restriction on the reduction of blood pressure in overweight hypertensive patients. N Engl J Med 1978; 298:1–6.
13. Tuck ML, Sowers J, Dornfeld L, et al. The effect of weight reduction on blood pressure, plasma renin activity, and plasma aldosterone levels in obese patients. N Engl J Med 1981; 304:930–933.
14. Barrett-Connor E, Khaw K-T. Is hypertension more benign when associated with obesity? Circulation 1985; 72:53–60.
15. Messerli FH. Obesity in hypertension: how innocent a bystander? Am J Med 1984; 77:1077–1082.
16. Reisen E, Messerli FH, Ventura HO, Frohlich ED. Renal hemodynamic studies in obesity hypertension. J Hypertension 1987; 5:397–400.
17. Raison JM, Safar ME, Cambien FA, London GM. Forearm haemodynamics in obese normotensive and hypertensive subjects. J Hypertension 1988; 6:299–303.
18. Egan BM, Schork NJ, Weder AB. Regional hemodynamic abnormalities in overweight men. Am J Hypertens 1989; 2:428–434.
19. Sowers JR, Whitfield LA, Catania RA, et al. Role of the sympathetic nervous system in blood pressure maintainance in obesity. J Clin Endocrinol Metab 1982; 54:1181–1186.
20. Tuck ML. Obesity, the sympathetic nervous system and essential hypertension. Hypertension 1992; 19(suppl I):I-67–lI-77.
21. Katzeff HL, Daniels R. The sympathetic nervous system in human obesity. Int J Obesity 1985; 9(suppl 2):131–137.
22. Troisi RJ, Weiss ST, Parker DR, et al. Relation of obesity and diet to sympathetic nervous system activity. Hypertension 1991; 17:669–677.
23. Weinsier RL, James D, Darnell BE, et al. Obesity-related hypertension: evaluation of the separate effects of energy restriction and weight reduction on hemodynamic and neuroendocrine status. Am J Med 1991; 90:460–468.
24. Rocchini AP, Katch V, Kveselis D, et al. Insulin and renal sodium retention in obese adolescents. Hypertension 1989; 14:367–374.
25. Bonora E, Zavaroni I, Alpi O, et al. Relationship between blood pressure and plasma insulin in non-obese and obese non-diabetic subjects. Diobetologia 1987; 30:719–723.
26. Hall JE, Brands MW, Hildebrandt DA, Mizelle HL. Obesity-associated hypertension: hyperinsulinemia and renal mechanisms. Hypertension 1992; 19(suppl I):I-45–I-55.
27. Kikuchi K, Iimura O, Yamaji I, et al. The pathophysiological role of water-sodium balance and renal dopaminergic activity in overweight patients with essential hypertension. Am J Hypertens 1988; 1:31–37.
28. Weinberger MH, Luft FC, Henry DP. The role of the sympathetic nervous system in the modulation of sodium excretion. Clin Exp Hypertens 1982; A4:719–735.
29. Kasiske BL, Crosson JT. Renal disease in patients with massive obesity. Arch Intern Med 1986; 146:1105–1109.
30. Schotte DE, Stunkard AJ. The effects of weight reduction on blood pressure in 301 obese patients. Arch Intern Med 1990; 150:1701–1704.

31. Cohen N, Flamenbaum W. Obesity and hypertension: demonstration of a "floor effect." Am J Med 1986; 80:177–181.
32. Haynes RB, Harper AC, Costly SR, et al. Failure of weight reduction to reduce mildly elevated blood pressure: a randomized trial. J Hypertens 1984; 2: 535–539.
33. Andersson B, Elam M, Wallin BG, et al. Effect of energy-restricted diet on sympathetic muscle nerve activity in obese women. Hypertension 1991; 18:783–789.
34. Fagerberg B, Andersson OK, Persson B, Hedner T. Reactivity to norepinephrine and effect of sodium on blood pressure during weight loss. Hypertension 1985; 7:586–592.
35. Maxwell MH, Kushiro T, Dornfeld LP, et al. BP changes in obese hypertensive subjects during rapid weight loss. Arch Intern Med 1984; 144:1581–1584.
36. Rissanen A, Pietinen P, Siljamake-Ojansuu U, et al. Treatment of hypertension in obese patients: efficacy and feasibility of weight and salt reduction programs. Acta Med Scand 1985; 218:149–156.
37. Beilin LJ. Diet and hypertension: critical concepts and controversies. J Hypertens 1987; 5(suppl 5):S447–S457.
38. Stamler R, Stamler J, Gos;ch FC, et al. Primary prevention of hypertension by nutritional-hygienic means. JAMA 1989; 262:1801–1807.
39. Hypertension Prevention Trial Research Group. The Hypertension Prevention Trial: three-year effects of dietary changes on blood pressure. Arch Intern Med 1990; 150:153–162.
40. The Trials of Hypertension Prevention Collaborative Group. The effects of nonpharmacologic interventions on blood pressure of persons with high normal levels. JAMA 1992; 267:1213–1220.
41. Blaufox MD, Lee HB, Davis B, et al. Renin predicts diastolic blood pressure response to nonpharmacologic and pharmacologic therapy. JAMA 1992; 267: 1221–1225.
42. Fagerberg B, Berglund A, Andersson OK, Berglund G. Weight reduction versus antihypertensive drug therapy in obese men with high blood pressure: effects upon plasma insulin levels and association with changes in blood pressure and serum lipids. J Hypertens 1992; 10:1053–1061.
43. Davis BR, Oberman A, Blaufox MD, et al. Effect of antihypertensive therapy on weight loss. Hypertension 1992; 19:393–399.
44. Frank S, Colliver JA, Frank A. The electrocardiogram in obesity: statistical analysis of 1029 patients. J Am Coll Cardiol 1986; 7:295–299.
45. Kannel WB, Castelli WP, Gordon T. Serum cholesterol lipoproteins, and risk of coronary heart disease: The Framingham Study. Ann Intern Med 1971; 24: 1–7.
46. Stamler J, Wentworth D, Neaton JD. Is relationship between serum cholesterol and risk of premature death from coronary heart disease continuous and graded? JAMA 1986; 256:2823–2828.
47. Anderson KM, Castelli WP, Levy D. Cholesterol and mortality: 30 years of follow-up from the Framingham Study. JAMA 1987; 257:2176–2180.

48. Gordon T, Castelli WP, Hjortland MC, et al. High density lipoprotein as a protective factor against coronary heart disease: The Framingham Study. Am J Med 1977; 62:707–714.
49. Castelli WP, Garrison RJ, Wilson PWF, et al. Incidence of coronary heart disease and lipoprotein cholesterol levels: The Framingham Study. JAMA 1986; 256:2835–2838.
50. Wilson PWF. High-density lipoprotein, low-density lipoprotein and coronary artery disease. Am J Cardiol 1990; 66:7A–10A.
51. Gordon DJ, Rivkind BM. High-density lipoprotein: the clinical implications of recent studies. N Engl J Med 1989; 321:1311–1316.
52. Brunzell JD, Austin MA. Plasma triglyceride levels and coronary disease. N Engl J Med 1989; 320:1273–1275.
53. Seed M, Hoppichler F, Reaveley D, et al. Relation of serum lipoprotein (a) concentration and apolipoprotein (a) phenotype to coronary heart disease in patients with familial hypercholesterolemia. N Engl J Med 1990; 322:1494–1499.
54. Williams RR, Hunt SC, Hopkins PN, et al. Familial dyslipidemic hypertension. JAMA 1988; 259:3579–3586.
55. Williams RR, Hopkins PN, Hunt SC, et al. Population-based frequency of dyslipidemia syndromes in coronary-prone families in Utah. Arch Intern Med 1990; 150:582–588.
56. Steinberg D, Parthasarathy S, Carew TE, et al. Beyond cholesterol: modifications of low-density lipoprotein that increase its atherogenicity. N Engl J Med 1989; 320:915–924.
57. Brown MS, Kovanen PT, Goldstein JL. Regulation of plasma cholesterol by lipoprotein receptors. Science 1981; 212:628–635.
58. Assmann G, Schulte H. The prospective cardiovascular Munster Study: Prevalence and prognostic significance of hyperlipidemia in men with systemic hypertension. Am J Cardiol 1987; 59:9G–17G.
59. Chobanian AV, Lichtenstein AH, Nilakhe V, et al. Influence of hypertension on aortic atherosclerosis in the Watanabe rabbit. Hypertension 1989; 14:203–209.
60. Samuelsson O, Wilhelmsen L, Andersson OK, et al. Cardiovascular morbidity in relation to change in blood pressure and serum cholesterol levels in treated hypertension. JAMA 1987; 258:1768–1776.
61. Chobanian AV, Haudenschild CC, Nickerson C, Drago R. Antiatherogenic effect of captopril in the Watanabe heritable hyperlipidemic rabbit. Hypertension 1990; 15:327–331.
62. Weinberger MH. Antihypertensive therapy and lipids: evidence, mechanisms and implications. Arch Intern Med 1985; 145:1102–1105.
63. Byington RP, Worthy J, Craven T, Furberg CD. Propranolol-induced lipid changes and their prognostic significance after a myocardial infarction: The beta-blocker heart attack trial experience. Am J Cardiol 1990; 65:1287–1291.
64. Modan M, Halkin H, Almog S, et al. Hyperinsulinemia: a link between hypertension, obesity and glucose intolerance. J Clin Invest 1985; 75:809–817.
65. Ferrannini E, Buzzigoli G, Bonadona R. Insulin resistance in essential hypertension. N Engl J Med 1987; 317:350–357.

66. Reaven GM, Hoffman BB. Hypertension as a disease of carbohydrate and lipoprotein metabolism. Am J Med 1989; 87(suppl 6A):2S–6S.
67. Morgan DA, Ray CA, Balon TW, Mark AL. Metformin increases insulin sensitivity and lowers arterial pressure in spontaneously hypertensive rats (abstr). Hypertension 1992; 20:421.
68. Pershadsingh HA, Szollosi J, Benson S, et al. Effects of ciglitazone on blood pressure and intracellular calcium metabolism. Hypertension 1993; 21(suppl): 1020–1023.

6

Therapy for the Black Hypertensive

IRIS R. KEYS and ELIJAH SAUNDERS
University of Maryland
Baltimore, Maryland

Hypertension occurs more frequently in the black population than in the nonblack population. In blacks hypertension develops at an earlier age and at all ages it is more severe than whites (1). Review of death rates from hypertensive disease and hypertensive heart disease from 1979 to 1985 shows a significantly higher death rate among the black group, especially the black males (2). This is shown further in the 9.5 year follow-up observation of persons aged 50 years and older who were selected as a representative sample of the adult U.S. population for the 1971 to 1975 National Health and Nutritional Examination Survey I (3) (Figure 1). Fewer black men and women survived than did white men and women at comparable levels of blood pressure, with the highest mortality rate in those with definite hypertension (Figure 1). Therefore, black hypertensives present a special challenge to the physician as hypertension is manifested at a younger age with greater severity, implying the necessity of more medication. Compliance becomes an important issue in management, as the cost and side effects rise with increased medication.

The severity and duration of disease predispose black hypertensives to more target organ damage, including coronary artery disease, congestive heart failure, cerebrovascular accident, peripheral vascular disease, and end stage renal disease. If they are successfully treated, however, they do obtain

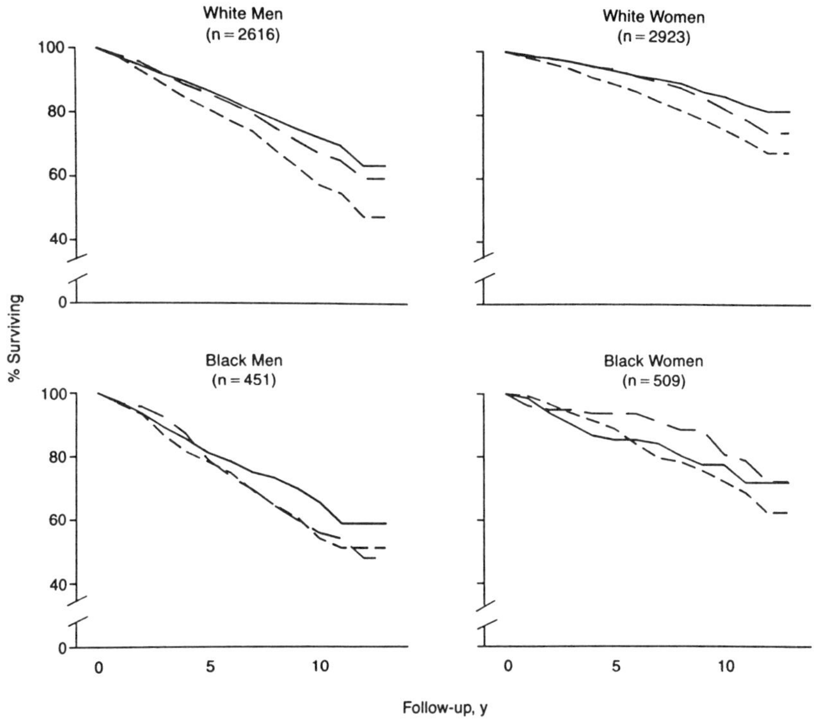

Figure 1 Probability of survival for up to 12 years according to blood pressure category (normal [solid line], borderline hypertension [long dashes], and definite hypertension [short dashes]) among persons aged 50 years and over (follow-up study [National Health Epidemiologic Follow-up Study (NHEFS)]). (From Ref. 3.)

protection from these hypertension-related diseases. The Hypertension Detection and Follow-up Program was the first large-scale epidemiological trial to include a large number of black participants and demonstrated a reduction in 5 year mortality rate in black hypertensives with therapy (4). As we will describe, studies have shown that there are racial differences in response to antihypertensive agents. Individualization of therapy for the black hypertensive should therefore be aimed at selecting a regimen which includes agents that have been shown to be most efficacious in this group.

I. NONPHARMACOLOGICAL MEASURES

As noted in the other populations described in previous chapters, many modifications in life-style have been advocated as adjunctive therapy in the management of hypertension. Patients are advised to lose weight, increase exercise, and use alcohol and salt in moderation. Other possible useful measures are increase in dietary potassium and possibly calcium and magnesium. Reduction of dietary fat and caffeine intake may also be beneficial. The Joint National Committee Report notes that the addition of these measures to any pharmacological regimen will improve the efficacy of the agents used (1). In addition to being definitive therapy for high normal and stage I–II hypertension, these measures may be useful in the primary prevention of hypertension.

A. Sodium Restriction

Of all these recommendations, the use of sodium has been most highly researched among black hypertensives. Black hypertensives exhibit more sodium sensitivity, relatively expanded plasma volume, lower plasma renin and prostaglandin levels, and increased peripheral and renal vascular resistance when compared to nonblacks (5). Large therapeutic trials demonstrate a fall in systolic blood pressure from 2.2 to 10 mm Hg for every 100 mmol reduction in dietary sodium intake (6). The individual response varies among populations, with blacks and the elderly showing the greatest sensitivity (7). Since the black population has the highest number of sodium sensitive individuals, it is essential to instruct patients on how to decrease sodium in the diet, including sources of hidden sodium. Emphasis must be placed on the high percentage, approximately 60% to 70%, of dietary sodium that comes from processed foods as opposed to that added in cooking or at the table. Also in the black community, fast foods and ethnic ("soul") menus are commonly consumed and are very high in sodium (and fat).

II. PHARMACOLOGICAL TREATMENT

Antihypertensive drugs produce varied responses in different ethnic groups. The knowledge of racial differences should aid the physician in selecting the treatment plan which will be the most effective. In recent years, many publications have compared the efficacy of a variety of agents in the hypertensive black patient (8–12). The 1993 Joint National Committee report recommends that initial therapy for patients with blood pressures from 140/90 to 179/109 (stage I and II) be monotherapy (1). The major classes which are listed as effective as monotherapy are diuretics, angiotensin converting enzyme (ACE) inhibitors, beta-blockers, calcium channel blockers, $alpha_1$-adrenergic blockers, and alpha-beta-blockers. The Joint National Committee recommends diuretics and beta-blockers as preferred agents for initial therapy because they have demonstrated reduced cardiovascular morbidity and mortality. Patients who have blood pressure from 180/110 to $>210/>120$ (stages III and IV) may require two or more agents.

A. Diuretic Agents

Thiazide and thiazidelike diuretics have traditionally been the cornerstone of therapy for the black hypertensive, either as monotherapy or as a part of combination therapy. Blacks have been shown to be very responsive to thiazide diuretics, in part because of their lower renin activity, expanded plasma volume, and sodium sensitivity. Studies also suggest that black hypertensives have reduced sodium–potassium–adenosine triphosphatase (Na^+-K^+-ATPase) activity with a higher intracellular sodium concentration (13).

Recently the use of diuretics has fallen out of favor because of the adverse metabolic and biochemical alterations as well as the side effect profile associated with their use. Diuretic usage may be associated with hypokalemia, hyperuricemia, as well as elevations in lipid and glucose levels. The presence of these changes may put the hypertensive at higher risk for development of cardiovascular complications.

An increase in cardiac mortality with long-term diuretic therapy despite good blood pressure control in the Multiple Risk Factor Intervention Trial (MRFIT) was suspected to be the result of arrhythmias induced by hypokalemia (14), although this has not been consistently demonstrated in other secondary prevention trials. Patients on diuretic therapy should be monitored closely for decreases in potassium, and levels maintained not just within the normal range, but as near the patient's pretreatment normal as possible. Frequency of hypokalemia can be diminished somewhat by using lower doses ranging from 12.5 to 25 mg of hydrochlorothiazide daily, although a few patients may require as much as 50 mg daily in order to achieve the desired effect on blood pressure.

Studies conducted to compare thiazides with loop diuretics have shown a smaller decline in blood pressure in the group receiving furosemide, making thiazides the diuretic of choice unless the patient has renal or cardiac failure.

Despite the associated metabolic side effects, if properly monitored, the thiazide diuretics are a safe, effective, and inexpensive option for monotherapy in the black hypertensive.

B. Calcium Channel Blockers

The controversy over thiazide therapy has caused clinicians to search for other agents which are comparable in effect in managing the hypertensive black patient. Although the Joint National Committee recommends the use of beta-blockers as one of the initial agents as monotherapy, numerous therapeutic trials comparing beta-blockers (BBs), ACE inhibitors (ACEIs), and calcium channel blockers (CCBs) in the black population have shown calcium channel blockers to be clearly more efficacious than beta-blockers in reducing both systolic and diastolic blood pressure. The CCB provides an option for therapy which considers the lower renin profile and higher peripheral resistance in these patients.

In a study comparing an ACEI, a BB, and a CCB, Saunders and colleagues demonstrated that the greatest decline in systolic and diastolic blood pressure was achieved with the CCB (Verapamil SR) when compared to the ACEI (captopril) and the BB (atenolol) (15) (Table 1). The VA Cooperative Studies Program published the results of a double blind 1 year trial which compared six antihypertensive agents (CCB, HCTZ, BB, alpha-blocker, central sympatholytic, and ACEI) used as monotherapy. The CCB, diltiazem, was the most effective in reducing blood pressure in the black hypertensive regardless of age, even more effective than the diuretic when used in adequate doses (16) (Figure 2). The reduction in diastolic blood pressure was 14/5 mm Hg in the under 60 age group and 15/5 in the over 60 group. The effectiveness of CCBs in the black hypertensive has been demonstrated repeatedly. The decision of which of the calcium blockers to select is a choice based on the individual patient's tolerance. The dihydropyridine CCBs tend to cause more ankle edema which does not respond to diuretic therapy and which female patients tend to find uncomfortable.

Table 1 Response to Treatment

	Atenolol	Captopril	Verapamil SR
Period 2[a] (N = 345)			
N[b]	118	112	115
Success[c] %	55.1	43.8	65.2
Failure %	44.9	46.3	34.8
Period 3 (low and high dose) (N = 307)			
N	109	98	100
Success %	59.6	57.1	73.0
Failure %	40.4	42.9	27
Period 3 (high dose only) (N = 157)			
N	56	47	54
Success %	58.9	61.7	83.3
Failure %	41.1	38.3	16.7

[a]Period 1 represented baseline (placebo lead-in); periods 2 and 3 are treatment periods.
[b]Numbers of patients given represent those for whom data could be evaluated.
[c]Success defined as supine diastolic blood pressure < 90 mm Hg and/or a drop of 10 mm Hg or more from baseline.
Source: Ref. 15.

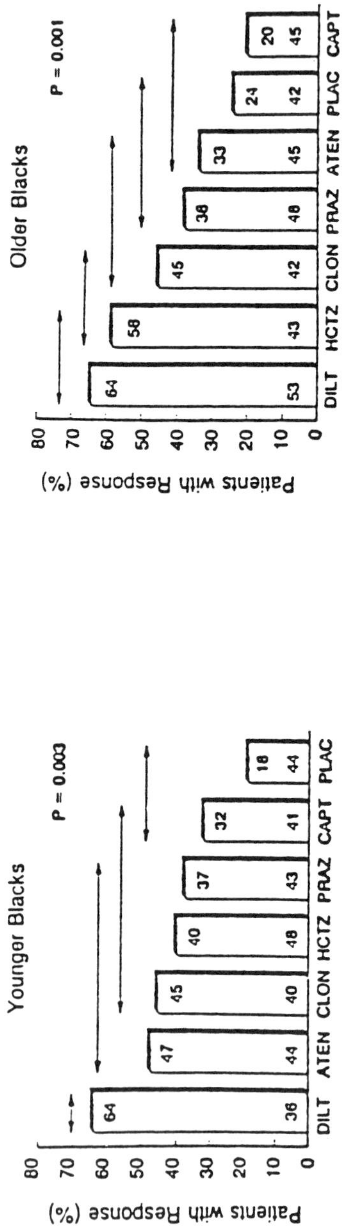

Figure 2 The percentage of younger black (left) and older black (right) patients who had a good response to a drug from one of six classes of antihypertensive agents in a VA Cooperative Trial. Dilt; diltiazem; aten; atenolol; clon; clonidine; HCTZ; hydrochlorothiazide; praz; prazosin; capt; captopril; plac; placebo. (From Ref. 16.)

The selection of an antihypertensive agent should also consider the benefit to the patient with evidence of target organ damage. As noted in Chapter 7, left ventricular hypertrophy (LVH) is a manifestation of severe uncontrolled hypertension, which is more frequently encountered in the black population (17). LVH is a major risk factor for cardiac death, myocardial infarction, and other morbid events (18). A clinical trial by Schulman and colleagues demonstrated regression of LVH in older hypertensives, many of whom were black, who were treated with a calcium channel blocker or a beta-blocker (19). Calcium channel blockers are effective agents in black hypertensives and demonstrate the desirable effect of reducing LVH, making these agents very attractive in the management of these patients.

C. Beta-Blockers

A substantial number of clinical trials previously cited have shown that blacks and the elderly display a less significant response to beta-adrenergic blockers when compared to white and younger individuals. The black hypertensive has approximately 60% of the usual response of the white hypertensive to a BB (20). Short-term studies conducted by the VA cooperative group comparing the response to beta-blockers in blacks and whites showed a blunted response in the black patients (16) (Figure 2). The same response was also demonstrated by Saunders and colleagues in their study comparing a CCB, BB, and ACEI (15) (Table 1).

Beta-blockers are believed to reduce blood pressure by blocking sympathetic effects on the heart, thereby decreasing heart rate and cardiac output as well as blocking adrenergic nerve-mediated release of renin from the juxtaglomerular cells. The lack of response to BBs in black hypertensives most likely reflects the racial difference in the pathophysiology of the disease. The mechanism of lowering plasma renin level would be less effective in low-renin and sodium-sensitive individuals. Nevertheless, it has been shown that the addition of a thiazide diuretic to the BB almost eradicates the differences in the two groups (20). In patients requiring BB because of concomitant illnesses, such as ischemic heart disease, racial response to blood pressure reduction should not be a reason to withhold the drug.

D. Angiotensin-Converting Enzyme Inhibitors

ACEIs lower blood pressure by preventing the formation of angiotensin II and the subsequent increase in total peripheral resistance caused by vasoconstriction. In addition, the decrease in vasoconstriction appears to cause an increase in renal perfusion and regression of LVH (11). ACEIs are effective in lowering blood pressure in a large portion of hypertensive patients; however, the recent VA study, as well as many others done in previous years, showed the ACEIs to be among the least effective agents in hypertensive blacks, especially the elderly (16) (Figure 2). In the same manner as that of the beta-blockers, the effectiveness of the ACEIs is enhanced with the addition of a thiazide diuretic or with the use of higher doses, thereby minimizing racial differences. ACEIs should be used with caution in a patient with preexisting renal disease as acute renal failure can be precipitated in some patients. Serum creatinine and potassium levels should be monitored when ACEI therapy is initiated in patients with mild renal insufficiency, diabetes, or the possibility of bilateral renal artery stenosis (1).

Recent studies (21) have suggested that ACEIs may preserve renal function better in diabetic patients than other antihypertensive drugs; this characteristic may broaden their indications even in black patients. A new generation of ACEIs which is reported to have high tissue penetration (e.g., quinapril and ramipril) may have a better efficacy profile in low-renin hypertensives such as blacks (22).

E. Alpha$_1$-Adrenergic Inhibitors

The side effect of sodium and water retention especially in the sodium-sensitive hypertensive patient may limit the use of alpha$_1$-blockers as single agents; however, they can be quite effective as second- and third-line agents in patients who remain uncontrolled on CCBs and diuretics. In the black hypertensive with high total peripheral resistance, alpha-blockers may be beneficial when combined with agents that block the reflex tachycardia (i.e., beta-blockers) and a diuretic to counteract fluid retention. This family of drugs may be associated with first dose syncope, which can be prevented by starting at a low dose and instructing the patient to take it at bedtime.

The comparative studies previously mentioned do not show any significant advantage to the use of alpha$_1$-blockers over any other agent, although they may have a very favorable impact on serum lipid levels. Additionally, studies have shown alpha$_1$-blocker monotherapy to be as effective in blacks as whites, although slightly higher doses may be required (23).

Labetalol is a nonselective beta-blocker with alpha$_1$-antagonist activity. The alpha$_1$ activity weakens after a few months of therapy; however, the black hypertensive may have a slightly better response to this agent than to the pure BB (20).

F. Direct Vasodilators

The direct acting vasodilators were among the earliest drugs to be used for the control of hypertension. Their use has declined with the discovery of other agents. Despite the availability of agents with fewer side effects, there is still a place for hydralazine and minoxidil in the management of hypertension in the black patient. These agents are associated with tachycardia and palpitations which may be prevented by administration of a CCB or BB, but many of the other side effects may limit their use. Precipitation of angina in patients with coronary artery disease may occur when the drug is given as a single agent, but this occurs infrequently when a BB is included. Hydralazine is well known to induce a lupuslike syndrome, but the incidence of this syndrome appears to be lower in blacks even at higher doses (24). The syndrome usually is characterized by arthralgias, malaise, weakness, or myalgias. Proteinuria and impaired renal function may occur. These signs and symptoms resolve slowly after the drug is discontinued (25).

Minoxidil is a potent vasodilator which is usually reserved for severe, refractory hypertension. Sodium retention is a prominent systemic effect of this agent. The severity of the edema usually cannot be managed by thiazide diuretics; most patients on minoxidil require large doses of a loop diuretic. Increased heart rate is universal and BB therapy should be started when this drug is initiated. Hair growth on the face and other parts of the body may have to be accepted as an unavoidable side effect.

III. SUMMARY

Individualization of therapy for the black hypertensive begins by having an awareness of the underlying hemodynamics and pathophysiology associated with this patient population (26) (Table 2). The selection of an antihypertensive agent should be based on correcting the existing abnormalities and taking advantage of known responses to available medications. In addition,

Table 2 Pathogenesis of Hypertension in Blacks

Genotype
Candidate genes unique to blacks
Intermediate phenotype
Enhanced sodium sensitivity
Altered cation transport
Suppressed renin-angiotensin-aldosterone
Lower kallikrein-kinin, prostaglandin
Increased adrenergic activity
Increased insulin resistance
Phenotype
Greater left ventricular hypertrophy
Increased peripheral vascular resistance
Advanced nephrosclerosis

Source: Ref. 26.

Table 3 A Treatment Plan for the Black Hypertensive

Nonpharmacological therapy
Sodium restriction
Weight reduction if obese
Potassium supplementation
Alcohol restriction if intake excessive
Pharmacological therapy
1. Start with a calcium channel blocker or diuretic.
2. Combine the two.
3. Add a direct vasodilator (hydralazine), alpha-blocker, ACE inhibitor, or beta-blocker.
4. Add minoxidil (plus an adrenergic inhibitor and adequate diuretic).
5. Consider testing for secondary causes.

the presence of other cardiovascular risk factors and concomitant diseases should be factored in.

One of the greatest needs for the black population is more education about hypertension. Weight loss, sodium restriction, reduction in alcohol consumption, and increased exercise should be a part of the treatment in all cases, even if pharmacological agents are required. Black patients usually have more severe hypertension, often more difficult to control. Financial constraints may become an important issue as dosages are increased.

The treatment algorithm shown in Table 3 is a suggested plan for achieving control based on the known response of black individuals to certain classes of drugs.

REFERENCES

1. Joint National Committee on Detection, Evaluation, and Treatment of High Blood Pressure. The fifth report of the Joint National Committee on Detection, Evaluation and Treatment of High Blood Pressure. Arch Intern Med 1993; 153: 154–183.
2. Gillum RF. Cardiovascular disease in the United States: an epidemiologic overview. In: Saunders E., ed. Cardiovascular Disease in Blacks. Philadelphia: F. A. Davis, 1991.
3. Cornoni-Huntley J, LaCroix AZ, Havlik RJ. Race and sex differentials in the impact of hypertension in the United States: the national health and nutrition examination survey I epidemiologic follow-up study. Arch Intern Med 1989; 149: 780–788.
4. Hypertension Detection and Follow-Up Program Cooperative Group. Five-year findings of the hypertension detection and follow-up program. II. Mortality by race, sex and age. JAMA 1979; 242:2572–2577.

5. Weir MR, Saunders E. Pharmacologic management of systemic hypertension in blacks. Am J Cardiol 1988; 61:46H–52H.
6. Law MR, Frost CD, Wald NJ. By how much does dietary salt reduction lower blood pressure? I. Analysis of observational data among populations. Br Med J 1991; 302:811–815.
7. Flack JM, Ensrud KE, Mascoli S, et al. Racial and ethnic modifiers of the salt blood pressure response. Hypertension 1991; 17(suppl I):I-115–I-121.
8. Hall WD. Pharmacologic therapy of hypertension in blacks. J Clin Hypertens 1987; 3(suppl):108S–113S.
9. Saunders E. Drug treatment considerations for the hypertensive black patient. J Fam Pract 1988; 26:659–664.
10. Hall WD. Hypertension in blacks. In: Wollam GL, Hall WD, eds. Hypertension Management: Clinical Practice and Therapeutic Dilemmas. Chicago: Year Book, 1988.
11. Weir MR. Impact of age, race, and obesity on hypertensive mechanisms and therapy. Am J Med 1991; 90:3S–14S.
12. Watkins LO. Racial differences in the management of hypertension. J Natl Med Assoc 1989; 81(suppl):17–24.
13. Aviv A, Gardner J. Racial differences in ion regulation and their possible links to hypertension in blacks. Hypertension 1988; 14:584–589.
14. Multiple Risk Factor Intervention Trial. Risk factor changes and mortality results. JAMA 1982; 248:1465–1477.
15. Saunders E, Weir MR, Kong BW, et al. A comparison of the efficacy and safety of a beta-blocker, a calcium channel blocker and a converting enzyme inhibitor in hypertensive blacks. Arch Intern Med 1990; 150:1707–1713.
16. Materson BJ, Reda DJ, Cushman WC, et al. Single drug therapy for hypertension in men: a comparison of six antihypertensive agents with placebo. N Engl J Med 1993; 328:914–921.
17. Frohlich ED, Apstein C, Chobanian AV, et al. The heart in hypertension. N Engl J Med 1992; 327:998–1008.
18. Levy D, Garrison RJ, Savage DD, et al. Prognostic implications of echocardiographically determined left ventricular mass in the Framingham Heart Study. N Engl J Med 1990; 322:1561–1566.
19. Schulman SP, Weiss JL, Becker LC. The effects of antihypertensive treatment of left ventricular hypertrophy in elderly patients. N Engl J Med 1990; 322:1350–1356.
20. Hall WD, Kong BW. Hypertension in blacks: nonpharmacologic and pharmacologic therapy. In: Saunders E, ed. Cardiovascular Disease in Blacks. Philadelphia: FA Davis, 1991:157.
21. Lewis EJ, Hunsicker LG, Bain RP, Rohde RD. The effect of angiotensin-converting enzyme inhibition on diabetic nephropathy. N Engl J Med 1993; 329:1456–1462.
22. Erman A, Winkler J, Chen-Gal B, et al. Inhibition of angiotensin converting enzyme by ramipril in serum and tissue of man. J Hypertens 191; 9:1057–1062.
23. Khoury AF, Kaplan NM. α-blocker therapy of hypertension: an unfilled promise. JAMA 1991; 266:394–398.

24. Hahn BH, Sharp GC, Irvin WS, et al. Immune responses to hydralazine and nuclear antigens in hydralazine-induced lupus erythematosus. Ann Intern Med 1972; 3:365–374.
25. Robinson BF, Benjamin N. Vasodilators. In: Laragh JH, Brenner BM, eds. Hypertension, Pathophysiology, Diagnosis and Treatment. New York: Raven Press, 1990:2263.
26. Falkner B. Differences in blacks and whites with essential hypertension: biochemistry and endocrine. Hypertension 1990; 15:681–686.

7

Hypertension in Patients with Cardiac Disease

ROBERT J. CODY
The Ohio State University Medical Center
Columbus, Ohio

Cardiovascular disorders are difficult to separate from systemic hypertension because of the considerable overlap of three key components: coronary artery disease, hypertension, and congestive heart failure. Large population studies indicate that hypertension carries with it a considerable risk of death, myocardial infraction, stroke, and congestive heart failure (1). It has been particularly difficult to separate cause and effect roles for these various components, as it is quite likely that they are closely interrelated. With this in mind, the present chapter will review the cardiovascular characteristics of hypertension, summarize the major group of antihypertensive agents relevant to cardiovascular disorders, and suggest treatment strategies for hypertension encountered in the more common forms of coexistent cardiovascular disorders.

I. CARDIOVASCULAR CHARACTERISTICS OF HYPERTENSION

Every patient with hypertension has a cardiovascular disorder. The spectrum and characteristics of ventricular remodeling in hypertension have been reviewed (2,3). Several factors, however, should be stressed. The majority of individuals with systemic hypertension have an inappropriate increase of vascular tone (4). This increase of vascular tone (systemic vascular resistance)

Table 1 Factors Producing Increased Vascular Resistance in Systemic Hypertension

Increased sympathetic nervous system activity and/or altered baroreceptor responsiveness
Activation of vasoactive pathways
1. True circulating endocrine effects
2. Paracrine/autocrine effects of the peptides/substances in 1
3. Locally produced vasoactive substances
4. Altered signal transduction or cell mediator function in response to 1 through 3.
Increased vascular turgor and stiffness due to sodium retention and volume expansion in sodium-sensitive essential hypertension and chronic renal failure.
Structural changes in vascular tissue
1. Increased elastic and collagen deposition
2. Altered contractile protein isoforms?

may be mediated by a number of factors (Table 1). These include enhanced sympathetic nervous system activity, activation of vasoconstrictor hormonal pathways, and excessive sodium content within the arterial wall and surrounding tissue. The heart itself may be a causal factor under certain conditions (5). However, hypertensive cardiomyopathy is actually a spectrum of disorders (Table 2). In most cases, the heart responds in an adaptive or maladaptive way to the increased wall stress resulting from increased vascular resistance and pressure in the arterial bed. Abnormalities of cardiac dysfunction in hypertension can be categorized into several groups: disorders of systolic function, diastolic function, chronotropic activity, and baroreceptor responsiveness. In addition, there may be hormone mediated disorders of the heart given the presence of atrial natriuretic factor within secretory granules of atrial and ventricular myocytes.

Systolic abnormalities are the most readily appreciated. This is because the heart must generate an enormous energy output in order to empty during systole against the increased resistance and pressure within the arterial bed. Ultimately, the persistence of this increased afterload will result in gross systolic dysfunction in hypertensive subjects. Hypertension, at one point, was one of the most common causes of congestive heart failure in the United

Table 2 Clinical Syndromes Often Defined as "Hypertensive Cardiomyopathy"

Left ventricular hypertrophy with diastolic dysfunction
Progressive hypertrophy and dilatation, with superimposed systolic dysfunction
Heart failure in the presence of coexistent hypertension and coronary artery disease
Heart failure occurring in the setting of accelerated hypertension/hypertensive crisis
Idiopathic cardiomyopathy with antecedent history of hypertension

States, and it remains a prodrome to the development of chronic congestive heart failure in many individuals.

The diastolic abnormalities of the heart have only received equal attention within the last decade, despite earlier reports that diastolic abnormalities could exist in the hypertensive population (6,7). There are both active and passive components to the relaxation of the ventricle in diastole. This is perhaps the pivotal portion of the cardiac cycle, in that compliance abnormalities may alter ventricular filling (stroke volume), and the majority of coronary blood flow occurs at this time. It is likely that diastolic abnormalities in hypertension are a direct reflection of abnormalities of coronary blood flow as well as abnormal ventricular mechanics. However, it is quite clear that these factors may contribute to the ischemic conditions identified in patients with hypertension in whom large vessel coronary disease is absent (2,8–11). Baroreceptor abnormalities may be part of a large constellation of sympathetic nervous system changes that characterize hypertension (12). If arterial and great vessel baroreceptors cannot respond appropriately to changes in arterial filling, this will produce an inappropriate enhancement of arterial tone and reduce chronotropic and inotropic suppression of the ventricle, thereby producing an inappropriate mismatch of vascular reactivity and cardiac responsiveness with a net result of increased blood pressure in systole. This mismatch may contribute to the incidence of pure systolic hypertension in the elderly.

The role for atrial natriuretic peptide has been identified (13). It is primarily secreted by atrial myocytes (14), but synthesis and release from ventricular myocytes can be recruited, particularly when the ventricle undergoes hypertrophy. This confers endocrine function to the heart, in addition to its other cardiovascular functions. One would anticipate that enhanced secretion of atrial natriuretic peptide with its natriuretic and vasodilator properties (14) would actually be favorable in hypertension. However, most studies demonstrate that atrial natriuretic peptide levels in hypertension have considerable overlap with the normal range (14,15,28). One can therefore reason that there is an inappropriately low production of atrial natriuretic peptide in many patients with hypertension, particularly in view of the tendency for an increased circulatory volume and cardiac output. Inadequate secretion of atrial natriuretic peptide would permissively contribute to the volume overload in hypertension that necessitates the extensive use of diuretics in this population. It should be noted that the atrial natriuretic peptide secretory response to increased atrial tension is preserved in hypertension (16) and heart failure (17) despite abnormally elevated basal levels in the latter.

Relatively less attention has been given to the abnormal status of the systemic vasculature in patients with hypertension, where abnormal vascular reactivity and structural changes contribute to the hypertensive process by increasing arterial resistance (4). The etiology for increased vascular resistance will vary for hypertension subgroups, and may vary from patient to patient. Studies performed under stress conditions such as exercise indicate that the arterial bed in hypertensive subjects does not dilate to the same extent as that of normal subjects (16,18,19).

Abnormalities of the lesser circulation, i.e., the pulmonary circulation, may also occur in patients with hypertension. Under resting conditions, pulmonary pressure and resistance are often normal, but can be increased in subsets of hypertensive subjects. Abnormal pulmonary hemodynamics may be more readily identified during maximal exercise (16,18,19), even in individuals with normal resting hemodynamics. The current literature does not establish the mechanism for abnormal pulmonary reactivity, nor does it address the issue of whether this represents a passive phenomenon due to left ventricular dysfunction. Irrespective of the mechanism(s), the right ventricle is placed under an inordinate stress as a result of increased pulmonary resistance and pressure. This may help to explain the development of independent right ventricular failure, or specific contribution to the bi-ventricular failure pattern of long-term hypertension, particularly where treatment is inadequate.

II. ANTIHYPERTENSIVE THERAPY AND ITS RELEVANCE TO PATIENTS WITH ASSOCIATED CARDIOVASCULAR DISORDERS

The broad indications of the major antihypertensive drug classes for patients with associated cardiovascular disorders should be considered. The goal of treatment in this group of patients is effective blood pressure control and, ideally, cotreatment of other existing diseases. This is not meant to be an exhaustive survey, as these drug classes are treated elsewhere in this text in greater detail. Specific indications for pharmacological classes are summarized in Table 3.

A. Diuretics

Diuretics are the most widely used antihypertensive therapy because of their low cost, their ease of administration, and the need for counterbalancing excessive sodium intake. However, in terms of their effectiveness in subsets of patients with coexistent cardiovascular disorders, their primary role is twofold: the rapid excretion of excess sodium and water, and the treatment of congestive heart failure. These two goals are often sought in the same individual. Specific benefits of diuretics relevant to patients with associated coronary artery disease, myocardial infarction, or peripheral vascular disease

Table 3 Specific Cardiovascular Indications for Antihypertensive Drug Classes

Diuretics
Congestive heart failure
Central sympatholytics
Aortic dissection
Beta-adrenergic blockers
Coronary artery disease
Aortic dissection
Some forms of heart failure
Some atrial/ventricular arrhythmias
Vasodilator agents
Congestive heart failure
Peripheral vascular disease
Some forms of coronary artery disease
ACE inhibitors
Left ventricular dysfunction and congestive heart failure
Myocardial ischemia/infarction
Ventricular arrhythmias?
Calcium channel antagonists
Symptomatic coronary artery disease
Peripheral vascular disease
Some forms of diastolic heart failure
Some atrial/ventricular arrhythmias

may be difficult to identify, beyond long-term blood pressure reduction. When used in moderate doses, diuretics are most readily effective in cases of hypertension associated with congestive heart failure. Here, diuretics reduce circulatory and tissue congestion and ultimately provide symptomatic relief.

Balanced against this are several potential adverse effects. These include induction of electrolyte depletion that promotes ventricular arrhythmias (20), or activation of hormonal pathways (e.g., the renin system) that may adversely influence the outcome of the disease. The latter can be identified in congestive heart failure, where sodium depletion activates the renin-angiotensin system and the sympathetic nervous system (21), which may be counterproductive in terms of the overall outcome.

B. Central Sympatholytics

The central sympatholytic agents generally consist of the central alpha-agonists, which reduce general sympathetic outflow. In cardiovascular disorders, these drugs are now less used, because of their tendency to induce somnolence.

Alpha-methyldopa is an effective agent for hypertensive emergencies and has a well established profile so that many physicians feel comfortable with its use. Clonidine is frequently used in hypertensive emergencies (22), where its limited efficacy is balanced by the fact that it normally is well tolerated and safe. However, clonidine does not have concomitant favorable effects in coexistent disorders such as coronary artery disease or congestive heart failure. In patients with cardiac disorders, it is difficult to identify discrete indications for central sympatholytics. In fact, the bradycardia and orthostatic hypotension which central sympatholytics produce may be detrimental in the presence of many cardiovascular disorders.

C. Beta- and Alpha-Adrenergic Blockade

Beta-adrenergic blockade has long been a standard approach to antihypertensive therapy (23). A further distinction applied to these agents is whether they block both $beta_1$ and $beta_2$ receptors, versus having selective effects on the $beta_1$ receptor. In addition, individual beta-blockers may demonstrate intrinsic sympathomimetic activity, producing partial beta-agonist effects. Beta-adrenergic blockers are readily effective in patients with several associated cardiovascular disorders including coronary artery disease. Beta-blockers limit symptoms, maintain a protective effect against myocardial ischemia, and actually improve survival among patients with myocardial infarction, thereby indicating that these drugs should be particularly effective when hypertension coexists with coronary artery disease. Beta-adrenergic blockade is particularly useful in patients with ongoing coronary ischemia and/or myocardial infarction. Blood pressure reduction occurs in the time frame of one to several hours rather than minutes, while the negative inotropic and chronotropic effects occur within a shorter time frame (23).

Beta-adrenergic blockade remains one of the treatments of choice for aortic dissection (22), particularly during the acute phase of aortic leakage, as beta-blockers lower ventricular dp/dt (thereby reducing shearing forces within the aorta), in addition to reducing systolic blood pressure.

Beta-blockade can be effective as an adjunct for controlling ventricular rate in subjects with atrial fibrillation. However, there are several disorders in which beta-adrenergic blockade may be detrimental. In patients with congestive heart failure, the predominant hemodynamic effect of beta-adrenergic blockade is a reduction of both chronotropy and inotropy, so that there is at least a moderate risk that congestive heart failure will be exacerbated in the course of therapy. While the results of multicenter trials of beta-blockade in heart failure are encouraging, they add a risk of decompensation in the presence of systolic dysfunction. When hypertension heart failure is primarily diastolic in origin (7) or when hypertension coexists with hypertrophic obstructive cardiomyopathy, beta-blockade is appropriate therapy. In patients with peripheral vascular disease, beta-adrenergic blockade may produce limb ischemia by central and peripheral mechanisms. Because of the negative chronotropic and inotropic effects of beta-blocking agents, their use in valvular heart disease, particularly aortic or mitral stenosis, is limited.

The clinical expression of alpha-adrenergic blockade is primarily vasodilation (23). Peripheral postsynaptic alpha-adrenergic blocking agents such as doxazosin and terazosin are potent vasodilators that reduce alpha-mediated vasoconstriction. As with the direct acting vasodilators, they are effective in the presence of a wide variety of cardiovascular disorders, as outlined later. In view of favorable reduction of the symptoms of urinary retention in elderly males with prostatic enlargement, they may be particularly effective in this subpopulation of hypertension.

Labetalol combines both alpha- and beta-adrenergic blockade (24). Its favorable profile in hypertensive emergencies is well documented (25). It is available in both intravenous and oral preparations. Because of its mechanisms of action, it is generally well tolerated for the treatment of hypertension associated with cardiovascular disorders.

D. Vasodilator Agents

There are several pharmaceutical classes with vasodilator properties that fall within the broad category of vasodilator agents, including the direct acting vasodilators nitroprusside, hydralazine, and minoxidil. ACE inhibitors and calcium channel antagonists are discussed separately. Direct-acting vasodilators reverse constriction of vascular smooth muscle. These drugs are potent and have rapid onset of vasodilation, so that they are particularly effective in hypertension that coexists with congestive heart failure, peripheral vascular disease, and, in some instances, coronary artery disease. Nitroprusside and hydralazine can be administered parenterally (see Chapter 13). Minoxidil is a potent vasodilator which may produce excessive fluid retention, compromising its use with coexistent congestive heart failure. Hydralazine is effective for the treatment of hypertensive emergencies wherein vasodilation is desired, such as with coexistent pulmonary edema or congestive heart failure.

Nitroglycerin compounds are often used for hypertensive emergencies, when prompt reduction of blood pressure is necessary. Although nitroglycerin is not considered to be an antihypertensive agent, it can be effective in the treatment of hypertension with coexistent coronary ischemia, myocardial infarction, or congestive heart failure.

E. Angiotensin-Converting Enzyme Inhibitors

Angiotensin-converting enzyme (ACE) inhibitors are highly effective for the treatment of hypertension and coexistent cardiovascular disorders. In patients with hypertension, blood pressure is reduced by a reduction of systemic vascular resistance, primarily as a result of inhibiting the formation of angiotensin II (26). There is little change of cardiac index, and minimal change in heart rate. During long-term studies, both mean pulmonary artery pressure and pulmonary capillary wedge pressure are reduced compared to baseline (27).

These agents are generally well tolerated in virtually all of the associated cardiovascular disorders discussed. Perhaps most notable are their efficacy, safety, and wide applicability in patients with congestive heart failure characterized by systolic dysfunction (28). As with severe renovascular hypertension, converting enzyme inhibitors can induce profound hypotension or progression of renal insufficiency in patients with coexistent heart failure.

Angiotensin-converting enzyme inhibitors provide effective treatment of hypertension in the setting of other cardiovascular disorders. There is now evidence that converting enzyme inhibitors prevent infarct expansion and progressive left ventricular dysfunction after myocardial infarction (29). However, they are not beneficial in the immediate setting of acute myocardial infarction (30).

F. Calcium Channel Antagonists

The chemically diverse class of calcium channel antagonists antagonizes the influx of calcium through the slow channels of cardiac and vascular muscle cells and decreases cytosolic calcium (31). Verapamil may have more of a negative inotropic effect, and both verapamil and diltiazem tend to reduce electrical conduction (31). The dihydropyridines may have a greater action on vascular smooth muscle and tend to increase heart rate (32). It is clear that they are all potent vasodilators and in the coronary circulation, dilate large and small vessels, thereby reducing angina. More recent data demonstrate that these agents can reverse small vessel spasm and improve ventricular compliance (31). The asset of the calcium channel antagonists is their ability to interrupt the increase of cytosolic calcium in vascular smooth muscle, thereby producing vasodilation (33).

The very first observations suggesting that calcium channel antagonists may have negative inotropic effect were performed over 20 years ago, when the negative inotropic effect of verapamil was inferred from a minimal increase of pulmonary diastolic pressure. Changes in contractility of the myocardium represent only one of several possible direct effects on the myocardium. There are also potential changes in heart rate that can affect myocardial function. Wall tension is substantially reduced by calcium channel antagonists as a result of reduction of systolic pressure and, to some extent, diastolic volume. Coronary filling, which influences oxygen supply to the myocardium, can be influenced in a number of ways. This can be due to direct effects on coronary artery diameter including the microcirculation, which increase in response to calcium channel antagonism, as well as indirect effects on vascular vasoactive substances, including catecholamines and endothelin (31). There is also an influence on myocardial perfusion, determined by the effect of calcium channel antagonists on relative aortic and left ventricular diastolic pressure gradient. Finally, the diastolic filling time can be greatly influenced by the heart rate change induced by these agents. This includes an increase of diastolic time produced by verapamil, to the potential reduction in diastolic filling time due to the effects of dihydropyridines. In patients with abnormal left ventricular function, calcium channel antagonists may reduce end-systolic pressure and volume as well as increase cardiac output. While it appears that the negative inotropic effects of the newer calcium channel antagonists are less striking, and that the overall negative inotropic effects of this class of drugs are less than that of beta-adrenergic blockade, this issue still poses a limitation for the utilization of these compounds in certain disorders. This is most obvious for patients with moderate to severe congestive heart failure.

In the majority of patients with essential hypertension, increased peripheral vascular resistance is the primary hemodynamic abnormality and cardiac performance is usually preserved until later stages of the disease. Similar favorable acute hemodynamic responses to intravenous therapy have been observed with both verapamil and the dihydropyridine nicardipine (32). Reduction of blood pressure is accompanied by reversal of vasoconstriction. Cardiac output is increased, primarily by an increase of heart rate. Pulmonary capillary wedge pressure is either unchanged or decreased.

This hemodynamic response to acute calcium channel antagonists is confirmed by invasive exercise hemodynamic studies (31). The pattern of pulmonary artery wedge pressure response to exercise may differ among calcium channel antagonists. With verapamil, there was no appreciable reduction of the exercise-induced increase of pulmonary wedge pressure (18), in contrast, nicardipine was associated with marked reduction (19). Thus, while calcium channel antagonists may share similar overall effects, the myocardial and vascular responses to therapy vary considerably for the individual agents.

Considerable blood pressure reduction results from the vasodilator effects of calcium channel antagonists, and this may mask much of the real or potential negative inotropic effect in the hypertensive population. Therefore, calcium channel antagonists for the treatment of hypertension associated with symptomatic coronary artery disease typically are well tolerated. Nonetheless, rapid blood pressure reduction in severe hypertension, particularly with associated cardiovascular disorders such as myocardial infarction, by the use of parenteral (intravenous or sublingual) calcium channel antagonist administration (34), is a potential risk which should be avoided. The favorable effect of these drugs can also be anticipated in the presence of peripheral vascular disease, through reversal of the vasospastic component of blood flow reduction (33), particularly in the resistance vessels. In the hypertensive population where there is a range of systolic and diastolic ventricular abnormalities, use of calcium channel antagonists can be highly effective, particularly in patients with left ventricular hypertrophy and diastolic dysfunction. However, the majority of current data suggest that calcium channel antagonists should not be used as first-line vasodilator therapy in heart failure. Calcium channel antagonists could produce adverse effects in severe valvular stenosis by either a negative inotropic or a chronotropic effect. Verapamil and diltiazem particularly should be used with caution in the presence of conduction disease or when a beta-adrenergic blocking agent is being used.

III. HEART AND CIRCULATORY ABNORMALITIES FREQUENTLY ENCOUNTERED IN PATIENTS WITH HYPERTENSION (Table 4)

A. Coronary Artery Disease

Perhaps the most common and important coexistent disorder in patients with hypertension is the spectrum of coronary artery disease, particularly in the aging adult population. Except under unusual circumstances, the presence of an asymptomatic noncritical coronary lesion may not impose a considerable stress on the myocardium. However, when one combines this lesion with systemic arterial hypertension, it is easy to envision abnormal perfusion in the targeted region of the myocardium. The reduction of perfusion pressure across such a coronary lesion, particularly when left ventricular

Table 4 Cardiac and Circulatory Abnormalities Frequently Encountered in Hypertension

Coronary artery disease/myocardial infarction
Congestive heart failure
Peripheral vascular disease
Valvular heart disease
Cardiac conduction abnormalities and arrhythmias
Obesity and lipid disorders

end-diastolic pressure (LVEDP) is increased, results in diminished coronary flow (8–11). Myocardial ischemia is likely to be more profound when LVEDP increases with exercise in hypertensive subjects (18,19). It is therefore readily apparent that the risk of severe ischemia or infarction is even greater when there is coexistent critical obstruction of one or more coronary arteries. This may be more than an additive risk. Considering the potential of enhanced sympathetic activity, increase of angiotensin II, and a propensity of vasospasm within the hypertensive population, the coexistence of hypertension and fixed coronary obstruction likely results in a synergistic progressive compromise of coronary perfusion. Ultimately, such patients may be more prone than their normotensive counterparts to a high incidence of myocardial infarction (2,9). Myocardial infarction therefore is an expected or predictable sequela to these coexistent disease processes.

One might predict that individuals who have systemic hypertension would be predisposed to a myocardial infarction of greater severity or deleterious outcome when compared to normotensive subjects. Abnormalities of platelet function and increased blood viscosity (35) may contribute to abnormal flow characteristics and hypertrophy within the hypertensive population. Such abnormalities contribute to the overall "resistance" to flow encountered in the hypertensive population and may contribute to the thrombotic events that typify acute myocardial infarction. The extent of the infarct zone relates to the speed and extent with which the acute thrombotic lesion resolves. In the hypertensive patient, underlying abnormalities of both platelet function and viscosity could impede clot resolution, resulting in myocardial infarction of much greater severity than in normotensive subjects. It is now well established that an infarcted myocardial segment may undergo a phase of expansion, contributing to overall deterioration of left ventricular function (29). Thus, in terms of rheological, hemodynamic, and structural phenomena, a greater tendency for severe complicated myocardial infarction could be anticipated in hypertensive subjects, compared with normotensive subjects.

In the last 20 years, it has been clear that antihypertensive therapy has provided effective control of blood pressure and a reduction of stroke (1). However, the full expected impact of antihypertensive therapy on the incidence of myocardial infarction has not been seen. The reasons for this are not clear. For instance, diuretics are the traditional first step in the standardized step care approach to therapy and have been the most widely used class of drugs for treating hypertension. Yet their mechanism of action does not produce a favorable direct physiological effect on coexistent coronary artery disease. However, the problem is likely to be more complex, and the lack of a greater impact of antihypertensive therapy on myocardial infarction may be the result of several characteristics of the hypertensive patient with coronary artery disease. First, the reduction of coronary blood flow produced by coronary artery disease is accentuated in the presence of increased left ventricular filling pressures and hypertrophy. Second, increased blood viscosity may be present, yielding a greater tendency for clot formation and coronary thrombosis. Third, relative dissociation of vascular stiffness and autonomic control of the heart emerges in the presence of hypertension. Fourth, increased neurohormonal activity exists, with a predominance of vasoconstriction and spasm. Fifth, there may be a greater proclivity to cardiac arrhythmias with this disease combination.

Diuretics may actually adversely affect these pathophysiological events (20). These possibilities carry several implications. First, the abnormalities of the heart in hypertension, particularly with coexistent coronary artery disease, must be more completely characterized. Second, the treatment of hypertension in the patient with coronary artery disease or ventricular dysfunction must be targeted to address the pathophysiological abnormalities in the heart more directly. Third, the design of large-scale antihypertensive treatment trials should identify specific cardiovascular endpoints to judge safety and efficacy.

The types of coronary disease that must be managed, in concert with antihypertensive therapy, include stable angina, unstable angina, acute myocardial infarction, and the clinical course following myocardial infarction. In patients with hypertension and stable angina, beta-blockade and nitrate therapy should be considered the cornerstone of therapy, with use of a diurctic as necessary. If either hypertension or angina remains uncontrolled, a calcium channel antagonist may be added. Special consideration of hypertension and unstable angina/acute infarction management depends upon the clinical setting. First, unless contraindicated, beta-blockade should be given by intravenous or oral route as necessary. Clinical experience and published data are not as supportive for calcium antagonists in the acute infarction stage, and they should not precede beta-blockade. Of course, unstable angina/myocardial infarction, associated with a diastolic blood pressure greater than 120 mm Hg, is a "hypertensive emergency" and should be treated accordingly.

In view of the results of the recent SAVE Trial (29), treating hypertension after myocardial infarction assumes even greater importance. The SAVE Trial demonstrates the clinical importance of preventing remodeling of the left ventricle from its standard ellipsoid shape to a more spherical configuration that predisposes to left ventricular dysfunction. In the presence of hypertension, the further excessive wall stress would hasten such a progression. Aggressive reduction of blood pressure to less than 130/70, rather than 150/90, may be warranted. In addition to beta-blockade, or if left ventricular dysfunction is severe, ACE inhibitors in full therapeutic dosage, combined with diuretic and other vasodilators, are warranted. Results of multicenter trials suggest an adverse outcome of use of calcium antagonists in this setting.

B. Congestive Heart Failure

Congestive heart failure is one of the most common cardiovascular sequelae in patients with hypertension. However, it has always been assumed that the majority of heart failure symptoms were due to systolic dysfunction. While this may be true, particularly in the era preceding the availability of vasodilator therapy, it is likely that a considerable amount of this "failure" is caused by stiffness of the left ventricle, or impaired diastolic relaxation. This assumption is based on several lines of evidence. It has been shown that abnormal diastolic filling characteristics occur frequently in patients with hypertension (2,3,6,7,11,12). While pulmonary wedge pressure is well within the normal range under resting conditions, marked increases of pulmonary wedge pressure occur during exercise (18,19). By the time that systolic abnormalities are apparent, systolic blood pressure is often attenuated or even normal, as a result of ventricular power failure; clinical observations show that patients who have "hypertensive cardiomyopathy" are frequently normotensive at the time of symptomatic presentation. The distinction between systolic versus diastolic dysfunction is important. In systolic dysfunction, one would treat with pharmacological classes similar to those used to treat chronic congestive heart failure. When systolic function is demonstrated to be normal (usually by echocardiography) and heart failure is presumed to be due to diastolic dysfunction, one should use alternate drug groups, such as beta-adrenergic blockers or calcium channel antagonists. An ACE inhibitor may still be a primary choice.

Hypertension associated with congestive heart failure may occur as an acute syndrome and should be treated as aggressively as any form of pulmonary edema. When arterial diastolic blood pressure is greater than 120 mm Hg, this is also considered a "hypertensive emergency." For hypertension and acute heart failure, diuretics and vasodilator therapy should be given. If rapid blood pressure reduction is desired, the single best agent is intravenous nitroprusside. Sublingual nifedipine should be avoided. When the clinical situation is controlled, clarification of systolic function by echo is appropriate to guide therapy. Certainly, a diuretic would be appropriate in virtually all cases.

Hypertension associated with chronic compensated congestive heart failure should combine therapies shown to be effective for each disorder. Of vasodilators, ACE inhibitors and hydralazine are most effective for heart failure, and the additional benefits of vasodilators such as alpha-blockers and minoxidil in hypertension should be considered. Calcium channel antagonists should be chosen only when heart failure is primarily due to diastolic dysfunction, pending results of further multicenter trials, such as VHEFT III and PRAISE. The key to therapy is aggressive blood pressure reduction. As left ventricular systolic function may be depressed, arterial systolic pressure may be relatively low (e.g., 130–160 mm Hg), whereas diastolic pressure is relatively high (e.g., 90–100 mm Hg). In this case, a blood pressure range of 100–110/70–80 should be targeted, as long as a symptomatic orthostatic blood pressure fall is not induced.

C. Peripheral Vascular Disease

Structural disease of the conduit and resistance vessels also commonly occurs in hypertension, often recognized as atherosclerotic disease of the great vessels of the neck. Furthermore, the tendency for intracranial hemorrhage from congenital or Charcot-Bouchard aneurysms (36) could be increased when arterial shearing stresses are increased by hypertension. This effect is also germane to aortic dissection and aneurysmal aortic dilatation (22). An obvious, yet critical association in many hypertensive patients is the presence of unitlateral or bilateral renal arterial occlusive disease. Occasionally drug-resistant hypertension occurs in a patient whose blood pressure was previously easy to control. Many of these patients may have secondary renal artery stenosis, superimposed upon essential hypertension, resulting in a combined cause of hypertension.

The experience with diuretic therapy in the elderly suggests that this class of treatment is effective and well tolerated in patients with peripheral vascular disease. Vasodilator therapy would also be most appropriate, as well as sympatholytic therapy. Beta-blockade should not be used for peripheral vascular disease, where it may increase symptoms of claudication. This class can be effective for hypertension associated with other forms of vascular disease: carotid stenosis, aortic dissection/aneurysm, and renovascular disease.

D. Valvular Heart Disease

Systemic arterial hypertension may be associated with valvular heart disease. The coexistence of regurgitant aortic or mitral lesions with arterial hypertension may produce a greater degree of eccentric ventricular hypertrophy and dilatation, thereby accelerating the progression to systolic ventricular dysfunction and failure. Formal studies of regurgitant fractions in relation to systemic hypertension are lacking. However, effective reduction of blood pressure, particularly with vasdilator therapy, will likely reduce regurgitant flow and improve overall ventricular performance in both aortic and mitral regurgitation. A similar effect may occur in the presence of pulmonary or tricuspid regurgitation, but these valvular lesions are very much dependent upon the pulmonary circulation and right ventricular geometry and function, which are less affected by systemic vasodilatation.

Stenotic aortic and mitral valve lesions have a different impact. Aortic stenosis accelerates concentric hypertrophy of the ventricle that may already be present as a result of hypertension. Both aortic and mitral stenosis mechanically limit cardiac output, thereby reducing stroke volume. When these valvular lesions are at early stages of progression, aggressive antihypertensive therapy may not have adverse circulatory effects. Coexistent hypertension and moderate to severe valvular stenosis should be considered resistance in series: the former cause is functional, while the latter is anatomical. Aggressive blood pressure reduction may result in untoward symptoms such as syncope or angina in the presence of valvular stenosis. Thus, when stenosis has progressed to clinically relevant valve area reduction, or even milder stages that nonetheless prevent appropriate blood pressure control, surgical correction of valvular stenosis is warranted.

When hypertension coexists with subvalvular obstruction (hypertrophic obstructive cardiomyopathy), vasodilators should be avoided, and therapy should center on beta-blockade or use of verapamil.

E. Cardiac Conduction Abnormalities/Arrhythmias

Conduction abnormalities must be considered in patients with hypertension, particularly in the elderly patient. Bradycardia and functional or structural block at any of several points in the conduction system may influence the choice of drugs to treat hypertension. In the presence of conduction abnormalities, dihydropyridines are preferable to verapamil and diltiazem, and beta-blockade should be used with caution. In addition, hypertensive patients may be prone to enhanced ventricular ectopy (37). The clinical relevance of the latter is not certain. As hypertension is often a cause of atrial fibrillation, hypertensive therapy with agents such as verapamil which control the ventricular response in atrial fibrillation is desirable.

F. Obesity and Lipid Disorders

As described in Chapter 5, obesity and lipid disorders may also affect, and be affected by, drug treatment. Obesity is one of the most compromising factors on the circulatory system of the hypertensive patient (38). Volume overload and eccentric hypertrophy act in tandem with hypertension, further impairing ventricular performance (2,3,6,7,11,12).

It has become popular to judge antihypertensive therapies by their effects on serum lipids. The effect of these agents on serum lipid levels is relatively small and the clinical significance of such changes has been questioned (39).

Whereas diuretics and beta-adrenergic blocking agents produce an increase of serum lipid levels and angiotensin converting enzyme inhibitors and alpha-blockers may reduce serum lipid levels, it is obvious that a much greater impact would be observed by patients' adhering to appropriate dietary measures directed at lipid reduction and normalization of weight.

IV. SUMMARY

This chapter has considered the treatment of hypertension with respect to individualized needs of patients with cardiovascular disorders. The management of hypertension in patients who have associated cardiovascular disorders will always be complex and difficult but will be most successful when blood pressure is optimally treated and normalized. However, treatment strategies must also be structured to address the pathophysiological abnormalities and characteristics of the coexistent cardiovascular disorder and the hemodynamic consequences of the antihypertensive treatment on the coexistent cardiovascular disorder.

REFERENCES

1. Shea S, Cook EF, Kannel WB, Goldman L. Treatment of hypertension and its effect on cardiovascular risk factors: data from the Framingham Heart Study. Circulation 1985; 71:22–30.
2. Strauer BE. Left ventricular hypertrophy, myocardial blood flow and coronary flow reserve. Cardiology 1991; 81:274–282.
3. Lavie CJ, Ventura HO, Messerli FH. Regression of increased left ventricular mass by antihypertensives. Drugs 1991; 42:945–961.
4. Cody RJ. Mechanisms of vasoconstriction in hypertension and chronic congestive heart failure. In: Dhalla NS, Singal PK, Beamish RE, eds. Pathophysiology of Heart Disease. Boston, Martinus Nijhoff, 1987:143–150.
5. Tarazi RC. The heart in hypertension. N Engl J Med 1985; 312:308–309.
6. Karliner JL, Williams D, Gorwit J, et al. Left ventricular performance in patients with left ventricular hypertrophy caused by systemic arterial hypertension. Br Heart J 1977; 39:1239–1245.
7. Hartford M, Wikstrand J, Wallentin I, et al. Diastolic function of the heart in untreated primary hypertension. Hypertension 1984; 6:329–338.
8. Cannon RO, Bonow RO, Bacharach SL, et al. Left ventricular dysfunction in patients with angina pectoris normal epicardial coronary arteries and abnormal vasodilator reserve. Circulation 1985; 71:18–26.
9. Fox KM, Levy RD, Mockus L, Wright C. Hypertension and the ischemic myocardium. J Hypertens 1987; 8(suppl 3):S17–S18.
10. Maron BJ, Wolfson JK, Epstein SE, Roberts WC. Intramural ("small vessel") coronary artery disease in hypertrophic cardiomyopathy. J Am Coll Cardiol 1986; 8:545–547.

11. Nichols AB, Sciacca R, Weiss MB, et al. Effect of left ventricular hypertrophy on myocardial blood flow and ventricular performance in systemic hypertension. Circulation 1980; 62:329–340.
12. Cody RJ, Bravo EL, Fouad FM, Tarazi RC. Cardiovascular reflexes during chronic converting enzyme inhibition and sodium depletion: the response to tilt in hypertensive patients. Am J Med 1981; 71:422–426.
13. Cody RJ, Atlas SA, Laragh JH, et al. Atrial natriuretic factor in normal subjects and heart failure patients: plasma levels and renal, hormonal, and hemodynamic responses to peptide infusion. J Clin Invest 1986; 78:1362–1374.
14. Cody RJ, Atlas SA, Laragh JH. Physiological and pharmacological studies of atrial natriuretic factor, a natriuretic and vasoactive peptide. J Clin Pharmacol 1987; 27:927–936.
15. Ganau A, Devereux RB, Atlas SA, et al. Plasma atrial natriuretic factor in essential hypertension: relationship to cardiac size, function and systemic hemodynamics. J Am Coll Cardiol 1989; 14:715–724.
16. Cody RJ, Kubo SH, Laragh JH, et al. Exercise-induced secretion of atrial natriuretic factor and its relation to hemodynamic and sympathetic stimulation in untreated essential hypertension. Am J Cardiol 1991; 68:918–924.
17. Cody RJ, Kubo SH, Laragh JH, Atlas SA. Exercise-induced myocardial secretion of atrial natriuetic factor in patients with chronic congestive heart failure. J Appl Physiol 1992; 73:1627–1643.
18. Cody RJ, Kubo SH, Covit AB, et al. Exercise hemodynamics and oxygen delivery in human hypertension: response to verapamil. Hypertension 1986; 8:3–10.
19. Cody RJ, Kubo SH, Ryman KS, et al. Systemic and pulmonary hemodynamic responses to nicardipine during graded ergometric exercise in patients with moderate to severe essential hypertension. J Am Coll Cardiol 1987; 10:647–654.
20. Poole-Wilson PA. Diuretics, hypokalemia and arrhythmias in hypertensive patients: still an unresolved problem. J Hypertens 1987; 5(suppl 3):S51–S55.
21. Kubo SH, Clark M, Laragh JH, et al. Identification of normal neurohormonal activity in mild congestive heart failure and the stimulating effect of upright posture and diuretics. Am J Cardiol 1987; 60:1322–1328.
22. Cody RJ. Hypertensive emergencies and aortic dissection. In: Parrillo JE ed. Current Therapy in Critical Care Medicine. Toronto, BC Decker, 1991:155–158.
23. Lund-Johansen P, Omvik P. Acute and chronic hemodynamic effects of drugs with different actions on adrenergic receptors: a comparison between alpha-blockers and different types of beta-blockers with and without vasodilating effect. Cardiovasc Drugs Ther 1991; 5:605–615.
24. Louis WJ, McNeil JJ, Drummer OH. Pharmacology of combined alpha-beta-blockade. Drugs 1984; 28:16–33.
25. Cressman MD, Vidt DG, Gifford RW Jr, et al. Intravenous labetalol in the management of severe hypertension and hypertensive emergencies. Am Heart J 1984; 107:980–985.
26. Cody RJ, Tarazi RC, Bravo EL, Fouad FM. Hemodynamics of orally active converting enzyme inhibitor (SQ 14225) in hypertensive patients. Clin Sci Mol Med 1978; 55:453–459.

27. Fagard R, Amery A, Reybrouckj T, et al. Acute and chronic systemic and pulmonary hemodynamic effects of angiotensin converting enzyme inhibition with captopril in hypertensive patients. Am J Cardiol 1980; 46:295–300.
28. Cody RJ. Hemodynamic responses to specific renin angiotensin inhibitors in hypertension and heart failure: a review. Drugs 1984; 28:144–169.
29. Pfeffer MA, Branunwald E, Moye LA. Effect of captopril on mortality and morbidity in patients with left ventricular dysfunction after myocardial infarction. N Engl J Med 1992; 327:669–677.
30. Swedberg K, Held P, Kjekshus J, et al. Effects of the early administration of enalapril on mortality in patients with acute myocardial infarction: results of the Cooperative New Scandinavian Enalapril Survival Study II (Consensus II). N Engl J Med 1992; 327:678–684.
31. Cody RJ. Vascular and myocardial responses to calcium antagonists: implications for hypertension and congestive heart failure. In: Epstein M ed. Calcium Antagonists in Clinical Medicine. Philadelphia, Hanley and Belfus, 1992:105–135.
32. Ryman KS, Kubo SH, Shaknovich A, Cody RJ. Influence of baseline hemodynamic status and sympathetic activity on the response to nicardipine, a new dihydropyridine, in patients with hypertension or chronic congestive heart failure. Clin Pharmacol Ther 1987; 41:483–489.
33. Cody RJ, Riew KD, Kubo SH. Reversal of a calcium-mediated vasoconstrictor component in patients with congestive heart failure. Clin Pharmacol Ther 1989; 46:291–296.
34. Ellrodt AG, Ault MJ, Riedinger MS, Murata GH. Efficacy and safety of sublingual nifedipine in hypertensive emergencies. Am J Med 1985; 79:19–24.
35. Devereux RB, Drayer J, Chien S, et al. Whole blood viscosity as a determinant of cardiac hypertrophy in systemic hypertension. Am J Cardiol 1984; 54:592–595.
36. Pickering G. Hypertension: definitions, natural histories and consequences. Am J Med 1972; 52:570–583.
37. Messerli FH, Ventura HO, Elizardi DJ, et al. Hypertension and sudden death: increased ventricular ectopic activity in left ventricular hypertrophy. Am J Med 1984; 77:18–22.
38. de Divitiis O, Fazio S, Petitto M, et al. Obesity and cardiac function. Circulation 1981; 64:477–488.
39. Burris JF. Beta-blockers, diplipidemia, and coronary artery disease. Arch Intern Med 1993; 153:2085–2092.

8

Hypertension with Cerebrovascular Disease

OLAF B. PAULSON
University Hospital, Rigshospitalet
Copenhagen, Denmark

SVEND STRANDGAARD
Herley Hospital
Herley, Denmark

I. INTRODUCTION

Hypertension has a profound influence on the cerebral circulation and is a major risk factor for cerebrovascular disease. Antihypertensive drugs, especially when given for emergency blood pressure lowering, can have a variety of unexpected effects in the cerebral circulation. Stroke prevention is the main benefit afforded by modern antihypertensive treatment, but occasionally overzealous clinical blood pressure lowering may lead to cerebral ischemia. These aspects of hypertension, its treatment, and the response of the cerebral circulation are reviewed in this chapter.

II. HYPERTENSIVE ADAPTATION OF CEREBRAL CIRCULATION

The absolute value of resting cerebral blood flow (CBF) is the same in hypertensive and normotensive humans when no neurological deficit is present and is of the order of 50 ml/100 g perfused tissue/min (1). This means that hypertension is associated with an increased vascular resistance in the brain, as in other parts of the vascular system. Hypertensive arterioles and small arteries are narrowed with thickened walls (Figure 1) (2) as a result of a complex process of vessel wall growth and remodeling (3). This causes a functional adaptation of CBF autoregulation in hypertension, most importantly a shift of autoregulation toward higher pressure.

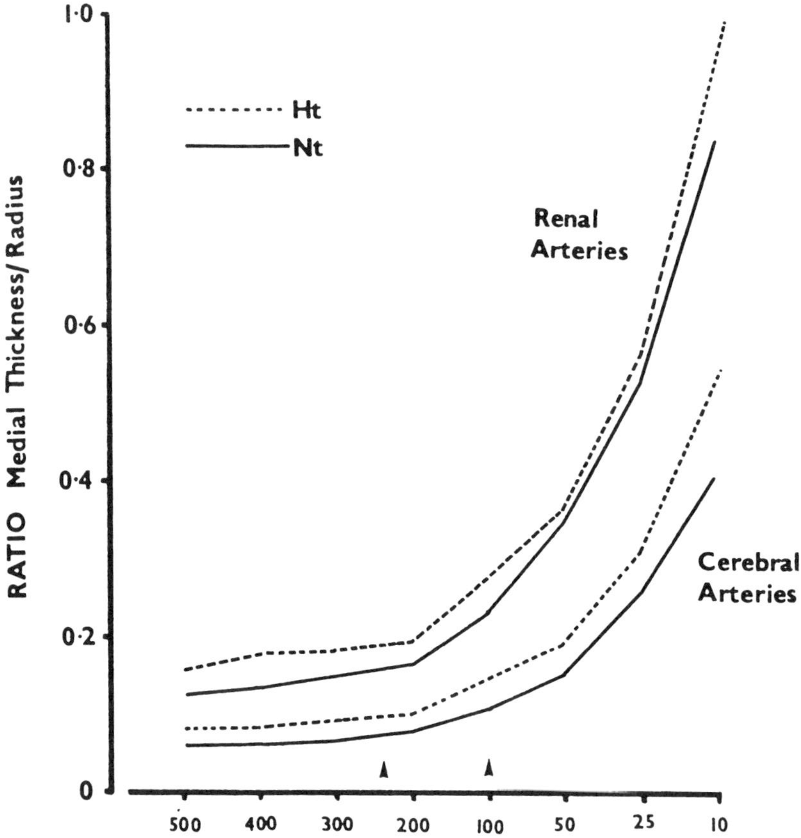

Figure 1 Increased wall thickness in hypertensive (Ht) as compared with normotensive (Nt) arteries and arterioles. (From Ref. 2.)

Autoregulation denotes the ability of an organ or a vascular system to maintain a constant blood flow in the face of changes in perfusion pressure. In the brain, perfusion pressure is the difference between blood pressure and intracranial pressure. Since the latter is mostly constant and rather low, CBF autoregulation in most cases operates in response to changes in blood pressure. Thus, when blood pressure falls (or intracranial pressure rises), the cerebral arterioles dilate, and when blood pressure rises, they constrict, attempting to keep CBF constant. Below a mean blood pressure around 50 mm Hg, autoregulatory vasodilatation becomes inadequate, and CBF decreases. The brain can compensate somewhat for this by extracting more oxygen from the blood, and only when the blood pressure and CBF are approximately halved are symptoms of brain hypoperfusion encountered. Beyond a mean blood pressure around 150 mm Hg, autoregulatory vasoconstriction gives way to pressure-forced vasodilatation.

In chronic hypertension, structural vascular changes cause a shift of the lower and upper blood pressure limits of autoregulation toward higher pressure (4–6) (Figure 2). Thus, vascular narrowing and wall thickening impair the tolerance to low blood pressure but improve the tolerance to high blood

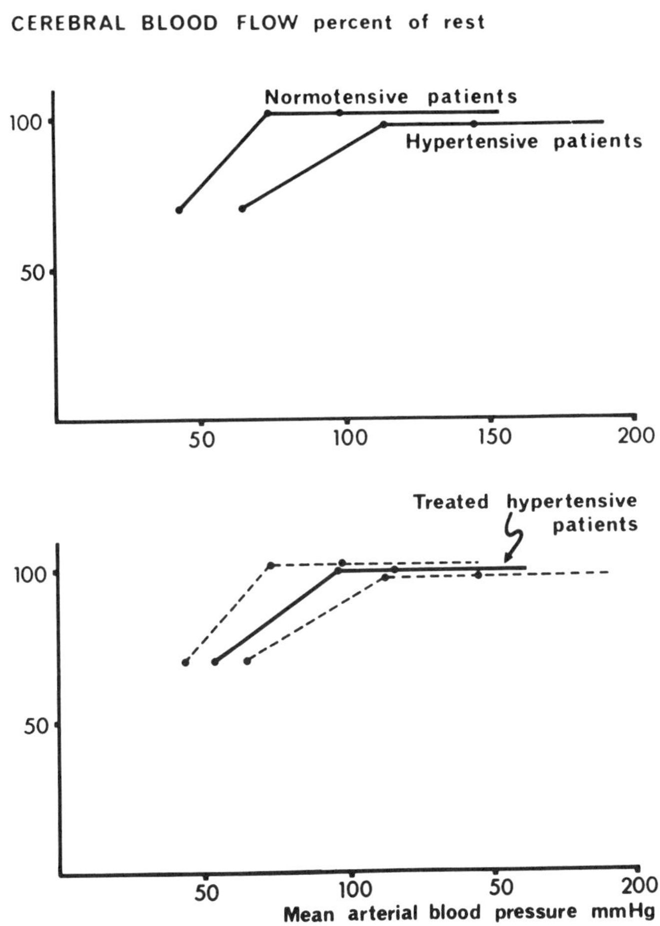

Figure 2 The lower limit of autoregulation of cerebral blood flow is shifted toward high blood pressure in untreated or poorly controlled hypertension. (From Ref. 4.).

pressure. Animal studies suggest that the hypertensive shift of CBF autoregulation is more pronounced for the upper limit than for the lower limit (6).

With long-term antihypertensive treatment, CBF autoregulation may readapt itself toward normal. Studies in middle-aged hypertensive patients have demonstrated that this may or may not happen in the course of 1 year's effective pressure lowering (4). In young rats with renovascular hypertension, CBF autoregulation may normalize completely during a few months of antihypertensive treatment (Figure 3) (7,8).

Antihypertensive treatment prevents strokes and does not normally cause cerebral ischemia. The reason for this may be that a gradual readaptation of CBF autoregulation takes place in many patients once treatment has been started. It may also be important that the brain, contrary to the myocardium, has the potential for extracting more oxygen from the blood passing through it, should CBF fall. In rare clinical settings, discussed later in the chapter, antihypertensive treatment may lower the blood pressure excessively and provoke cerebral ischemia. It is however important to understand that the hypertensive changes in cerebrovascular physiology do not normally lead to reservations about clinical antihypertensive treatment, known from clinical trials to protect patients against cerebrovascular catastrophes.

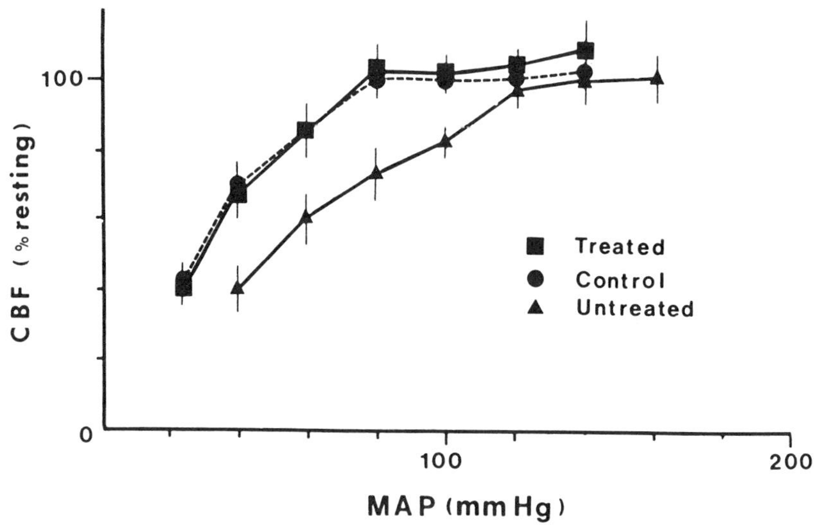

Figure 3 Effect of chronic antihypertensive treatment with hydrochlorothiazide, hydralazine, and reserpine on the lower limit of autoregulation of cerebral blood flow (CBF) in young rats with renal hypertension and normotensive Wistar Kyoto rats. The lower limit is shifted markedly toward high pressure in hypertensive rats, but is normalized during treatment. (From Ref. 7.).

III. STROKE AND HYPERTENSION

Hypertension is associated with an increased incidence of both cerebral infarcts (large vessels), lacunar lesions (small vessels), and hemorrhages (9–14). In the Framingham study a linear correlation was found between blood pressure, both systolic and diastolic, and the incidence of stroke (9,11). In contrast, other studies have demonstrated that there is no relation between blood pressure and stroke incidence at low pressure levels, but an exponential increase of stroke at high pressure levels (Figure 4) (13). Antihypertensive treatment reduces or eliminates this increased risk of stroke, but over-

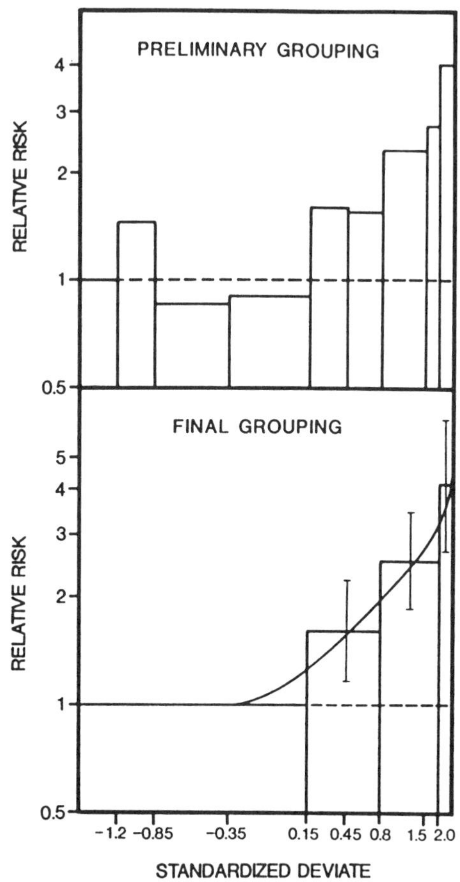

Figure 4 Estimated effect of systolic blood pressure on stroke risk. Standardized deviate was obtained by subtracting the average from the systolic blood pressure and dividing by the standard deviation of systolic blood pressure for 10-year age and sex group. (From Ref. 13.)

zealous antihypertensive treatment may occasionally provoke a stroke. In acute stroke the blood pressure is frequently transiently increased (15) and about half of the patients have preexisting hypertension (16–18). These important aspects of interaction between hypertension and stroke are discussed in the following sections.

A. Hypertension and the Various Types of Stroke

Large vessel disease (atherothrombotic) ischemic stroke is caused by thrombosis or embolism of cerebral arteries and constitute the majority of strokes. Hypertension increases the risk of these strokes as it accelerates the development of arteriosclerosis. The formation of a thrombosis may suddenly accelerate and aggravate a stenosis or form an arterial occlusion. Emboli may originate from ulcerated plaques in larger arteries or from the heart. A minor part of the large vessel ischemic strokes are of a hemodynamic nature, where a fall in blood pressure (e.g., orthostatic or induced by overzealous antihypertensive treatment) may cause a critical fall in perfusion of a brain area nourished by a functional end artery stenosed by atheroma.

Transient ischemic attacks (TIAs) are strokes in which the symptoms clear completely within the first 24 hours of onset. They are ordinarily caused by the same large vessel disease as those underlying the previously mentioned strokes, but for the TIA small cerebral emboli are lysed spontaneously before tissue damage becomes irreversible. Occasionally permanent tissue damage may be visualized by computed tomography (CT) or magnetic resonance imaging after a TIA as a result of an infarction of cerebral tissue in an area in which no significant neurological deficits occur. As with strokes, a small fraction of TIAs are of a hemodynamic nature. Interestingly, endothelial-derived vasospasm has also been postulated to be the pathogenetic mechanism in some cases of TIA (19). Antihypertensive treatment has been shown to prevent TIA (20), indirectly confirming the nonhemodynamic nature of most cases.

The hemodynamic mechanism can also be considered as a condition of chronic threatening ischemia which occurs if a stenosing or occluding lesion of an artery supplying the brain reduces the local blood pressure to such an extent that the perfusion is reduced or threatened but the tissue or most of it is still structurally intact and alive. In the normal brain blood flow is autoregulated: that is, cerebral blood flow remains constant despite rather large changes in the arterial blood pressure. But in the region threatened by ischemia the local blood pressure is at or below the lower limit of the normal autoregulation (21,22). The blood flow may consequently be somewhat reduced already in the resting condition and decreases further with even a slight reduction of the blood pressure. The application of cerebral vasodilator stimuli such as intravenous acetazolamide may reveal a "steal syndrome" in which the flow in the ischemic region is further reduced simultaneously with a normal flow increase in the other parts of the brain (23). TIA of hemodynamic origin and chronic threatening ischemia are uncommon but still of importance as these patients may be at special risk when placed on antihypertensive treatment and may be candidates for bypass surgery.

Cerebral hemorrhages are considered to be a result of small vessel disease if they are not a consequence of a ruptured larger vascular malformation. They constitute a minor percentage of strokes but are rather closely related to hypertension. Hemorrhages can occur anywhere in the cerebrum, cerebellum, or brain stem, but are most commonly located deep in the hemispheres. Cerebral hemorrhages may or may not be caused by rupture of Charcot-Bouchard microaneurysms. These microaneurysms have a diameter of 1 to 2 mm and are seen predominantly in hypertensive individuals (24,25). They must not be confused with the larger saccular aneurysms that cause subarachnoid hemorrhage. Recently the importance of microaneurysms in the pathogenesis of cerebral hemorrhage has been challenged (26). Cerebral hemorrhages may be small to massive lesions that may cause a life-threatening rise in intracranial pressure. In general, clinical symptoms allow only a limited bedside distinction between hemorrhagic and ischemic stroke. The increased use of CT has allowed in vivo diagnosis of more cerebral hemorrhages than previously possible, particularly to small lesions (27).

Lacunar strokes result from small vessel disease. They are due to degenerative changes in penetrating small arteries that cause small lesions, sometimes multiple, and often located deep in the white matter of the hemispheres (28). They may be related to Charcot-Bouchard microaneurysms and have several probable causes: small ischemic lesions, small hemorrhages which have been resorbed, or localized hypertensive damage due to hypertensive episodes with disturbed blood-brain barrier function.

Border-zone infarcts are a type of ischemic brain lesion that occurs in the "watershed" area between the three major cerebral arteries: anterior, medial, and posterior. These lesions may occur if systemic blood pressure falls drastically, for example, as a result of cardiac arrest or when emergency blood pressure lowering is out of control.

Multi-infarct dementia, formerly called atherosclerotic dementia, and Alzheimer's disease are the most common cause of gradual loss of cognitive function. Multi-infarct dementia in hypertensive patients should to some extent be preventable by antihypertensive treatment, though no study appears to have dealt with this question.

Binswanger's encephalopathy (*leukoarariosis*) causes white matter lesions that can be demonstrated in many hypertensive patients by MRI or advanced CT scans. The nature of these often rather discrete changes and their relation to the level of blood pressure and duration of hypertension are unknown. More severe lesions of this type, sometimes called Binswanger's encephalopathy, appear to be a cause of dementia in hypertension; they were described in autopsy studies a century ago. A more recent term is "leukoaraiosis," or thinning of white matter (29). The lesions appear to have some relation to lacunes. They are different from the gray matter lesions of experimental hypertensive encephalopathy (30) and from the infarcts of multi-infarct dementia. Significant periventricular atrophy has been demonstrated by MR imaging in elderly, well-treated hypertensives with no cognitive impairment and no other signs of hypertensive target organ damage (31). Clearly, further studies are needed to elucidate the nature and consequences of leukoaraiosis.

B. Antihypertensive Treatment and Stroke Prevention

Antihypertensive treatment decreases or eliminates a lifetime's increased risk for stroke in the course of 3 to 5 years (32). In animal models of stroke, chronic antihypertensive treatment appears to diminish the infarct size after medial cerebral artery occlusion. This has been shown in stroke-prone spontaneously hypertensive rats (SHRs), in which the converting enzyme inhibitor cilazapril has been more effective in this respect than a combination of hydralazine, reserpine, and hydrochlorothiazide (33). Possibly, this effect is due to regression of hypertensive vascular remodeling, which improves the tolerance to low blood pressure and hence tends to prevent ischemia in the brain tissue. Placebo-controlled trials in humans generally have not reported on the severity of stroke, beyond distinguishing between nonfatal and fatal cases. A mitigating effect of antihypertensive treatment on cerebral infarct size in humans is thus likely but unproven.

In large-scale epidemiological studies of hypertension and stroke, diagnostic imaging with MRI and CT generally has not been done, and hence the term "atherothrombotic stroke," used, for example, in the reports of the Framingham study, should be regarded with some caution. It is thus uncertain to what extent large and small vessel disease or infarcts, hemorrhage, and lacunar lesions are prevented by antihypertensive treatment. Probably they are all prevented, though maybe not to the same extent. Only a few epidemiological studies have made it possible to differentiate between the different stroke types by using more extensive evaluation, including CT scan and/or autopsy. In a Finnish community study the incidence and mortality rates of stroke in 1972–73 and 1978–80 were compared. A decline in the incidence of hemorrhages but not of ischemic lesions was observed, and this difference was attributed to improved treatment of hypertension. Lacunar lesions were not reported as a separate entity (34). Spence found that from 1977 to 1984 a change occurred in the diagnostic pattern of stroke patients admitted to a major Canadian referral hospital. All patients had CT scans, and while the number of admitted cases declined by about 50% in the observation period, the proportion of lacunar and hemorrhagic stroke declined from 59% to 10% and the proportion of cerebral infarcts rose from 50% to 70%. This finding has, however, not been confirmed in larger series, and it is still generally accepted that about 10% of all strokes are intracerebral hemorrhage and 30% are lacunage. Therefore, further epidemiological investigation is definitely warranted before more firm conclusions can be drawn.

C. High Blood Pressure in Acute Stroke

In acute stroke, blood pressure is often transiently elevated and returns to the prestroke level in the course of a few days (15). It has been hotly debated whether pharmacological blood pressure lowering should be attempted in the early phase of stroke (35–37). In ischemic stroke, the infarcted tissue may be surrounded by a zone of underperfused but vital tissue, and lowering the pressure may jeopardize the perfusion of this "penumbra" zone. If a cerebral vascular embolus is spontaneously lysed, as occurs frequently, formerly ischemic tissue may become hyperemic, and with high pressure, hemorrhage into the infarct may occur. Leaving the blood pressure high in this situation may be risky. Unfortunately, spontaneous thrombolysis with changes from cerebral ischemia to hyperemia in acute stroke is not clinically obvious and requires sequential CBF and brain imaging studies for demonstration. On balance, as the blood pressure falls spontaneously in most stroke patients, it would seem prudent to leave all but the highest pressures untreated in the acute phase of a stroke. Prestroke antihypertensive treatment should in most cases be continued. Thus, the authors would recommend a period of observation of hours to days before embarking on blood pressure reduction in acute stroke and restriction of treatment in the acute phase to cases of blood pressures that remain at or above around 130 mm Hg. This probably also applies in lacunar stroke.

In cerebral hemorrhages most authorities recommend cautious lowering of diastolic blood pressures over 120 mm Hg, but whether this is justified is unproved. If imaging studies such as CT are not done in acute stroke, many intracerebral hemorrhages remain undiagnosed, and it would seem prudent to assume that all such patients have ischemic stroke and to manage their blood pressure accordingly.

It is possible that treatment with calcium antagonists may have a beneficial pharmacological effect in acute stroke. Thus, in acute rat experiments, the calcium antagonist isradipine caused a reduction in infarct size when given before or up to 4 hours after middle cerebral artery occlusion (38).

Interestingly this protective effect was not seen with a stereoisomeric form of isradipine that does not cross the blood-brain barrier (39). In stroke patients, though, another calcium antagonist given acutely caused an undesirable steal of blood from ischemic to normal brain tissue (40). This suggests that the beneficial effect of isradipine seen in the rat studies may be of a cytoprotective rather than a hemodynamic nature. Clinical trials of calcium antagonists in acute stroke have given conflicting results, some showing better patient outcome, others not (41,42).

D. Antihypertensive Treatment in Stroke Survivors

It has been somewhat controversial whether antihypertensive treatment should be given to stroke survivors, once the acute phase of the stroke is over. Theoretically, the patients are at risk of having stenotic lesions in the arteries to the brain with chronic threatening ischemia. Lowering the blood pressure by antihypertensive treatment may then provoke TIA or a manifest stroke; that is, provoke the same disease that the treatment is aimed at preventing. However, since the majority of ischemic strokes are thromboembolic and not hemodynamic, the risk of provoking a stroke is probably rather slight. Clinical observations on antihypertensive treatment in hypertensive stroke survivors have confirmed the beneficial effect of treatment (43).

The overall statistically beneficial effect of antihypertensive treatment in hypertensive stroke survivors does, however, not eliminate the potential risks and hazards in the individual. Careful clinical evaluated should be performed in all patients; in selected cases more sophisticated evaluation of cerebral hemodynamics may be needed.

E. Ischemic Stroke Precipitated by Antihypertensive Treatment

As briefly mentioned, antihypertensive treatment may occasionally precipitate cerebral ischemia. This may occur if transient hypertension in acute stroke is treated aggressively, as described previously. Overzealous antihypertensive treatment may also cause a stroke in severely hypertensive patients, elderly hypertensives, the rare patients who have hemodynamically mediated transitory ischemic attacks, and the occasional patient who has hypotensive anesthesia. These clinical situations are discussed in the following sections.

1. Initial or Intensified Treatment of Severe Hypertension

A number of cases have been published in which emergency blood pressure lowering was excessive and caused ischemic cerebral damage (Figure 5) (44–46). Symptoms have included blindness or pareses, and the ischemic lesions have sometimes been located in the border zones or watershed regions in the

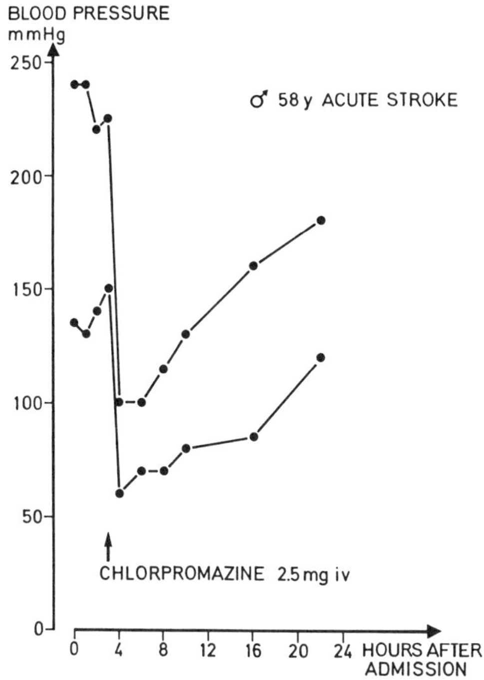

Figure 5 Drastic fall in blood pressure caused by a small dose of chlorpromazine in a severely hypertensive patient with acute stroke. The patient's hemiparesis fortunately did not worsen during the hypotensive episode.

brain between the territories supplied by the three major arteries (47). Many of the early reported cases were given bolus-dose diazoxide, but all kinds of hypotensive regimens have been involved; the common denominator is that too low a blood pressure was maintained for too long. Clearly, treatment of very high blood pressure should be very cautious, because the risk of overtreatment in many cases is as great as or greater than the risk of the very high blood pressure itself. The cerebrovascular pharmacological characteristics of the various antihypertensive drugs recommended for emergency blood pressure lowering are discussed later in this chapter.

2. Treatment of Hypertension in the Elderly

Recent controlled clinical trials have shown that antihypertensive treatment is beneficial in elderly patients, even in cases of isolated systolic hypertension (20,48,49). Treatment prevents stroke as effectively as in younger patients, and even has a protective effect on coronary disease. Actually, since the incidence of stroke increases markedly with age, more strokes can be prevented by antihypertensive treatment in the elderly than in the young and middle-aged. In spite of this, the risk of overtreating elderly patients is real, in particular if the results of the trials in fit elderly people are interpreted uncritically in favor of lowering blood pressure in the more frail elderly. Reports of overtreatment of elderly hypertensives are of necessity anecdotal. It appears however that postural hypotension, which is sometimes present in a mild, asymptomatic form in old age, is a risk factor for overtreating hypertension and causing cerebral ischemic lesions (Figure 6) (50, 51). Clearly, blood pressure lowering in the elderly should be done with caution, with supine and standing pressure measurement before and after start of treatment.

3. *Transitory Ischemic Attacks of a Hemodynamic Nature*

As described earlier, most TIAs are nonhemodynamic and are to some extent prevented by chronic antihypertensive treatment. A few cases, however, may be precipitated by blood pressure lowering, which causes ischemia in a brain region nourished by a stenotic end artery. In such cases, antihypertensive treatment should obviously be modified to alleviate symptoms, and vascular surgery should be considered.

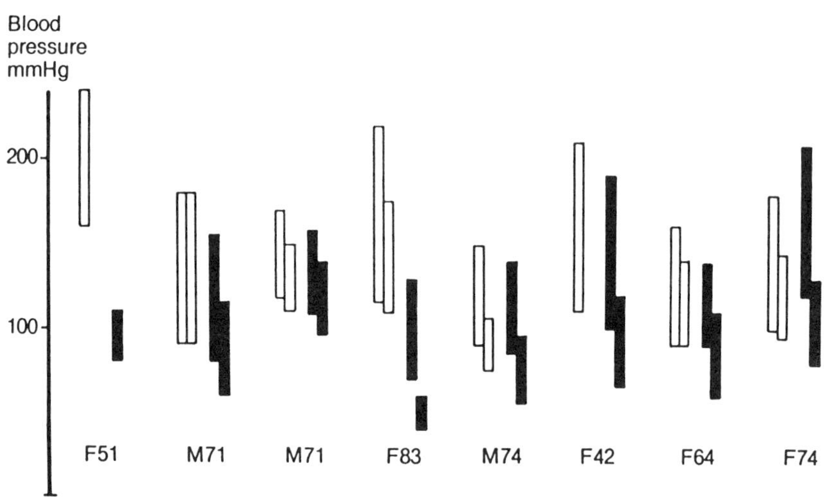

Figure 6 Supine and erect blood pressure in eight mostly elderly patients in whom ischemic stroke developed during overtreatment with antihypertensive drugs. Solid bars denote pressures upon admission with acute stroke; open bars denote pressures before the stroke or after treatment had been discontinued. Even when asymptomatic, many of the patients had postural hypotension, which in the elderly limits the tolerance to antihypertensive treatment. Supine and erect blood pressures (□ asymptomatic; ■ symptomatic). (From Ref. 51.)

4. *Hypotensive Anesthesia*

Cerebral ischemia may develop unnoticed during hypotensive anesthesia when the patient's neurological status cannot be adequately monitored. The risk may be highest in effectively treated middle-aged or elderly patients who may have retained structural hypertensive vascular remodeling and hence an impaired tolerance to low pressure. Such cases, though, have only been reported occasionally and are probably rare (46).

IV. SUBARACHNOID HEMORRHAGE AND HYPERTENSION

Subarachnoid hemorrhages occur directly into the subarachnoid space. There is some overlap with the intracerebral hemorrhages discussed previously. The cause of the subarachnoid hemorrhage is in about 70% of cases a ruptured saccular arterial aneurysm at the bifurcation of the larger cerebral arteries, in 10% bleeding from an arteriovenous malformation, and in the remaining 20% a rupture of a seemingly normal vessel. The subarachnoid hemorrhage in most instances occurs in situations with episodes of physiological increase of the blood pressure, such as coitus and isometric exercise. It should be noted that the saccular arterial aneurysms and the vascular malformations are not protected by cerebral autoregulation against episodes of increased blood pressure since they most often arise from the larger resistance vessels.

It would be expected that chronic arterial hypertension would also increase the risk of subarachnoidal hemorrhage and of the formation of the saccular intracranial aneurysms. Epidemiological studies support this assumption. A clear correlation between rupture of intracranial aneurysms and hypertension was observed in the Framingham study (52) and in a large Danish multicenter study (53). The risk of subarachnoid hemorrhage was also found to be increased in hypertensive patients in a case-control population study (54). Human kidney donors dying of subarachnoid hemorrhage have higher relative heart weights than donors dying of head injury, suggesting a higher blood pressure level in the former (Figure 7) (55). The outcome of subarachnoid hemorrhage has been found to be worse in hypertensive than in normotensive patients (53,56).

V. ACUTE HYPERTENSIVE ENCEPHALOPATHY

Acute hypertensive encephalopathy in the strict sense is now a rare condition, undoubtedly prevented by the widespread use of antihypertensive treatment. It is a stormy clinical syndrome with severe headache, nausea, vomiting, blurred consciousness, and eventually convulsions and coma (see Chapter 13). The pathogenesis of this condition has been attributed to hypertensive "vasospasm," or pathological vasoconstriction, but is more likely the opposite: forced cerebral vasodilatation beyond the upper limit of autoregulation

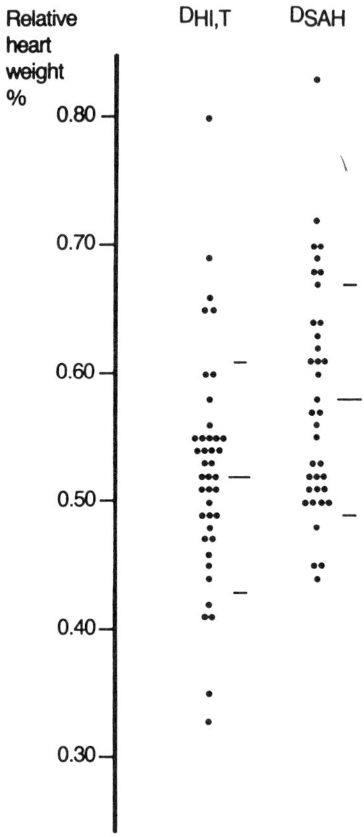

Figure 7 Relative heart weight (i.e., heart weight as percentage of body weight) as registered at autopsy in human kidney donors. Relative heart weight was significantly higher in donors dying of subarachnoid hemorrhage (DSAH) than in those dying of head injury or brain tumor (D-HI,T). (From Ref. 55.)

57–59). Hypertensive autoregulatory failure may be associated with blood-brain barrier dysfunction and the formation of brain edema (60,61) and may be accompanied by a rise in intracranial pressure. With careful, gradual pressure lowering, the patient with acute hypertensive encephalopathy can recover to a surprising extent. As discussed later, overtreatment with immediate "normalization" of blood pressure carries a severe risk of precipitating irreversible ischemic brain damage.

VI. THE CEREBROVASCULAR PHARMACOLOGY OF ANTIHYPERTENSIVE DRUGS

A. Acute Blood Pressure Lowering

When the blood pressure is lowered acutely with a drug, a limited number of responses can be anticipated in the cerebral circulation. On the basis of experimental studies and observations in patients, drugs used for emergency blood pressure lowering can conveniently be classified into the following groups.

1. Drugs with No Pharmacological Effect in the Cerebral Circulation

Diazoxide is the best studied example of these drugs. If the blood pressure is lowered acutely with diazoxide, and the blood pressure remains above the lower limit of autoregulation, CBF remains unchanged. If the drug takes the blood pressure below the lower limit, CBF falls (Figure 8). This does not necessarily cause clinical symptoms, since the brain responds by extracting more oxygen from the blood. If a pressor drug is subsequently given, CBF autoregulation will be found to be intact (62,63).

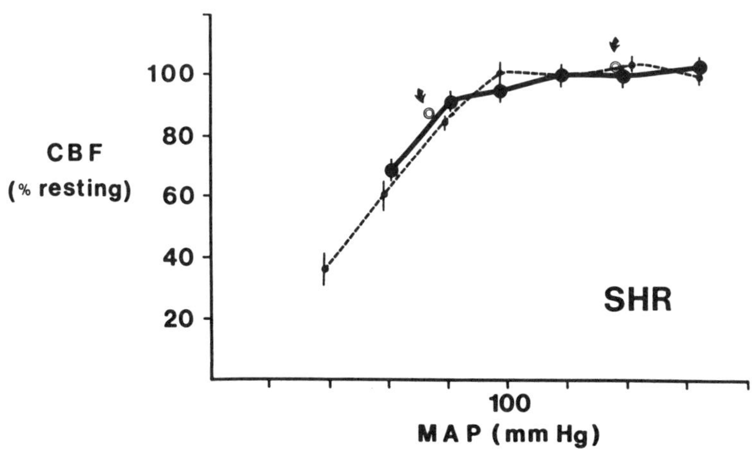

Figure 8 Effect of diazoxide on cerebral blood flow (CBF) in spontaneously hypertensive rats (SHRs). A dose of 5 mg/kg given as an intravenous bolus caused a fall in CBF as the blood pressure fell below the lower limit of autoregulation (open circles and arrows). With subsequent blood pressure manipulation by controlled bleeding or norepinephrine infusion, autoregulation was found to be intact (solid line) when compared to that in a group of control animals (dotted line). (From Ref. 62.)

2. Cerebral Vasodilators

If the blood pressure is lowered acutely with a cerebral vasodilator such as dihydralazine or sodium nitroprusside, the fall in blood pressure may be accompanied by a rise in CBF (64) and intracranial pressure (30, 65–69). CBF may remain at normal levels well below the lower limit of autoregulation (67). In dihydralazine-induced hypotension in rats, infusion of a pressor drug caused a massive rise in CBF, demonstrating paralysis of autoregulation (Figure 9) (63). In malignant hypertension and hypertensive encephalopathy, cerebral vasodilators may add to the preexisting rise in intracranial pressure

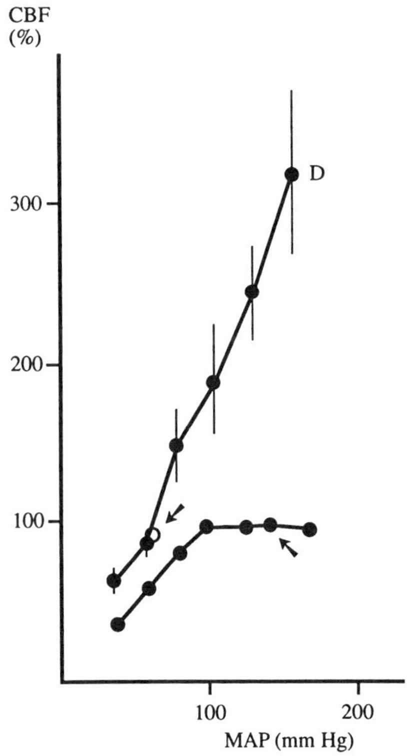

Figure 9 Effect of dihydralazine on cerebral blood flow (CBF) in spontaneously hypertensive rats (SHRs). With repetitive incremental doses of dihydralazine(D), the blood pressure fell below the lower limit of autoregulation with no fall in CBF, signifying cerebral vasodilatation (arrows and open circle). With subsequent infusion of norepinephrine, CBF rose massively, demonstrating paralyzed autoregulation. Autoregulation in a group of SHRs not given dihydralazine is shown for comparison. (From Ref. 63.)

(70). This questions the rather widespread clinical practice of treating patients with eclampsia with intravenous hydralazine or dihydralazine and using sodium nitroprusside for emergency blood pressure lowering. When cerebral vasodilators are given in such clinical settings, patients must be observed with the utmost care for signs of progressive cerebral dysfunction.

3. Calcium Antagonists

With calcium antagonists, some intracerebral vasodilatation may occur. When nifedipine was given orally to severely hypertensive patients, blood pressure fell markedly while CBF was unchanged; a comparable fall in blood pressure induced with clonidine was associated with a fall in CBF (71). In SHRs, nifedipine caused a fall in blood pressure and a marked rise in CBF (72). Nitrendipine in patients caused a fall in blood pressure with no change in CBF (71). With nimodipine, no change in CBF but a rise in intracranial pressure has been demonstrated in patients with normal-pressure hydrocephalus (73). The effect of calcium antagonists in acute stroke is still controversial, as discussed earlier in this chapter.

4. Angiotensin Converting Enzyme Inhibitors

Angiotensin converting enzyme (ACE) inhibitors such as captopril given acutely to hypertensive rats shift the lower limit of autoregulation toward lower pressure (67), an effect also suggested in humans by studies in heart failure patients (Figure 10) (74) and demonstrated in patients with normal-pressure hydrocephalus (75); in the latter, captopril had no effect on intracranial pressure. Probably, the ACE inhibitors have a preferential dilatory effect in the larger cerebral resistance vessels. Surprisingly, in healthy normotensive volunteers and hypertensive patients the effect of captopril on the lower limit of CBF autoregulation was at the limit of statistical significance (76). It is likely that the ACE inhibitors have a dilatory effect on the larger cerebral resistance vessels. In humans, they do not impair autoregulation to moderate blood pressure increases (75,76). In experimental cerebral infarction in stroke-prone SHRs, pretreatment with the ACE inhibitor cilazapril was more effective in restricting infarct size than lowering of the pressure with hydrochlorothiazide, reserpine, and hydralazine (33).

An interaction can be shown between the renin-angiotensin system and the sympathetic nervous system. Thus the downward shift of the upper limit of autoregulation is attenuated by simultaneous stimulation of the superior cervical sympathetic ganglion in the rat (77). This observation is obviously of major interest for the treatment of hypertensive patients with converting enzyme inhibitors since spontaneous increases of the systemic blood pressure always involve enhanced sympathetic activity. The effect of captopril on the limits of autoregulation in the rat is still present after chronic sympathetic denervation (78). This demonstrates that the renin-angiotensin sys-

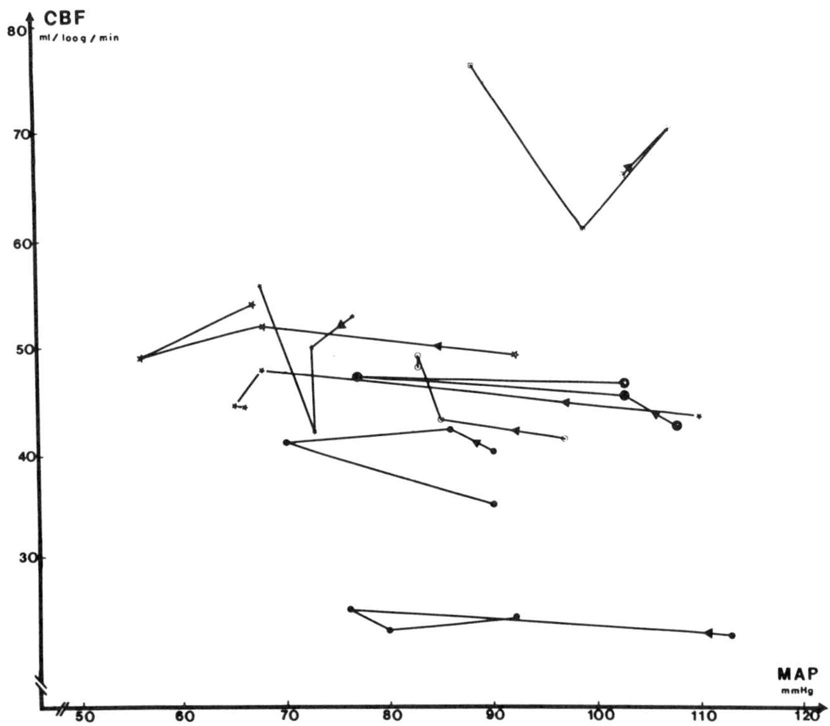

Figure 10 Effect of captopril 6–25 mg orally in eight patients with congestive heart failure on cerebral blood flow (CBF) and mean arterial pressure (MAP). CBF is given in ml/100g/min. The arrows are between the resting CBF measurement and the study undertaken 15 min after administration of captopril. The following signs on the individual patients' curves indicate the third and fourth CBF measurements performed 60 min and 180 min after captopril administration. (From Ref. 84.)

tem influences cerebral blood flow autoregulation independently of the sympathetic nervous system.

5. Alpha-Blockers and Ganglionic Blockers

Alpha-blockers and ganglionic blockers, like ACE inhibitors, exert a weak dilatory effect on the larger cerebral resistance vessels. Labetalol, which is used rather widely for clinical emergency blood pressure lowering, does not influence intracranial pressure (79). Labetalol would be expected to improve autoregulation to low blood pressure, but this has not been well studied.

From the point of view of the cerebral circulation, the ideal drug for emergency pressure lowering would be an alpha-blocker which has the potential for improving the brain's tolerance to low pressure, does not increase intracranial pressure, and does not cause unpredictable drastic pressure falls. In the view of the authors, the alpha-beta blocker labetalol comes close to being such a drug. The ACE inhibitors, which have approximately the same cerebrovascular hemodynamic effects as the alpha-blockers, are less suitable for emergency pressure lowering, as they may cause a drastic pressure fall in some cases of unrecognized renovascular hypertension.

B. Chronic Antihypertensive Treatment

The effect of chronic antihypertensive treatment on the cerebral circulation has been less extensively investigated than the effect of acute blood pressure lowering. Apart from the autoregulatory response and pharmacological effects on the cerebral vessels, chronic treatment may also cause regression of hypertenive vascular remodeling and hence a readaptation of CBF autoregulation toward lower pressure. This has been demonstrated during drug treatment of short-term renal hypertension in the rat (7,8) and may or may not occur during treatment in hypertensive humans (4), as discussed earlier.

It has been shown in hypertensive patients that CBF is unchanged before and after some weeks to months of treatment with a diuretic (80), a diuretic plus the alpha-blocker prazosin (81), the vasodilatating beta-blocker carvedilol (82), the calcium antagonists nitrendipine and verapamil (71), and the ACE inhibitor enalapril (83). The fall in blood pressure in these studies generally has been slight, on the order of 5 to 15 mm Hg, and while major drug-induced vasodilatation has been ruled out, the studies give no information on more subtle cerebrovascular effects of the drugs, if any. One hypothetical beneficial effect of ACE inhibitors or alpha-blockers, for instance, might be a better cerebrovascular tolerance of nocturnal drug-induced hypotension. Thus chronic treatment with ACE inhibitors appears to shift the lower limit of CBF autoregulation toward lower pressure in both rats and heart failure patients (84). This would explain why heart failure patients treated with ACE inhibitors can tolerate very low blood pressure without clinical symptoms of cerebral ischemia.

The headache sometimes seen during long-term treatment with hydralazine and calcium antagonists would suggest a state of chronic cerebral vasodilatation and possibly a tendency toward a somewhat raised intracranial pressure. This, however, has not been studied.

REFERENCES

1. Kety SS, Hafkenschiel JH, Jeffers WA, et al. The blood flow, vascular resistance, and oxygen consumption of the brain in essential hypertension. J Clin Invest 1948; 27:511–514.

2. Cook TA, Yates PO. A histometric study of cerebral and renal arteries in normotensives and chronic hypertensives. J Pathol 1972; 108:129–135.
3. Heagerty AM, Aalkjaer C, Bund SJ, et al. Small artery structure in hypertension: dual processes of remodeling and growth. Hypertension 1993; 21:391–397.
4. Strandgaard S. Autoregulation of cerebral blood flow in hypertensive patients. The modifying influence of prolonged antihypertensive treatment on the tolerance to acute, drug-induced hypotension. Circulation 1976; 53:720–727.
5. Strandgaard S, Jones JV, Mackenzie ET, Harper AM. Upper limit of cerebral blood flow autoregulation in the baboon with experimental renovascular hypotension. Circ Res 1975; 37:164–167.
6. Harper SL, Bohlen HG. Microvascular adaptation in the cerebral cortex of adult spontaneously hypertensive rats. Hypertension 1984; 6:408–419.
7. Vorstrup S, Barry DI, Jarden JO, et al. Chronic antihypertensive treatment in the rat reverses hypertension-induced changes in cerebral blood flow autoregulation. Stroke 1984; 15:312–318.
8. Muller F, Lartaud I, Bray L, et al. Chronic treatment with the angiotensin I converting enzyme inhibitor, perindopril, restores the lower limit of autoregulation of cerebral blood flow in the awake renovascular hypertensive rat. J Hypertens 1990; 8:1037–1042.
9. Shurtleff D. Some characteristics related to the incidence of cardiovascular disease and death: The Framingham Study. 18 year follow-up. In: Kannel WB, Gordon T, eds. The Framingham Study, an Epidemiologic Investigation of Cardiovascular Disease. Section 30. Washington D.C.: U.S. Department of Health, Education, and Welfare, 1974:74–599.
10. Herman B, Schmitz PIM, Leyten ACM, et al. Multivariate logistic analysis of risk factors for stroke in Tilburg, The Netherlands. Am J Epidemiol 1983; 118: 514–525.
11. Wolf PA, Kannel WB, Verter J. Current status of risk factors for stroke. Neurol Clin 1983; 1:317–343.
12. Davis PH, Dambrosia JM, Schoenberg BS, et al. Risk factors for ischemic stroke: a prospective study in Rochester, Minnesota. Ann Neurol 1987; 22:319–327.
13. Boysen G, Nyboe J, Appleyard M, et al. Stroke incidence and risk factors for stroke in Copenhagen, Denmark. Stroke 1988; 19:1345–1353.
14. MacMahon S, Peto R, Cutler J, et al. Blood pressure, stroke and coronary heart disease. Part 1. Prolonged differences in blood pressure: prospective observational studies corrected for the regression dilution bias. Lancet 1990; 335:765–774.
15. Britton M, Carlsson A, de Faire U. Blood pressure course in patients with acute stroke and matched controls. Stroke 1986; 17:861–864.
16. Brott T, Thalinger K, Hertzberg V. Hypertension as a risk factor for spontaneous intracerebral hemorrhage. Stroke 1986; 17:1078–1083.
17. Schulte BP, Leyten AC, Herman B. Pre-stroke and immediate post-stroke hypertension: neuroepidemiological data. Br J Clin Pract 1985; 39(Symp Suppl): 31–33.
18. Roberts WC. Frequency of systemic hypertension in various cardiovascular diseases. Am J Cardiol 1987; 60:1E–8E.

19. Williams JK, Baumbach GL, Armstrong ML, Heistad DD. Hypothesis: vasoconstriction contributes to amaurosis fugax. J Cereb Blood Flow Metab 1989; 9:111–116.
20. SHEP Cooperative Research Group. Prevention of stroke by antihypertensive drug treatment in older persons with isolated systolic hypertension: final results of the Systolic Hypertension in the Elderly Program. JAMA 1991; 265:3255–3264.
21. Shima T, Nishida M, Okada Y, Uozumi T. Cortical artery pressure and anastomotic blood flow during bypass surgery. J Cereb Blood Flow Metab 1983; 3 (suppl 1):620–621.
22. Spetzler RF, Roski RA, Zabramski J. Middle cerebral artery perfusion pressure in cerebrovascular occlusive disease. Stroke 1983; 14:512–515.
23. Vorstrup S, Brun B, Lassen NA. Evaluation of the cerebral vasodilatory capacity by the acetazolamide test before EC-IC bypass surgery in patients with occlusion of the internal carotid artery. Stroke 1986; 17:1291–1298.
24. Charcot JM, Bouchard CH. Nouvelles recherches sur la pathogénie de l'hémorragie cérébrale. Arch Physiol Norm Path 1868; 1:110–127, 643–665, 725–735.
25. Russell RW. Pathological changes in small cerebral arteries causing occlusion and haemorrhage. J Cardiovasc Pharmacol 1984; 6:S691–S695.
26. Challa VR, Moody DM, Bell MA. The Charcot-Bouchard aneurysm controversy: impact of a new histologic technique. J Neuropathol Exp Neurol 1992; 51:264–274.
27. Rowe CC, Donnan GA, Bladin PF. Intracerebral haemorrhage: incidence and uses of computed tomography. Br Med J 1988; 297:1177–1178.
28. Fisher CM. The arterial lesions underlying lacunes. Acta Neuropathol (Berlin) 1969; 12:1–15.
29. Hachinski VC, Potter P, Mershey H. Leuko-araiosis. Arch Neurol 1987; 44: 21–23.
30. Johansson BB, Linder LE. The blood-brain barrier in renal hypertensive rats. Clin Exp Hypertens 1980; 2:983–993.
31. Salerno JA, Murphy DGM, Horwitz et al. Brain atrophy in hypertension: a volumetric magnetic resonance imaging study. Hypertension 1992; 20:340–348.
32. Collins R, Peto R, MacMahon S, et al. Blood pressure, stroke and coronary heart disease. Part 2. Short-term reductions in blood pressure: overview of randomised drug trials in their epidemiological context. Lancet 1990; 335:827–838.
33. Fujii K, Weno BL, Baumbach GL, Heistad DD. Effect of antihypertensive treatment on focal cerebral infarction. Hypertension 1992; 19:713–716.
34. Kotila M. Declining incidence and mortality of stroke? Stroke 1984; 15:255–259.
35. Yatsu FM, Zivin J. Hypertension in acute ischemic strokes: not to treat. Arch Neurol 1985; 42:999–1000.
36. Spence JD, del Maestro RF. Hypertension in acute ischemic strokes: Treat. Arch Neurol 1985; 42:1000–1002.
37. Bannan LT, Beevers DG, Jackson SD, Wright N. ABC of blood pressure reduction: special problems. Br Med J 1980; 281:1200–1202.
38. Sauter A, Rudin M, Wiederhold KH. Cytoprotective characteristics of dihydropyridine calcium antagonists in a rat model of stroke: implications for clinical

trials. In: Hartmann A, Kuschinsky W, eds. Cerebral Ischaemia and Calcium. New York: Springer, 1989:282–291.
39. Sauter A, Rudin M. Prevention of stroke and brain damage with calcium antagonists in animals. Am J Hypertens 1991; 4:121S–127S.
40. Vorstrup S, Andersen A, Blegvad N, Paulson OB. Calcium antagonist (PY 108–068) treatment may further decrease flow in ischemic areas in acute stroke. J Cereb Blood Flow Metab 1986; 6:222–229.
41. Gelmers HJ, Gorter K, de Weerdt CJ, Wiezer HJA. A controlled trial of nimodipine in acute ischemic stroke. N Engl J Med 1988; 318:203–207.
42. The American Nimodipine Study Group. Clinical trial of nimodipine in acute ischemic stroke. Stroke 1992; 23:3–8.
43. Beevers DG, Fairman MJ, Hamilton M, Harpur JE. Antihypertensive treatment and the course of established cerebral vascular disease. Lancet 1973; 1:1407–1409.
44. Ledingham JGG, Rajagopalan B. Cerebral complications in the treatment of accelerated hypertension. Q J Med 1979; 48:25–41.
45. Cove BH, Seddom M, Fletcher RF, Dukes DC. Blindness after treatment for malignant hypertension. Br Med J 1979; 2:245–246.
46. Strandgaard S, Andersen GS, Ahlgreen P, Nielsen PE. Visual disturbances and occipital brain infarct following acute, transient hypotension in hypertensive patients. Acta Med Scand 1984; 216:417–422.
47. Graham DI. Ischaemic brain damage of cerebral perfusion failure type after treatment of severe hypertension. Br Med J 1975; 4:739.
48. Dahlöf B, Lindholm LH, Hansson L, et al. Morbidity and mortality in the Swedish trial in old patients with hypertension (STOP-hypertension). Lancet 1991; 338:1281–1285.
49. MRC Working Party. Medical Research Council trial of treatment of hypertension in older adults: principal results. Br Med J 1992; 304:405–412.
50. Jackson G, Pierscianowski TA, Mahon W, Condon J. Inappropriate antihypertensive therapy in the elderly. Lancet 1976; 2:1317–1318.
51. Hankey GJ, Gubbay SS. Focal cerebral ischaemia and infarction due to antihypertensive therapy. Med J Aust 1987; 146:412–414.
52. Sacco RL, Wolf PA, Bharucha NE, et al. Subarachnoid and intracerebral hemorrhage: natural history, prognosis, and precursive factors in the Framingham Study. Neurology 1984; 34:847–854.
53. Eskesen V, Rosenorn J, Schmidt K, Ronde F. Pre-existing arterial hypertension in subarachnoidhaemorrhage: an unfavourable prognostic factor. Br J Neurosurg 1987; 1:455–461.
54. Bonita R. Cigarette smoking, hypertension and the risk of subarachnoid hemorrhage: a population-based case-control study. Stroke 1986; 17:831–835.
55. Strandgaard S, Hansen U. Hypertension in renal allograft recipients may be conveyed by kidneys from donors with subarachnoid haemorrhage. Br Med J 1986; 292:1041–1044.
56. Ohman J, Servo A, Heiskanen O. Risks factors for cerebral infarction in goodgradepatients after aneurysmal subarachnoid hemorrhage and surgery: a prospective study. J Neurosurg 1991; 74:14–20.

57. Byrom FB. The Hypertensive Vascular Crisis: An Experimental Study. London: Heinemann, 1969.
58. Lassen NA, Agnoli A. The upper limit of autoregulation of cerebral blood flow: on the pathogenesis of hypertensive encephalopathy. Scand J Clin Lab Invest 1973; 30:113–116.
59. Farrar JK, Jones JV, Graham DI, et al. Evidence against cerebral vasospasm during acutely induced hypertension. Brain Res 1976; 104:176–180.
60. Johansson B. Blood-brain barrier dysfunction in acute arterial hypertension after papaverine-induced vasodilatation. Acta Neurol Scand 1974; 50:366–376.
61. Westergaard E, van Deurs B, Brøndsted H. Increased vesicular transfer of horseradish peroxydase across cerebral endothelium, evoked by acute hypertension. Acta Neuropath (Berlin) 1977; 37:141–152.
62. Barry I, Strandgaard S, Graham DI, et al. Effect of diaxozide induced hypotension on cerebral blood flow in hypertensive rats. Eur J Clin Invest 1983; 13: 201–207.
63. Barry DI, Strandgaard S. Acute effects of antihypertensive drugs on autoregulation of cerebral blood flow in spontaneously hypertensive rats. Prog Appl Microcirc 1985; 8:206–212.
64. Schroeder T, Sillesen H. Dihydralazine induces marked cerebral vasodilatation in man. Eur J Clin Invest 1987; 17:214–217.
65. Rowe GG, Maxwell GM, Crumpton CW. The cerebral haemodynamic response to administration of hydralazine. Circulation 1962; 25:970–972.
66. Overgaard J, Skinhøj E. A paradoxical cerebral haemodynamic effect of hydralazine. Stroke 1975; 6:402–404.
67. Barry DI, Jarden JO, Paulson OB, et al. Cerebrovascular effects of converting enzyme inhibition. I. Effects of intravenous captopril in spontaneously hypertensive and normotensive rats. J Hypertens 1984; 2:589–597.
68. Turner JM, Powell D, Gibson RM, McDowall DG. Intracranial pressure changes in neurosurgical patients during hypotension induced with sodium nitro prusside or trimetaphan. Br J Anaesthesiol 1977; 49:419–420.
69. Henriksen L, Thorshauge C, Harmsen A, Christensen P, et al. Controlled hypotension with sodium nitroprusside: effects of cerebral blood flow and cerebral venous blood gases in patients operated for cerebral aneurysms. Acta Anaesthesiol Scand 1983; 27:62–67.
70. Kincaid-Smith P, McMichael J, Murphy EA. The clinical course and pathology of hypertension with papilloedema (malignant hypertension). Q J Med 1958; 27: 117–153.
71. Conen D, Rüttmann S, Noll G, et al. Short- and long-term cerebrovascular effects of nitrendipine in hypertensive patients. J Cardiovasc Pharm 1988; 12(suppl 14):S64–S68.
72. Ooboshi H, Sadoshima S, Fujii K, et al. Acute effects of antihypertensive agents on cerebral blood flow in hypertensive rats. Eur J Pharmacol 1990; 179:253–261.
73. Schmidt JF, Albeck M, Gjerris F. The effect of nimodipine on intracranial pressure and cerebral blood flow in patients with normal-pressure hydrocephalus. Acta Neurochir 1990; 102:11–13.

74. Paulson OB, Jarden JO, Godtfredsen J, Vorstrup S. Cerebral blood flow in patients with congestive heart failure treated with captopril. Am J Med 1984; 76 (5B):91–95.
75. Schmidt JF, Andersen AR, Paulson OB, Gjerris F. Angiotensin converting enzyme inhibition, CBF autoregulation and ICP in patients with normal-pressure hydrocephalus. Acta Neurochir 1990; 106:9–12.
76. Waldemar G, Schmidt JF, Andersen AR, et al. Angiotensin converting enzyme inhibition and cerebral blood flow autoregulation in normotensive and hypertensive man. J Hypertens 1989; 7:229–235.
77. Waldemar G, Paulson OB, Barry DI, Knudsen GM. Angiotensin converting enzyme inhibition and the upper limit of cerebral blood flow autoregulation: effect of sympathetic stimulation. Circ Res 1989; 64:1197–1204.
78. Waldemar G. Acute sympathetic denervation does not eliminate the effect of angiotensin converting enzyme inhibition on CBF autoregulation in spontaneously hypertensive rats. J Cereb Blood Flow Metab 1990; 10:43–47.
79. van Aken H, Puchstein C, Schweppe ML, Heinecke A. Effect of labetalol on intracranial pressure in dogs with and without intracranial hypertension. Acta Anaesth Scand 1982; 26:615–619.
80. Traub YM, Shapiro AP, Dujovny M, Nelson D. Cerebral blood flow changes with diuretic therapy in elderly subjects with diastolic hypertension. Clin Exp Hypertens 1982; A4:1193–1201.
81. Ram CVS, Meese R, Kaplan NM, et al. Antihypertensive therapy in the elderly: effects on blood pressure and cerebral blood flow. Am J Med 1987; 82 (suppl 1A):53–57.
82. Kuriyama Y, Nakamura M, Kyougoku I, Sawada T. Effects of carvedilol on cerebral blood flow and its autoregulation in previous stroke patients with hypertension. Eur J Clin Pharmacol 1990; 38:S120–S121.
83. Frei A, Müller-Brand J. Cerebral blood flow and antihypertensive treatment with enalapril. J Hypertens 1986; 4:365–367.
84. Paulson OB, Jarden JO, Vorstrup S, et al. Effect of captopril on the cerebral circulation in chronic heart failure. Eur J Clin Invest 1986; 16:124–132.

9

Hypertension with Renal Disease

ROBERT J. HEYKA
Cleveland Clinic Foundation
Cleveland, Ohio

DONALD G. VIDT
Ohio State University
and Cleveland Clinic Foundation
Cleveland, Ohio

In this chapter we review the evaluation and care of patients with hypertension (HTN) and chronic renal failure (CRF). Hypertension with chronic renal failure is the most common cause of secondary hypertension (1). Its importance lies in two areas: the risk for cardiovascular disease that is (presumed) to be common to any form of hypertension and the unique risk for progressive CRF in which hypertension is possibly the most important factor. By no means a homogeneous entity, hypertension in CRF varies by specific renal disease and among specific groups of patients. The pathogenesis of hypertension in CRF is intimately related to the pathophysiological changes of CRF, but the mechanisms involved may be identical to those in essential hypertension. We will also review the assessment of renal function, nonpharmacological and pharmacological treatment, appropriate target levels of control, and whether any class of agents offers specific advantages in the prevention or postponement of progressive renal disease. Finally we will offer guidelines for the approach to the individual patient with hypertension and chronic renal failure.

I. IMPORTANCE OF HYPERTENSION WITH CHRONIC RENAL FAILURE

A. Hypertension and Renal Disease

Hypertension and CRF can be related in several ways. First, essential hypertension may develop and damage the kidneys, leading to CRF and possibly end-stage renal disease (ESRD). The kidney may well play a part in this process related to its central role in salt, water, and hemodynamic balance. Thus, the kidney can be a villain in the initiation of essential hypertension (2,3). Second, primary renal diseases, especially those involving the small blood vessels or glomeruli (4), may lead to new or worsening secondary hypertension. Here the kidney is more a victim of its own dysfunction. A third group of diseases, the actual frequency of which is unknown, has been named "masqueraders" of essential hypertension (5,6,7) (Table 1). This group have in common a lack of precise definition and thus an unclear prevalence rate. Since national ESRD registries (United States and other countries) require neither tissue for pathological diagnosis nor rigid criteria for clinical diagnosis, the exact cause of much ESRD is, in fact, unknown. Many studies that have provided epidemiological data are likewise based on incomplete clinical or

Table 1 Hypertension with Chronic Renal Failure

- Secondary to essential hypertension
  - Stage I and II
  - Severe (stage III and IV)
  - Accelerated or malignant
- With renal parenchymal disease
  - Common (glomerular diseases)
    - Diabetes mellitus, membranous glomerulonephritis, lupus nephritis, vasculitis, rapidly progressive glomerulonephritis
  - Common (tubular-interstitial diseases)
    - Autosomal dominant polycystic kidney disease (ADPKD)
    - Analgesic abuse nephropathy
  - Uncommon
    - Immunoglobulin A nephropathy, membranoproliferative glomerulonephritis, chronic pyelonephritis
- Misdiagnosed masqueraders
  - Lead nephropathy
  - Renovascular hypertension
  - Atheroembolic disease
  - Toxic exposure nephropathy
  - Human immunodeficiency virus nephropathy

Source: Refs. 3–7.

tissue diagnosis. For example, undetected ischemic nephropathy may lead to CRF and ESRD but be labeled as essential hypertension. We must await better delineation of study and national data bases to determine the exact size of this latter category.

The prevalence and severity of hypertension increase as the glomerular filtration rate (GFR) falls and approach 80% to 90% in pre-ESRD patients (8). In some renal diseases, such as poststreptococcal glomerulonephritis, hypertension is short-lived and probably contributes little as a long-term risk factor. In other diseases, such as insulin-dependent diabetes mellitus (IDDM), vasculitis, and autosomal dominant polycystic kidney disease (ADPKD), hypertension—both systemic and intraglomerular—plays a crucial role in disease progression and patient survival.

B. Risk of Cardiovascular Disease

Once present, hypertension with CRF is clinically important because of two considerations. First is the risk of cardiovascular disease secondary to hypertension. It is presumed (but not proved) that the same risk factors identified in studies such as Framingham apply to patients with CRF and ESRD (9). The Hypertension Detection and Follow-up Program (HDFP) reported that elevated serum creatinine level (above 150 μmol/l or 1.7 mg/mg/dl) was an important marker of cardiovascular and all-cause mortality (10). Cardiovascular disease remains the most common cause of mortality in the ESRD population (11). A prospective evaluation of risk factor modification in the CRF population and the identification of (any) risk factors unique to the uremic milieu is sadly lacking. However, a recent report found the amount of dialysis given and level of mean arterial pressure (MAP) to be the best indices of survival in a center reporting the lowest mortality rates in the world (12). Patients with MAP below 99 mm Hg had a significantly greater survival rate than patients with higher MAP levels.

C. Risk of Progressive Chronic Renal Failure

The second consideration in the importance of HTN with CRF relates to disease progression. Clinicians have long noted the tendency for CRF to progress to ESRD. Renal diseases of different causes tend to progress at different rates (4), as do individual patients with the same disease. A discussion of the mechanisms involved in the progression of renal disease is beyond the scope of this review, but several factors are intertwined with blood pressure control. Recent reviews on this topic have appeared emphasizing the pathophysiological characteristics (13) and the difficulty of extrapolation from animal studies to the human situation (14).

1. Dietary Factors

The role of dietary protein and phosphorus intake in the progression of CRF has proved a fertile ground for animal and human experimentation. The Modification of Diet in Renal Disease (MDRD) study has reported findings of its feasibility study (15). The rate of decline of GFR was inversely correlated to MAP over the entire range of blood pressure readings.

Blood pressure goals in the full-scale trial will be as low as MAP of 92 mm Hg (~125/75). In addition, an antihypertensive regimen that includes a converting enzyme inhibitor or calcium antagonist will be encouraged with or without the addition of diuretics (15).

2. Lipids

Hyperlipidemia present before renal disease begins, initiated with renal disease, or induced by choice of antihypertensive agents may have an impact on progression of CRF. Dyslipidemias in renal disease may lead directly to progressive glomerular structural damage or interact with hemodynamic or other factors to worsen renal function (16). A recent study showed that therapy to decrease proteinuria in patients with type II diabetic nephropathy was effective in improving the dyslipidemia of renal disease (17). As we learn more about the role of lipids, especially of subtypes such as oxidized low-density lipoproteins (LDLs) or lipoprotein a (LPa), pharmacological therapy of lipid disorders may become part of our therapy to slow the progression of CRF.

3. Proteinuria

Proteinuria may identify patients with HTN and CRF at increased risk for progression. Microalbuminuria, defined as 30 to 300 μg/min or 20 to 200 mg/day of albumin excretion, is just above the normal range of albumin excretion (up to 20 mg/day). Patients with untreated essential hypertension may have microalbuminuria that is proportional to the blood pressure level and tends to decrease with treatment (18). Microalbuminuria may reflect a change in glomerular hemodynamics secondary to elevated pressures, altered handling of protein by renal tubules, or structural changes in the kidney and may identify patients at increased risk for atherosclerotic vascular disease (18). In diabetics, microalbuminuria, if present with hypertension and impaired creatinine clearance, indicates established abnormalities in glomerular structure (19) and is a predictor of those patients at risk of development of diabetic nephropathy (20).

Overt proteinuria (along with age and diastolic blood pressure) was associated with progression of renal disease among the HDFP study population (10). The recently completed MDRD trial found that baseline proteinuria was the strongest predictor of decline in GFR regardless of initial GFR (21). Converting enzyme inhibitors (CEIs) can dramatically decrease proteinuria and may confer renal protection. The Trial of Converting Enzyme Inhibitors in type I diabetic nephropathy showed an association between better blood pressure (BP) control using CEI and spontaneous remission of nephrotic range proteinuria with stable serum creatinine levels (22). Macromolecules like albumin and lipids may, in fact, have a common pathological mechanism wherein the increased trafficking of macromolecules due to altered membrane permselectivity in a damaged kidney leads to progressive glomerulosclerosis (23).

4. Renal Hemodynamics

Another potentially controllable factor in the progression of CRF is intrarenal hemodynamics, specifically glomerular hyperfiltration and hypertension (13). Classically, autopsy findings in patients with HTN and CRF showed arterial and arteriolar obliteration that was thought to result in decreased renal blood flow and renal ischemia (24). More recently, it has been shown that decreased resistance of the afferent arterioles combined with a loss of autoregulation leads to an increased transmission of flow and pressure to the glomerulus. The effect of this glomerular hyperfiltration and hypertension is to accelerate renal injury in a previously damaged kidney (24). There continues to be tremendous research in this area, but skepticism regarding the applicability of animal hyperfiltration models to human renal disease also persists (14). Converting enzyme inhibitors (CEIs) and calcium antagonists (CAs) may selectively decrease glomerular hyperfiltration and hypertension secondary to their hemodynamic effects (25). It is possible that these intrarenal hemodynamic effects can occur divorced from systemic blood pressure changes. Thus, two different therapies that lower blood pressure to the same degree may have different renal protective effects (26).

5. Epidemiology

Large gaps exist in our knowledge of the epidemiology of hypertension and chronic renal failure. The most recent United States Renal Data System (USRDS) reports four diseases as responsible for 80% of all ESRD. Diabetes mellitus accounts for 34%, hypertension for 29%, chronic glomerulonephritis for 14%, and cystic disease (primarily ADPKD) for 3% (11). These diseases are all associated with the early onset of hypertension (4). There are approximately 250,000 patients with ESRD in the United States. It is expected that this number will continue to rise beyond the year 2000 (27). The cost to Medicare increases by at least $1 billion every 5 years (27). The ESRD population has grown disproportionately among the African-American, Hispanic, and Native American populations, and in patients over the age of 60 (11) (Table 2). These groups have a higher incidence of hypertensive ESRD as well (28). Additional risk factors for progressive CRF include cigarette smoking, age, diagnosis of hypertension (earlier diagnosis leads to less ESRD), severity of

Table 2 Populations at High Risk for Progressive Renal Failure

African-Americans with hypertension
Hispanic and Mexican Americans with hypertension
Elderly with hypertension
Preexistent chronic renal failure, especially diabetic nephropathy, ADPKD
Accelerated or severe hypertension

Source: Refs. 28–31.

HTN, income under $10,000, proportion of county residents who complete high school, number of missed office visits, employment as a laborer, family history of renal disease, and geographic location (29–31). Therefore, information is available to identify populations at increased risk for intensive study and intervention. Although the manner in which these risk factors influence the progress of renal damage is often unknown and causation cannot be inferred, risk may arise from different susceptibilities at similar levels of blood pressure, different renal functional and hemodynamic characteristics, or undiagnosed concomitant renal disease. The greatest aggregate risk in terms of total numbers, however, is likely similar to that seen with essential hypertension (32).

II. PATHOGENESIS OF RENAL HYPERTENSION

It is unclear whether different pathological mechanisms exist with CRF, or whether both renal and essential hypertension arise from similar disturbances. Putative factors including impaired sodium and water excretion, volume expansion, altered intrarenal pressor systems, and abnormal sympathetic nervous system activity have been recently reviewed (8,33).

A. Salt, Water, and Volume

With decreased GFR comes impairment in sodium excretion and the tendency to salt and water retention. However, any attempt to explain the pathophysiological process of renal hypertension must account for the finding that an increased total peripheral resistance (TPR), not an increased cardiac output, is the predominant abnormality in fixed renal hypertension (34). As renal function worsens, there is a better correlation of blood pressure (especially diastolic blood pressure) and sodium intake (35). Once a patient reaches ESRD, the association of sodium and volume with hypertension is strong. An early study of dialysis patients found that the blood pressure was controlled in 35/40 patients simply by ultrafiltration to target weight. These patients were thus labeled (perhaps simplistically) as having "volume-dependent" hypertension (36).

B. Renal Pressors

Despite continual functional deterioration, the renin-angiotensin-aldosterone (RAA) axis remains active even in patients with ESRD (37). Plasma renin activity (PRA) levels are probably inappropriate given the degree of volume overload (38). In fact, early investigations showed that the best correlation with MAP was with a factor that included both total body sodium and the log of PRA (38). Pharmacological blockade with CEI, therefore, continues to be a treatment option even in dialysis patients. In early studies, those patients whose blood pressure did not fall in response to volume removal responded to bilateral nephrectomy and were thus labeled as having "renin-dependent" hypertension (36). Bilateral nephrectomy to control hypertension has become largely unnecessary with the introduction of more potent antihypertensive medication.

C. Sympathetic Nervous System

The sympathetic nervous system also remains active even with worsening renal function and likely contributes to renal hypertension. Direct effects include increased cardiac output and TPR. Indirect effects include increased activity of the RAA axis, increased sodium reabsorption, and increased barosensitivity (33) in both renal and systemic receptors (39).

III. TREATMENT OF RENAL HYPERTENSION

A. Assessment of Renal Function

Treatment of the patient with hypertension and renal failure presupposes establishment of the diagnosis of chronic renal failure and evaluation of the degree of renal dysfunction. Diagnosis of CRF requires evidence that the patient has chronic, nonreversible disease: that is, the exclusion of acute (reversible) renal failure or spurious elevation in laboratory values (40). A history of nocturia, edema, infections, hematuria, or family renal disease can be very helpful. Prior records of urinalyses or serum creatinine level measurements likewise are useful. Associated medical conditions such as diabetes mellitus and ADPKD identify patients at high risk for CRF. On examination, objective findings can be misleading. Perhaps the best indicator of CRF is renal ultrasonic evidence of shrunken kidneys with increased echogenicity (40). Only a few diseases, such as diabetes or infiltration with amyloid, lymphoma, or multiple myeloma, are associated with enlarged kidneys and CRF. Evidence of secondary hyperparathyroidism with elevated PTH levels and characteristic radiographic changes can also help establish chronicity.

Once the presence of CRF is confirmed, it is important to know the exact degree of impairment to estimate salvagibility and prognosis and to guide pharmacological dosing. Serum creatinine level is most commonly used in the clinical estimation of renal function. Since creatinine undergoes tubular secretion with decreased GFR, serum creatinine level underestimates the impairment in renal function (41). Derivations based on serum creatinine level such as 1/serum creatinine level or the Cockcroft and Gault estimation can be highly variable and have the same problems with interpretation as serum creatinine level (42,43). Two procedures offer the greatest accuracy in determination of renal function. Radionuclide determinations of GFR give highly accurate and reproducible determinations of renal function (42). Twenty-four-hour urine collection for combined urea and creatinine clearances (44) has long been known to correlate very closely with inulin clearance. GFR determined with iothalmate radionuclide in more than 4000 patients showed that a creatinine level above 150 mmol/l (1.3 mg/dl) in females, or 141 mmol/L (1.6 mg/dl) in males, was always associated with GFR below 50 ml/min/1.73 m^2. In patients above the age of 60 years, a creatinine level above 400 mmol/L (4.6 mg/dl) was always associated with GFR below 10 ml/m/1.73 m^2 (i.e., ESRD) (42) (Table 3).

An individualized approach to the treatment of hypertension in a patient with CRF is mandated by the diverse clinical presentations of these patients. For example, the patient with postinfectious glomerulonephritis may have short-lived (2 to 3 months) but severe hypertension associated with dramatic

Table 3 Relationship Between Iothalamate GFR and Serum Creatinine Levels According to Age and Sex

	Age					
	15–30 yr		40–50 yr		60–70 yr	
GFR	Male (297 tests)	Female (334 tests)	Male (297 tests)	Female (256 tests)	Male (388 tests)	Female (225 tests)
10	6.6 ± 4.6	5.4 ± 3.2	5.8 ± 3.9	4.7 ± 2.5	4.6 ± 3.5	5.1 ± 3.2
25	3.0 ± 1.3	2.6 ± 1.9	3.0 ± 1.6	2.4 ± 1.2	2.6 ± 1.7	2.2 ± 1.5
50	1.8 ± 0.9	1.4 ± 0.6	1.7 ± 0.7	1.4 ± 0.5	1.6 ± 0.6	1.3 ± 0.5
100	1.2 ± 0.4	0.9 ± 0.3	1.2 ± 0.4	0.9 ± 0.3	1.1 ± 0.4	0.9 ± 0.3

[a]Serum creatinine values done on SMA (Technicon). GFR values in units of ml/min/1.73 m^2.
Source: Ref. 42.

fluid retention. A patient with interstitial disease secondary to a chronic pyelonephritis or analgesic abuse nephropathy may have minimal proteinuria, only stage I to II hypertension, and a low risk of progressive CRF. Patients with chronic glomerulonephritis, such as membranous glomerulonephritis or diabetic nephropathy, may have significant edema secondary to nephrotic range proteinuria, stage III to IV hypertension, a grossly abnormal lipid profile with increased LDL subfraction and inevitably progress to ESRD.

B. Level of Control

Diurnal variations seen in primary hypertension tend to be lost in patients with CRF who instead have an elevated nocturnal blood pressure profile (45). The inference from this finding is the necessity of adequate blood pressure control over the entire 24-hour period. Preliminary reports from the MDRD trial show that loss of GFR in patients with proteinuria greater than 1 g/a day can be slowed by control of blood pressure to MAP of 92 mm Hg (~ 125/75) (21). Three recent consensus statements made recommendations on target levels of blood pressure in patients with CRF. The National High Blood Pressure Education Program Report on Hypertension and Chronic Renal Failure recommended blood pressure levels of 130/85 mm Hg or lower (MAP of 100 mm Hg) for patients with established renal disease (27). The Working Group on Hypertension in Diabetes (46) recommended blood pressure of 140/90 mm Hg or lower if tolerated by the patient. The NIH Consensus Conference on the Morbidity and Mortality of Dialysis reasserted the importance of aggressive therapy of hypertension in patients with CRF and recommended a goal for therapy of "normal systolic and diastolic pressure" (47). JNC-V reiterated that cardiovascular risk increases with blood pressure above 120/80 mm Hg and defined "normal" blood pressure as 130/85 mm Hg (48). These recommendations must be balanced by concerns about a possible nadir for effective protection against cardiovascular disease: that is, does a J curve exist for diastolic blood pressure below which mortality rate increases in patients with renal disease (49)? Recent data, particularly in elderly patients with systolic hypertension, seem to show decreased cardiovascular morbidity and mortality rates with lowered systolic blood pressure and no J curve effects for diastolic blood pressure (50), but prospective studies to answer this critical question in patients with HTN and CRF are unavailable at this time. There is a growing body of evidence from JNC-V, the MDRD trial, and consensus statements that prior target blood pressure goals were too high. Blood pressure levels of 135/85 and possibly to 120/80 are reasonable goals in patients with HTN and CRF and may have a significant impact on progression of CRF.

C. Life-Style Modification

Nonpharmacological therapy, or life-style modification, is effective in patients with primary hypertension (51). Although no specific guidelines for life-style modification in patients with HTN and CRF have appeared, general recommendations can be inferred. Life-style factors that may worsen HTN include low intake of potassium, physical inactivity, excessive alcohol consumption, excessive consumption of calories, and high sodium intake (51). Each of these life-style modifications, however, needs to be tailored for patients with CRF. Potassium restriction is mandatory as renal function deteriorates, especially if medications such as converting enzyme inhibitors or nonsteroidal anti-inflammatory drugs are necessary since either can increase potassium retention.

Physical activity can be limited by fatigue secondary to uremia or anemia of chronic disease. Other causes of anemia, such as cryptic blood loss or preexistent iron deficiency, must be explored and corrected if present. Treatment of anemia with recombinant erythropoietin (EPO) can significantly increase exercise capacity (52) but may increase blood pressure as well (53). However, there is no evidence that the use of EPO accelerates progression of CRF (53).

Restricted sodium consumption is important for control of volume status as well as blood pressure, especially as renal function worsens. For each patient a "target" weight needs to be determined above which symptoms and signs of volume overload such as shortness of breath, orthopnea, or edema occur, and below which symptoms of volume depletion become evident (3). In a patient with established peripheral neuropathy and orthostatic hypotension, this can be extremely difficult, and at times mild fluid retention and supine hypertension must be allowed to prevent the symptoms of orthostatic hypotension (46). More elaborate procedures such as radionuclide determination of plasma volume or ultrasonic measurements of inferior vena cava diameter (54) are available if target weight determinations are problematic. Rather than attempt to measure input and output of fluid on a long-term basis, we generally instruct patients to weigh themselves daily—at the same time and wearing the same clothing. Should patients notice an increase or decrease in weight of approximately 5 pounds (different limits can be set in individual cases), they are instructed to call. This is effective in preventing both dehydration and fluid overload, is much easier to follow than daily intake and output records, and allows patient participation in care plans.

Most patients are able to increase their fractional excretion of sodium (FENa) markedly as GFR decreases. In fact, FENa must double for each 50% decrement in GFR in order to maintain salt balance. This has been called "adaptive natriuresis" (55). However, the renal adaptation to rapid changes in sodium intake is blunted with CRF. Patients are, therefore, at increased risk either for acute fluid overload with dietary indiscretion or for dehydration from nausea, vomiting, diarrhea, or increase in diuretic doses. With a gradual decrease in sodium intake over several weeks, most patients are able to undergo a "deadaptation" and decrease their renal sodium excretion on a low-sodium diet (55). Once a patient lowers his or her sodium and fluid intake over several weeks, the patient must be counseled about the increased risk of "flash" pulmonary edema with dietary indiscretion (beer and pizza pulmonary edema). Reasonable starting guidelines for sodium are 1500 to 2000 mg/day (i.e., no added salt) with fluid intake to keep weight steady. There is certainly a trade-off, as the more severe the fluid and sodium restriction, the less likely is continued good compliance. As GFR decreases, dietary therapy becomes ineffective and other treatment modalities must be added. Effective long-term control of sodium intake and volume status usually requires a multidisciplinary approach that includes the services of a renal dietician.

D. Pharmacological Treatment

Most patients with hypertension and CRF require medication at some point. An individualized approach requires a knowledge of the pharmacological properties of each agent. For both parent compounds and metabolites, the half-life, bioavailability, primary site of metabolism (renal or hepatic), and extent of protein binding (which decreases with worsening renal function) are important considerations. Some of these data are presented in Table 4 and a more expanded discussion is available (56). Concomitant target organ damage, comorbid diseases, and other cardiovascular risk factors must also be considered in the choice of antihypertensive therapy (48).

1. Diuretics

Given the central role of sodium in the pathophysiological process of hypertension, either directly via increased extracellular volume (ECV) or indirectly via other vasopressor mechanisms, therapy for renal hypertension often requires the use of diuretics (3). If ECV overload is present, diuretics may be necessary as first-line drugs. They also increase the effectiveness of other agents (especially CEI and central agonists) when used in combination. Diuretics produce a diuresis and natriuresis and thus decrease ECV. They can cause a mild decrease in GFR and renal blood flow (RBF), especially with overly vigorous diuresis (57). Neither volume depletion nor reduction in renal function is seen with long-term use (56). For thiazide diuretics, ECV tends to return toward normal, and chronic antihypertensive effects are due mostly to a decrease in TPR (3).

Table 4 Antihypertensive Agents and Dosing Information in Chronic Renal Failur

Drug	Dose range[a] (mg/day) (normal renal function)	Adjustment with renal failure	Precautions
Diuretics			
Thiazides			
Hydrochlorothiazide	12.5–50	None with GFR > 30 ml/min	Avoid if GFR < 30 ml/min; volume depletion; hypokalemia; diuresis required for effect
Metolazone	0.5–10	None Effective to GFR approximately 10 ml/min	
Loop agents[a]			
Bumetanide	1–5	None	Volume depletion; hypokalemia; interstitial nephritis; ototoxicity; diuresis required for effect
Furosemide	20–320	None	
Ethacrynic acid	25–100	None	
Potassium-sparing agents (usually in combination diuretics)			
Amiloride	5–10	Major dosage reduction; usually avoided	Hyperkalemia if GFR < 30 ml/min
Triamterene	50–150		
Spironolactone	25–100		
Beta-blockers without ISA			
Atenolol	25–100	50% if GFR 10–50 25% if GFR < 10 Removed with HD	Accumulation of active parent compound and metabolites Hyperkalemia
Metoprolol	50–200	None	Hyperkalemia
Nadolol	20–240	As with atenolol	As with atenolol
Propranolol[a]	40–240	None	Hyperkalemia
Timolol[a]	20–40	None	Hyperkalemia
Beta-blockers with ISA			
Acebutolol	200–1200	50% if GFR 10–50	As with atenolol
Pindolol[a]	10–60	As with acebutolol	As with atenolol
Alpha-beta-blocker			
Labetolol[a]	200–120	None	Hyperkalemia
Alpha-blockers			
Prazosin[a]	1–20	Probably requires lower doses	First dose effect Start with low doses Prolonged hypotension

Table 4 Continued

Drug	Dose range[a] (mg/day) (normal renal function)	Adjustment with renal failure	Precautions
Terazosin	1–20	Same	Same
Doxazosin	1.0–16	Same	Same
Central agents			
Methyldopa[a]	250–2000	Active metabolites accumulate	Dry mouth Drowsiness
Clonidine[a]	0.1–1.2	Half dose if GFR < 20	Pseudotolerance Orthostasis
Guanabenz[a]	4–64	None	
Guanfacine	1–3	None	
ACE inhibitors			
Benazepril[a]	10–40	50% if GFR 20–50 25% if GFR < 10 Removed with HD	Reduce or stop diuretics prior to starting ACE inhibitors
Captopril[a]	12.5–150	Half dose if GFR 20–50 Quarter dose if GFR < 10	Increased incidence of side effects with decreased GFR; rash; leukopenia; dysgeusia; hyperkalemiia; acute renal insufficiency with bilateral renal artery stenosis
Enalapril	2.5–40	Same	Same
Fosinopril	10–40	No change	Same Hepatic metabolism Increases with fall in GFR
Lisinopril	5.0–40	As with Captopril	As with Captopril
Quinapril	5.0–80	As with Captopril	As with Captopril
Ramipril	1.25–20	As with Captopril	As with Captopril
Calcium antagonists			
Diltiazem	90–360	None	Constipation
Verapamil	120–480	None	Constipation
Dihydropyridines			
Amlodipine	2.5–10	None	None
Felodipine	5–20	None	None
Isradipine[a]	2.5–10	None	None
Nicardipine	60–120	None	None
Nifedipine	30–120	None	Possible hemodynamic worsening of renal function

continues

Table 4 Continued

Drug	Dose range[a] (mg/day) (normal renal function)	Adjustment with renal failure	Precautions
Vasodilators			
Hydralazine[a]	50–300	Increase dosage with GFR < 10	Sodium and fluid retention Reflex tachycardia Prolonged hypotension
Minoxidil[a]	2.5–80	None	As above
Diazoxide		Lower and slower doses	Decreased protein binding may precipitate angina Prolonged hypotension

[a]Requires multiple doses per day.
Source: Refs. 3, 56, 67.

a. Thiazides and Related Compounds. Thiazide diuretics are useful agents when the GFR is greater than 30 ml/min, that is, serum creatinine level below 177 mmol/L (2 mg/dl). Hydrochlorothiazide at 25 to 50 mg/day, or chlorthalidone in equivalent doses, is the usual choice. Once the GFR falls below 30 ml/min, three factors act to decrease the effectiveness of thiazide diuretics: (1) less sodium is filtered and thus, less sodium reaches the distal tubules, where thiazides act; (2) the proximal tubular organic anion transport mechanism that is necessary to transport both thiazides and loop diuretics into the tubular lumen is less effective in CRF since other organic and inorganic cations and anions, such as ketoacids, phosphates, and urates, lead to competitive inhibition of tubular secretion; (3) more avid reabsorption of sodium and chloride occurs in the medullary thick ascending loop of Henle, which is proximal to the site of action of thiazide diuretics (but is the site of action of loop diuretics). As a result, less total administered dose of medication arrives at the site of activity at the same time that higher doses of medication are required as a result of decreased filtered load of sodium (3).

b. Loop Diuretics. Once the GFR falls below approximately 30 ml/min, loop diuretics become a necessary component in the control of ECV and hypertension. The response to loop diuretics is dependent on the delivery of the drug to its site of action (pharmacokinetics) and the initiation of the desired response once the drug reaches the medullary thick ascending limb (pharmacodynamics) (58). Brater and Voelker have described a two-step dosage titration process in the use of loop diuretics (58). First, it is necessary to establish a threshold dose that will elicit the desired diuresis and natiuresis. Upward dosage titration best achieves this goal. Dosing can be either via the intravenous route or orally at home. For example, in an acute setting, furosemide is administered intravenously in doses of 40, 80, 160, and 320 mg until a response is obtained. A study of patients with creatinine clearance values less than 20 ml/min showed that an intravenous furosemide dose of 160 mg was sufficient to reach threshold levels in all patients who responded. The time course of response as determined by the onset of natiuresis was less intense but more prolonged compared to that in patients with normal renal function (59). When given orally, this maximal dose is equivalent to 320 to 400 mg of furosemide since furosemide has a bioavailability of approximately 40%. For bumetanide, the equivalent oral dose is approximately 4 to 5 mg since bumetanide has a higher bioavailability but more extensive extrarenal metabolism with CRF (60). Second, the best program to obtain a sustained response should be determined. Usually the effective dose must be given at least twice daily. Since the half-life of loop diuretics is approximately 6 hours, we generally tell patients to take their medication in the morning at breakfast and around suppertime—that is, 4:00 p.m. to 6:00 p.m. This schedule allows most diuresis to occur before 10:00 p.m. to midnight and lessens the disruption of sleep. Patients may continue to have nocturnal diuresis secondary to impaired concentrating ability of the damaged kidney, but this will not be worsened by concurrent medication effects. Patients also should be counseled against nocturnal fluid intake. As mentioned, should a patient's weight vary over a short period, adjustments either upward or downward in the diuretic dose are often necessary. The addition of either hydrochlorothiazide (50 to 100 mg/day) or metolazone (2.5 to 10 mg/day) to a loop diuretic increases the likelihood of response. There appears to be a synergistic effect of these two classes of diuretics in the distal renal tubule (61). Problems can occur with combination therapy or with larger doses of a single agent. The risk of toxicity, especially ototoxicity and hyponatremia, increases, and at some point the low filtered load of sodium renders diuretic use ineffective (62).

c. Potassium Sparing Agents. Potassium excretion decreases as GFR falls, and the risk of hypokalemia from diuretic use is less than in patients with normal renal function. Serum potassium level should be monitored and supplements given only if necessary. The potassium sparing diuretics, alone or in combination with hydrochlorothiazide, are usually not necessary to maintain potassium homeostasis and should be avoided. Hyperkalemia can be problematic in patients taking converting enzyme inhibitors (CEIs) or nonsteroidal anti-inflammatory drugs (NSAIDs) that also tend to interfere with potassium excretion.

2. Beta-Blockers

Beta-blockers have been used with good results in patients with CRF. Their effects include decreased heart rate, cardiac output, mean arterial pressure, central sympathetic discharge, and peripheral norepinephrine release. They also inhibit renin release and thus interfere to a variable degree with the RAA axis (63). Total peripheral resistance is acutely increased with most beta-blockers but probably returns toward pretreatment values with chronic therapy (56). The effects of individual beta-blockers on renal function are variable, but they rarely cause appreciable changes. They have little or no clinical effect on GFR, renal blood flow (RBF), renovascular resistance (RVR), or urinary sodium and potassium excretion. Although investigators have observed decreased RBF with propranolol and increased RBF with nadolol, it is unclear whether these effects continue on a chronic basis (56). An important consideration in the use of beta-blockers in CRF is the relative lipophilicity/hydrophilicity of an individual agent. Hydrophilic agents such as atenolol, acebutolol, and nadolol are excreted in the urine, have a longer serum half-life, and require significant dosage adjustment with progressive renal failure. Lipophilic agents such as metoprolol, propranolol, pindolol, and timolol require little dosage adjustment with CRF. Most beta-blockers raise triglyceride levels and lower high-density lipoprotein (HDL) levels. Only agents with intrinsic sympathomimetic activity (ISA), such as acebutolol and pindolol, do not produce these lipid changes (56). Other considerations in the selection of beta-blockers are the same as for any patient. The cardioprotective effect of beta-blockers in patients with coronary artery disease is a strong consideration for use of these drugs in this patient population.

3. Blocker-Dilator

Combined alpha- and beta-blockade with the blocker dilator agent labetalol leads to a greater decrease in TPR than is seen with beta-blockers alone. Labetalol is a nonselective beta-blocker and a postsynaptic alpha$_1$-receptor blocker. There is no dose adjustment necessary with CRF (64) and no untoward effects on RBF or GFR. Labetalol also is effective when given intravenously and, as described in Chapter 13, can be used in the treatment of hypertensive urgencies or emergencies via either minibolus administration or continuous infusion. Labetalol does not appear to affect plasma lipid levels adversely.

4. Alpha-Blockers

The three available alpha-blockers are prazosin, doxazosin, and terazosin. Little or no dosage adjustment is necessary with CRF since they are metabolized in the liver. None of these agents appears to have deleterious effects on plasma lipids (56). GFR and RBF are not significantly affected by either agent, but an increased sensitivity to prazosin has been reported in patients with CRF (65), making it prudent to begin with small doses. Doses of prazosin in the range of 3 to 8 mg/day have been as effective as or more effective than higher doses in patients with CRF (66).

5. *Central Agonists*

The available centrally acting agonists include methyldopa and the related drugs clonidine, guanabenz, and guanfacine. They have little or no effect on GFR or RBF and decrease RVR. Methyldopa has been available since 1963 with extensive clinical experience in CRF patients. There is an accumulation of active metabolites as renal function worsens and dosage adjustment is necessary (67). Pseudotolerance may develop with any central agonist secondary to salt and water retention and can be problematic in patients with impaired renal function. Conversely, the antihypertensive effect of these drugs is increased with control of volume status by diet or diuretics (56). As with any central agent, typical side effects are dry mouth (which may increase fluid intake), drowsiness, increased risk of orthostatic hypotension, and weakness. There is probably no significant effect on plasma lipid levels.

Clonidine has no significant effect on GFR or RBF (56). There are no active metabolites, but the parent compound does accumulate and dosage adjustment is necessary, especially with a GFR below 20 ml/min. There does not appear to be any loss of effectiveness with higher serum drug levels as was once suspected ("therapeutic window" effect) (68). Guanabenz is a central agonist with a structure similar to that of clonidine. Less than 1% of the parent drug is excreted in the urine and no significant accumulation occurs with CRF. As with all central agonists, it is best to begin with low doses and slowly increase the dosage. Guanfacine is a clonidine-related drug that undergoes both hepatic and renal metabolism with no significant accumulation in CRF (56). No dosage adjustment is necessary, but small starting doses are prudent. Guanficine acutely decreases GFR and RBF (69), although chronic effects are less clear.

6. *Calcium Antagonists*

Calcium antagonists (CAs) are a chemically diverse group with a similar mechanism of action. There are three major subgroups of CAs: (1) diltiazem, (2) verapamil, and (3) the dihydropyridine derivatives. These agents interfere with voltage-dependent calcium channels in vascular and cardiac smooth muscle. CAs differ in their relative specificity for cardiac or vascular smooth muscle although all produce some degree of peripheral vasodilitation (56). CAs can influence GFR, renal vascular tone, hormonal secretion, and epithelial transport (70). These observed effects on renal function may be present acutely, with initial administration but not with continued chronic administration of the drug (56). Acutely, CAs increase RBF, with the degree of vasodilatation related to the initial resting tone of the vascular smooth muscle. There is also an increase in urinary sodium excretion and plasma renin levels. Long-term studies generally show no deleterious effects on renal function in patients with hypertension (56,70). Although rare, nifedipine-induced renal dysfunction has been reported, possibly secondarily to acute alterations in renal hemodynamics (71). The mechanism producing this renal dysfunction is unclear and it has been reported only in elderly patients with atherosclerotic disease and CRF. It is reversible with discontinuation of the drug. In the rat remnant model of CRF, verapamil has been shown to be protective against progression of renal damage (72). Additional benefits with these agents include a cardioprotective effect in patients with atherosclerotic heart disease and no adverse effects on lipid profile. Dosage adjustment is not required with CRF (56). In patients taking phosphorus binders that may lead to constipation, the tendency for verapamil and diltiazem to worsen constipation can be problematic.

7. *Converting Enzyme Inhibitors*

Converting enzyme inhibitors (CEIs) appear to have a common mechanism of action. Their effects are not limited to converting enzyme inhibition and probably involve multiple hormonal systems (73). CEIs maintain or improve GFR and RBF and decrease RVR; most side effects are class-specific. All CEIs are excreted at least in part by the kidney. With chronic renal failure, significant delay occurs in peak concentrations and in excretion rates (56). Consequently, blood levels increase. Dosage reduction is necessary, especially with GFR below 50 ml/min. Hyperkalemia can be a significant side effect, especially with worsening renal function. Hypotension may occur, especially with concomitant diuretic use, dehydration, or large initial doses. When starting CEI, it is prudent to begin with one-quarter to one-half the usual dose and to discontinue or at least decrease the dose of any diuretics (73). Rapid deterioration in renal function leading to acute renal failure can occur if hypertension is related to hemodynamically significant bilateral renal artery stenosis or significant stenosis of the artery to a solitary kidney. The likelihood of this complication's occurring is increased with associated salt and water depletion (74).

8. *Vasodilators*

Although several of the medications mentioned can be considered vasodilators as they decrease TPR, hydralazine and minoxidil are the classic vasodilators. Both are third-line drugs. Neither agent significantly affects GFR although both increase RBF (56). Concomitant use of a sympatholytic agent to blunt reflex tachycardia and a diuretic to prevent salt and water accumulation is usually required. Hydralazine undergoes acetylation in the liver but has a longer duration of action in patients with renal failure because active metabolites are renally excreted (56). Historically, the use of minoxidil made bilateral nephrectomy unnecessary for the vast majority of patients with CRF and uncontrolled hypertension (75). It is metabolized in the liver and only about 10% is excreted in the urine. There is no significant dosage adjustment required with CRF. The risk of pericardial effusion may be increased in patients with CRF (76). Hirsutism is to be expected and can limit the acceptance of this medication particularly in children and women.

E. Calcium Antagonists Versus Converting Enzyme Inhibitors

1. Current Information

Interest in calcium antagonists and converting enzyme inhibitors has increased with the possibility that either or both may protect renal function and decrease proteinuria in patients with CRF (77,78) or those with primary hypertension who are at increased risk for eventual renal damage (79). Protection of renal function (and structure) may be secondary to favorable intrarenal hemodynamic effects (26), alteration of membrane permselectivity, protection of cellular function, inhibition of growth factors, or other mechanisms (25). A potential bias in many studies is that progression of CRF may be slowed simply by involvement in a clinical trial with more frequent follow-up observation and better control of blood pressure regardless of the antihypertensive regimen used (80). Thus randomized, prospective multicenter trials are necessary to determine the exact role of either of these classes of drugs in patients with HTN and CRF. Several clinical studies are in progress or recently completed and, it is hoped that exciting and useful information will be forthcoming. Both the NHBPEP Report on Chronic Renal Failure and Hypertension (27) and the report of the Working Group on Hypertension and Diabetes (46) have recommended either of these classes as preferred first-line agents with potential renal protective advantages.

2. Effects on Proteinuria

As discussed, the reduction of proteinuria per se may have a beneficial effect on renal function. Both CEIs and CAs have been shown to decrease proteinuria in patients with CRF (17,22,78). This effect can be seen even in patients with normal blood pressure, although it is not observed in all patients and there does tend to be a further decrease in blood pressure (even when initially normal) associated with the decline in proteinuria.

Different effects have been observed among the different CA subgroups. For example, Demarie et al. in a short-term crossover study of diabetic patients with proteinuria noted a decrease in proteinuria with diltiazem but an increase in proteinuria with nifedipine that was also associated with a worsening in renal function as measured by creatinine clearance (81). However, the Melbourne Diabetic Nephropathy Study Group compared the CEI perindopril with the CA nifedipine in 50 diabetic patients with microalbuminuria (82) and found similar beneficial effects on urinary protein excretion and preservation of renal function with either agent. A recent review of CEIs in nondiabetic renal disease (83) found that 20 of 23 short-term (less than 12 months) studies showed a decrease in proteinuria with CEIs. However, only 6 of 15 long-term (more than 12 months) studies showed similar results.

Several important questions remain unanswered: (1) Is there a difference in long-term reduction of microalbuminuria or proteinuria between CEIs and CAs or among individual agents in these classes? (2) Is the decrease in proteinuria mediated by decreased blood pressure alone, or are there independent intrarenal effects causing the decrease? (3) Most importantly, is the decrease in proteinuria independently important in the preservation of renal function?

3. *Use in Nondiabetic Renal Disease*

The recent review by ter Wee and Epstein (83) of 35 short-term and 17 long-term studies using CEIs in nondiabetic renal disease allowed few clear-cut conclusions. The two long-term studies that were random, were prospective, and used radionuclide determinations of renal function gave different results. A study in 70 patients with chronic renal failure that compared enalapril with a vasodilator-beta-blocker-diuretic combination showed a slower progression (but not preservation) of renal failure in the enalapril group. The rate of progression in the enalapril group was −0.20 (0.18 to −7.11) ml/min per 1.73 m^2 versus 0.31 (+0.01 to −1.97) ml/min per 1.73 m^2 (target blood pressure levels were 130 to 140/80 to 90 mm Hg) (84). A comparison of captopril with nifedipine in 121 patients followed for up to 4 years after a 1-year prerandomization on their usual blood pressure medications showed no difference between the two agents in rate of progression of CRF. MAPs obtained were between 100 and 103 mm Hg. The rate of progression was slowed (but not halted) in either group compared to prerandomization rate of progression, but the prerandomization blood pressures were higher than the blood pressures achieved during the study period (85).

4. *Use in Diabetic Renal Disease*

The choice of antihypertensive medications in diabetic nephropathy is becoming clearer. Prior reports had often involved few patients, been short-term only, and used creatinine clearance as the marker of renal function. A recent meta-analysis of 100 studies, both controlled and uncontrolled, showed that CEI use decreased proteinuria and preserved renal function independent of any effect on systemic blood pressure (86). Several other agents were found to decrease proteinuria but only when blood pressure was also decreased (86). A prospective randomized study with enalapril, however, showed no beneficial effect of CEIs in decreasing proteinuria independent of its effect on lowering blood pressure (87). The Angiotensin Converting-Enzyme Inhibitor in Diabetic Nephropathy trial has just been reported (88). Eligible patients were between 18 and 49 years old, with proteinuria above 500 mg/dl and serum creatinine level below 221 μmol/L (2.5 mg/dl). Patients received captopril 25 mg t.i.d. or non-CEI treatment (that also excluded CAs). Several important findings were reported in this study. Blood pressure control was very good with median levels of 128 to 136 mm Hg for systolic and 77 to 84 mm Hg for diastolic in both groups. The captopril group had a lower blood pressure but the difference was less than 4 mm Hg between the groups with MAP of 98 $\pm$ 8 mm Hg and 100 $\pm$ 8 mm Hg in captopril and placebo groups, respectively. However, there was a significant slowing of time to doubling of serum creatinine level and time to death, dialysis, or transplantation in the captopril group (primary and secondary end points) (88). Thus, independent of blood pressure changes (or perhaps in combination with very good blood pressure control), CEI (captopril) afforded significant protection in the progression of diabetic nephropathy that was evident at all values of serum creatinine level. With CAs, some authors have maintained that only certain classes of CAs, specifically excluding the dihydropyridine group, confer renal protection to diabetic patients (89).

Thus it may be that different strategies for intervention are necessary and different definitions of success are to be expected depending on (1) the level of blood pressure control, (2) the amount of proteinuria (either normal, microalbuminuria, or overt proteinuria), and (3) the amount of renal damage already present. The majority of studies with favorable results have used CEIs. On the basis of preliminary data and the recommendations of two consensus groups, it seems prudent to use either CEIs or CAs in patients with CRF whose blood pressure is elevated and to maintain blood pressure at a maximum of 130/85 mm Hg barring significant orthostatic hypotension. Recent studies such as the Angiotensin Converting Enzyme Inhibition in Diabetic Nephropathy Trial also provide compelling evidence that CEI use, even in normotensive patients with diabetic nephropathy, may offer renal protection.

IV. CONCLUSIONS

The approach to patients with hypertension and chronic renal failure begins with an assessment of patient status. Initial evaluation should include documentation of the presence of hypertension, chronic renal failure, and severity of renal dysfunction. If the patient has potentially reversible disease, all efforts should be made to treat the primary disease. If disease is not treatable or if the patient is beyond a "point of no return" where treatment will not correct the initial problem (primary prevention), then secondary prevention measures are begun. Additional cardiovascular risk factors should be identified and treated. If the patient falls into a high-risk group, as defined by epidemiological factors, primary disease, presence of microalbuminuria or proteinuria, or worsening renal function, then more intense treatment of blood pressure is necessary. Attempts to control blood pressure to 135/85 mm Hg or possibly lower with avoidance of orthostatic hypotension are prudent, using CEIs or CAs as primary agents. Further special care efforts include modification of diet, restriction of protein intake, control of lipid abnormalities, and tight metabolic control of diabetes mellitus and renal osteodystrophy. Volume status should be controlled with frequent reassessment of renal function. This intense approach is best begun as a team effort with primary and consulting physicians, nurses, dieticians, and social workers. It is hoped that in the next few years we will have a better understanding of basic pathological features, which factors are predictive and modifiable, and which agents offer advantages to patients with hypertension and chronic renal failure.

REFERENCES

1. Kaplan NM. Clinical Hypertension. 6th ed. Baltimore: Williams & Wilkins, 1994:299–317.
2. Klahr S. The kidney in hypertension: villain and victim. N Engl J Med 1989; 320(11):731–732.
3. Heyka RJ, Vidt DG. Control of hypertension in patients with chronic renal failure. Cleve Clin J Med 1989; 56:65–76.
4. Blythe WB. Natural history of hypertension in renal parenchymal disease. Am J Kidney Dis 1985; 5:A50–A56.
5. Weisstuch JM, Dworkin LD. Does essential hypertension cause end-stage renal disease? Kidney Int 1992; 41(suppl 36):S-33–S-37.
6. Steenland NK, Thun MJ, Ferguson CW, Port FK. Occupational and other exposures associated with male end-stage renal disease: a case/control study. Am J Public Health 1990; 80:153–159.
7. Staessen JA, Lauwerys RR, Buchet JP, et al. Impairment of renal function with increasing blood lead concentrations in the general population. N Engl J Med 1992; 327:151–156.
8. Acosta JH. Hypertension in chronic renal disease. Kidney Int 1982; 22:702–712.
9. Ma KW, Greene EL, Raij L. Cardiovascular risk factors in chronic renal failure and hemodialysis and hemodialysis populations. Am J Kidney Dis 1992; 19(6): 505–513.

10. Shulman NB, Ford CE, Hall WB, et al. Prognostic value of serum creatinine and effect of treatment of hypertension on renal function. Hypertension 1989; 13(suppl I):I-80–I-93.
11. United States Renal Data System. 1993 Annual Data Report. Bethesda, MD. National Institutes of Health, Natl Institute of Diabetes & Digestive & Kidney Diseases 1993.
12. Charra B, Calemard E, Ruffet M, et al. Survival as an index of adequacy of dialysis. Kidney International 1992; 41:1286–1291.
13. Klahr S, Schreiner G, Ichikawa I. The progression of renal disease. N Engl J Med 1988; 318(25):1657–1666.
14. Fine LG, Woolf AS, Gallego C. Of rats and men: the need for more convincing clinical studies on progression of renal diseases. Am J Kidney Dis 1991; 17:258–260.
15. Luke RG. The modification of diet in renal disease study: design, methods, and results from the feasibility study. Am J Kidney Dis 1992; 20:18–33.
16. Keane WF, O'Donnell MP, Kasiske BL, Schmitz PG. Lipids and the progression of renal disease. J Am Soc Nephrol 1990; 1:S69–S74.
17. Keilani T, Schlueter WA, Levin ML, Batlle DC. Improvement of lipid abnormalities associated with proteinuria using fosinopril, an angiotensin-converting enzyme inhibitor. Ann Intern Med 1993; 118:246–254.
18. Ljungman S. Microalbuminuria in essential hypertension. Am J Hypertens 1990; 3:956–960.
19. Clavers BM, Bilous RW, Ellis EN, et al. Glomerular lesions and urinary albumin excretion in Type I diabetes without overt proteinuria. N Engl J Med 1989; 320:966–970.
20. Mogensen CE, Christensen CK. Predicting diabetic nephropathy in insulin-dependent patients. N Engl J Med 1984; 311:89–93.
21. Peterson JC, Burkart J, Greene T, et al. The effect of blood pressure control on progression of renal disease depends on level of proteinuria (P) at baseline evaluation (abstr). J Am Soc Nephrol 1993; 4(3):254.
22. Hebert LA, Bain RP, Cattran D, et al. Remission (RM) of nephrotic-range proteinuria (NRP) in Type I diabetes: experience of the NIH multicenter controlled trial (T) of captopril (CAP) therapy in diabetic nephropathy (DN) (abstr). J Am Soc Nephrol 1993; 4(3):303.
23. Remuzzi G, Bertani T. Is glomerulosclerosis a consequence of altered glomerular permeability to macromolecules? Kidney Int 1990; 38:384–394.
24. Baldwin DS, Neugarten J. Treatment of hypertension in renal disease. Am J Kidney Dis 1985; 5:A57–A70.
25. Linas S. Calcium channel blockers versus angiotensin-converting enzyme inhibitors: renal effects. Am J Kidney Dis 1990; 16(4)(suppl 1):15–19).
26. Anderson S, Rennke HG, Brenner BM. Therapeutic advantage of converting enzyme inhibitors in arresting progressive renal disease associated with systemic hypertension in the rat. J Clin Invest 1986; 77:1993–2000.
27. National High Blood Pressure Education Program. National High Blood Pressure Education Program Working Group Report on Hypertension and Chronic Renal Failure. Arch Intern Med 1991; 151:1280–1287.
28. Feldman HI, Klag MJ, Chiapella AP, Whelton PK. End-stage renal disease in US minority groups. Am J Kidney Dis 1992; 19(5):397–410.

29. Whittle JC, Whelton PK, Seidler AJ, Klag MJ. Does racial variation in risk factors explain black-white differences in the incidence of hypertensive end-stage renal disease? Arch Intern Med 1991; 151:1359–1364.
30. Rostand SG, Brown G, Kirk A, et al. Renal insufficiency in treated essential hypertension. N Engl J Med 1989; 320:684–688.
31. Foxman B, Mounton LH, Wolfe RA, et al. Geographic variation in the incidence of treated end-stage renal disease. J Am Soc Nephrol 1991; 2:1144–1152.
32. Perneger TV, Klag MJ, Feldman HI, Whelton PK. Projections of hypertension-related renal disease in middle-aged residents of the United States. JAMA 1993; 269:1272–1277.
33. Smith MC, Dunn MJ. Hypertension due to renal parenchymal disease. In: Brenner BM, Rector FC, eds. The Kidney. 4th ed. Philadelphia: WB Saunders, 1992:1968–1996.
34. Brod J, Bahlmann J, Cachovan M, Pretschner P. Development of hypertension in renal disease. Clin Sci 1983; 64:141–152.
35. Koomans HA, Roos JC, Boer P, et al. Salt sensitivity of blood pressure in chronic renal failure. Hypertension 1982; 4:190–197.
36. Vertes V, Cangiano JL, Berman LB, Gould A. Hypertension in end-stage renal disease. N Engl J Med 1969; 280:978–981.
37. Weidmann P, Maxwell MH, Lupu AN, et al. Plasma renin activity and blood pressure in terminal renal failure. N Engl J Med 1971; 285:757–762.
38. Davies DL, Beevers DG, Briggs JD, et al. Abnormal relation between exchangeable sodium and the renin-angiotensin system in malignant hypertension and in hypertension with chronic renal failure. Lancet 1973; 1:683–687.
39. DiBona GF. The kidney in the pathogenesis of hypertension: the role of renal nerves. Am J Kidney Dis 1985; 5:A27–A31.
40. Yager HM, Harrington JT. Evaluation of serum electrolytes, creatinine, and blood urea nitrogen. In: Jacobson HR, Striker GE, Klahr GE, eds. The Principles and Practice of Nephrology. Philadelphia: BC Decker, 1991:163–166.
41. Shemesh O, Golbetz H, Kriss JP, Myers BD. Limitations of creatinine as a filtration marker in glomerulopathic patients. Kidney Int 1985; 28:830–838.
42. Rolin H, Hall PM. Evaluation of glomerular filtration rate and renal plasma flow. In: Jacobson HR, Striker GE, Klahr GE, eds. The Principles and Practice of Nephrology. Philadelphia: BC Decker, 1991:158–162.
43. Levey AS. Assessing the effectiveness of therapy to prevent the progression of renal disease. Am J Kidney Dis 1993; 22:207–214.
44. Lubowitz H, Slatopolsky E, Shankel S, et al. Glomerular filtration rate: Determination in patients with chronic renal disease. JAMA 1967; 199:100–104.
45. Portaluppi F, Montanari L, Massari M, et al. Loss of nocturnal decline of blood pressure in hypertension due to chronic renal failure. Am J Hypertens 1991; 4:20–26.
46. The Working Group on Hypertension in Diabetes. Statement on hypertension in diabetes mellitus. Arch Intern Med 1987; 147:830–842.
47. Morbidity and Mortality of Dialysis. NIH Consensus statement 1993. Nov 1–3; 11(2):1–33.

48. The Fifth Report of the Joint National Committee on Detection, Evaluation, and Treatment of High Blood Pressure (JNC V). Arch Intern Med 1993; 153: 154–183.
49. Fletcher AE, Bulpitt CJ. How far should blood pressure be lowered? N Engl J Med 1992; 326:251–255.
50. SHEP Cooperative Research Group. Prevention of stroke by antihypertensive drug treatment in older persons with isolated systolic hypertension. JAMA 1991; 265:3255–3264.
51. National High Blood Pressure Education Program Working Group Report on Primary Prevention of Hypertension. Arch Intern Med 1993; 153:186–208.
52. Macdougall IC, Lewis NP, Saunders MJ, et al. Long-term cardiorespiratory effects of amelioration of renal anaemia by erythropoietin. Lancet 1990; 335: 489–493.
53. Eschbach JW, Kelly MR, Haley NR, et al. Treatment of the anemia of progressive renal failure with recombinant human erythropoietin. N Engl J Med 1989; 321:158–163.
54. Cheriex EC, Leunissen KML, Janssen JHA, et al. Echography of the inferior vena cava is a simple and reliable tool for estimation of "dry weight" in haemodialysis patients. Nephrol Dial Transplant 1989; 4:563–568.
55. Bricker NS. Sodium homeostasis in chronic renal disease. Kidney Int 1982; 21: 886–897.
56. Bauer JH, Reams GP. Antihypertensive Drugs. In: Brenner BM, Rector FC, eds. The Kidney. 4th ed. Philadelphia: WB Saunders, 1991:2148–2185.
57. Kaufman AM, Levitt MF. The effect of diuretics on systemic and renal hemodynamics in patients with renal insufficiency. Am J Kidney Dis 1985; 5:A71–A78.
58. Brater DC, Voelker JR. Use of diuretics in patients with renal disease. In: Bennett WM, McCarron DA, Brenner BH, Stein JH, eds. Pharmacotherapy of Renal Disease and Hypertension. New York: Churchill Livingstone, 1987:115–147.
59. Brater DC, Anderson SA, Brown-Cartwright D. Response to furosemide in chronic renal insufficiency: rationale for limited doses. Clin Pharmacol Ther 1986; 40:134–139.
60. Voelker JR, Cartwright-Brown D, Anderson S, et al. Comparison of loop diuretics in patients with chronic renal insufficiency. Kidney Int 1987; 32:572–578.
61. Brater DC, Pressley RH, Anderson SA. Mechanisms of the synergistic combination of metolazone and bumetanide. J Pharmacol Exp Ther 1985; 233:70–76.
62. Wollam GL, Tarazi RC, Bravo EL, Dustan HP. Diuretic potency of combined hydrochlorothiazide and furosemide therapy in patients with azotemia. Am J Med 1982; 72:929–938.
63. Wilkinson R. β blockers and renal function. Drugs 1982; 23:195–206.
64. McNeil JJ, Louis WS. Clinical pharmacokinetics of labetalol. Clin Pharmacokinet 1984; 9:157–167.
65. Vincent J, Meredith PA, Reid JL, et al. Clinical pharmacokinetics of prazosin-1985. Clin Pharmacokinet 1985; 10:144–144.

66. Onesti G. Prazosin kinetics and effectiveness in renal failure. Clin Pharmacol Ther 1980; 27:779–283.
67. Myhre E, Rugstad HE, Hansen T. Clinical pharmacokinetics of methyldopa. Clin Pharmacokinet 1982; 7:221–233.
68. Lowenthal DT, Affrime MB, Meyer A, et al. Pharmacokinetics and pharmacodynamics of clonidine in varying stages of renal function. Chest 1983; 83(suppl): 386–390.
69. Roeckel A, Heidland A II. Acute and chronic renal effects of guanfacine in essential and renal hypertension. Br J Clin Pharmacol 1980; 10:141S–149S.
70. Romero JC, Raij L, Granger JP, et al. Multiple effects of calcium entry blockers on renal function in hypertension. Hypertension 1987; 10:140–151.
71. Diamond JR, Cheung JY, Fang LST. Nifedipine-induced renal dysfunction: alterations in renal hemodynamics. Am J Med 1984; 77:905–909.
72. Harris DCH, Hammond WS, Burke TJ, Schrier RW. Verapamil protects against progression of experimental chronic renal failure. Kidney Int 1987; 31:41–46.
73. Williams GH. Converting-enzyme inhibitors in the treatment of hypertension. N Engl J Med 1988; 319:1517–1525.
74. Hricik DE, Dunn MJ. Angiotensin-converting enzyme inhibitor-induced renal failure: causes, consequences, and diagnostic uses. J Am Soc Nephrol 1990; 1:845–858.
75. Pettinger WA, Mitchell HC. Minoxidil: an alternative to nephrectomy for refractory hypertension. N Engl J Med 1973; 289:167–173.
76. Campese VM. Minoxidil: a review of its pharmacological properties and therapeutic use. Drugs 1981; 22:257–278.
77. Keane WF, Anderson S, Aurell M, et al. Angiotensin converting enzyme inhibitors and progressive renal insufficiency. Ann Intern Med 1989; 111:503–516.
78. Epstein M. Calcium antagonists and renal protection. Arch Intern Med 1992; 152:1573–1584.
79. Bauer JH, Reams GP. Renal protection in essential hypertension: how do angiotensin-converting enzyme inhibitors compare with calcium antagonists? J Am Soc Nephrol 1990; 1:S80–S87.
80. Bergstrom J, Alvestrand A, Bucht H, Gutierrez A. Progression of chronic renal failure in man is retarded with more frequent clinical follow-ups and better blood pressure control. Clin Nephrol 1986; 25(1):1–6.
81. Demarie BK, Bakris GL. Effects on different calcium antagonists on proteinuria associated with diabetes mellitus. Ann Intern Med 1990; 113:987–988.
82. Melbourne Diabetic Nephropathy Study Group. Comparison between perindopril and nifedipine in hypertensive and normotensive diabetic patients with microalbuminuria. Br Med J 1991; 302:210–216.
83. ter Wee PM, Epstein M. Angiotensin-converting enzyme inhibitors and progression of nondiabetic chronic renal disease. Arch Intern Med 1993; 1749–1759.
84. Kamper AL, Strandgaard S, Leyssac PP. Effect of enalapril on the progression of chronic renal failure. Am J Hypertens 1992; 5:423–430.

85. Zucchelli, Zuccala A, Borghi M, et al. Long-term comparison between captopril and nifedipine in the progression of renal insufficiency. Kidney Int 1992; 42:452–458.
86. Kasiske BL, Kalil RSN, Ma JZ, et al. Effect of antihypertensive therapy on the kidney in patients with diabetes: a meta-regression analysis. Ann Intern Med 1993; 118:129–138.
87. Bauer JH, Reams GP, Hewitt J, et al. A randomized, double-blind, placebo-controlled trial to evaluate the effect of enalapril in patients with clinical diabetic nephropathy. Am J Kidney Dis 1992; 20:443–457.
88. Lewis EJ, Hunsicker LG, Bain RP, Rohde RD. The effect of angiotensin-enzyme inhibition on diabetic nephropathy. N Engl J Med 1993; 329:1456–1462.
89. Valentino VA, Wilson MD, Weart W, Bakris GL. A perspective on converting enzyme inhibitors and calcium channel antagonists in diabetic renal disease. Arch Intern Med 1991; 151:2367–2372.

10

Hypertension in Pregnancy

PHYLLIS AUGUST
Cornell University Medical College
New York, New York

MARSHALL D. LINDHEIMER
University of Chicago
Chicago, Illinois

I. INTRODUCTION

Managing pregnant hypertensives challenges obstetricians and internists alike. The former are reluctant to prescribe medications because of concern about fetal well-being, while the latter may be uncertain of whether or how to apply principles used to treat hypertension in nonpregnant populations to pregnant patients. These dilemmas intensify when practitioners are unfamiliar with the alterations in cardiovascular physiological processes of normal gestation. On the other hand, awareness of pregnancy-related hemodynamic changes, their effect in gravid women with preexisting hypertension, familiarity with the pathophysiological features of certain specific forms of high blood pressure peculiar to pregnancy, and appreciation of how disease and therapy may influence fetal well-being enhance a physician's ability to manage hypertensive gravidas. This awareness leads to a realization that therapeutic goals of treating hypertension in pregnancy differ from those in nonpregnant individuals, as well as to a strategy in which the primary goal is delivery of a healthy, mature fetus, without compromising maternal well-being, rather than the usual focus on long-term prevention of cardiovascular disease. This outcome is best accomplished by close maternal and fetal surveillance, nonpharmacological therapy, judicious use of antihypertensive medication, and timely delivery of the fetus.

This chapter commences with a basic overview of the physiological changes in normal pregnancy, focusing on alterations pertinent to hypertension. Next, problems of classification and diagnosis, as well as current concepts of the pathophysiological characteristics of the diverse hypertensive disorders of pregnancy, will be discussed. Then prevention and management will be addressed in considerable detail. It will become apparent, at every step of the way—prevention, diagnosis, and treatment—that individualized therapy is essential to appropriate management of hypertension during pregnancy.

II. UNIQUE PHYSIOLOGICAL ADJUSTMENTS OF PREGNANCY

A. Hemodynamic Changes

Cardiac output rises in pregnant women to values 30% to 40% above the nonpregnant resting state (1). This increase, apparent by the 12th gestational week, becomes maximal by midpregnancy. There is also generalized vasodilatation, resulting in a decreased afterload, as well as an increased plasma volume. Heart rate increases slightly, mainly in the last half of gestation, but stroke volume rises as a result of the changes in intravascular volume and peripheral resistance. Hypervolemia in combination with increases in cardiac output would be expected to raise blood pressure, but mean arterial pressure actually falls in gestation. The decrease is apparent during the first trimester, reaches a nadir by the end of the second trimester, and then usually increases gradually and often approaches prepregnancy levels at term, and may even rise transiently above nonpregnant levels in the puerperium (2).

Though aware the decreases in blood pressure are primarily the result of the generalized vasodilatation characteristic of pregnancy, we have much to learn about hormonal and cellular mechanisms responsible for these marked decrements in peripheral resistance. Prostaglandins, estrogens, and progesterone have all been implicated as possible mediators (3,4), and more recently exciting data have suggested that changes in the metabolism of endothelial derived relaxing factor(s) (EDRF, nitric oxide) during pregnancy play an important role in the observed vasodilatation (5).

B. Renal Changes

Both glomerular filtration rate (GFR) and renal blood flow increase dramatically in pregnancy (6). Midpregnancy increments are as great as 50% to 60%, with a slight fall apparent in the third trimester. These striking changes have been attributed to the increased cardiac output and fluid volume, as well as to concurrent endocrine changes, although many such alterations only appear after the GFR has risen. Micropuncture studies of single nephron GFR in the pregnant rat indicate that the increase in GFR is due to increased glomerular plasma flow, which in turn is a result of renal vasodilatation (7). Clinically, the alterations in renal hemodynamics result in a lowering of the normal values for serum creatinine and urea nitrogen levels, compared to nonpregnant levels.

There are several other renal adaptations to pregnancy. These include increased uric acid clearance, decreased plasma osmolality, increased urinary calcium excretion, and cumulative retention of sodium.

C. Endocrine Changes

Dramatic endocrine adaptations to pregnancy include changes in hormonal systems which may influence volume regulation and vascular reactivity. The fetus, placenta, and maternal ovary and adrenal gland participate in the production of large amounts of estradiol-17 beta, estriol, progesterone, aldosterone, deoxycorticosterone, human placental lactogen, and (hCG) as well as other pregnancy specific peptide hormones and prostaglandins. Both estrogen and progesterone have been shown to have hemodynamic and renal effects; therefore, it is likely that these hormones interact with other regulatory systems in the control of blood pressure during pregnancy.

Normal pregnancy is characterized by marked stimulation of all components of the renin-angiotensin-aldosterone system (RAAS) (8), apparent as early as the first trimester. Reasons for the stimulated RAAS during pregnancy are unclear, though the hemodynamic alterations (lower blood pressure and decreased systemic vascular resistance) likely contribute. In addition, estrogens stimulate the liver to produce angiotensinogen and there may be alteration of normal feedback suppression by angiotensin II (AII) (as occurs with contraceptive pill use). It is also hypothesized that intravascular volume, though increased, is "sensed" as suboptimal (decreased "effective volume"). Of note, levels of the RAAS change appropriately when gravidas are volume loaded, salt restricted, diuresed, or changed from a supine to an upright posture, all evidence that the "high" levels in pregnancy are physiologically appropriate (8).

Stimulation of the RAAS in pregnancy is associated with a marked refractoriness to the pressor effects of All (9). This decreased pressor sensitivity may be due, in part, to down regulation of vascular angiotensin receptors due to increased circulating All levels. Supporting this are observations of decreased ^{125}I-angiotensin binding to platelets in early pregnancy, which parallels the decrease in pressor response to All (10). Other hypotheses are that decreased vascular resistance may reflect enhanced basal or stimulated EDRF or alterations in neural reflex control of blood pressure in gestation (5).

III. THE HYPERTENSIVE DISORDERS OF PREGNANCY

A. The Importance of Accurate Diagnosis

The important diagnostic issue in pregnancy hypertension is the identification of preeclampsia, as it is this disorder which is associated with the greatest maternal and fetal morbidity and mortality. Moreover, important interventions, such as a decision to deliver, are often based on clinical impressions of the disease responsible for the hypertension. Thus the appropriate diagnosis may have significant implications for the future of the fetus.

B. Terminology

Although there are many proposed classification schemes for the hypertensive disorders of pregnancy, we use the Committee on Terminology of the American College of Obstetricians and Gynecologist's 1972 report (11), believing it the most practical of all those proposed. In this nosology, women with hypertension in pregnancy are classified into four groups: (1) chronic hypertension, (2) preeclampsia-eclampsia, (3) chronic hypertension with superimposed preeclampsia, or (4) transient hypertension.

Preeclampsia, the disorder unique to pregnancy, occurs primarily in primigravidas after the 20th week of gestation and is characterized by elevated blood pressure, proteinuria, generalized edema, and at times coagulation and/or liver function abnormalities. There is vasospasm, at times severe, which may lead to reduced perfusion of multiple organs including uterus, placenta, kidney, brain, and liver. Indeed, although elevated blood pressure and proteinuria are clinically useful ways of diagnosing preeclampsia, they are usually late manifestations of a subclinical process that has been present since early pregnancy. Preeclampsia may progress rapidly, at times without warning, to a convulsive phase, eclampsia, a dramatic and life-threatening complication.

Chronic hypertension is hypertension that precedes conception and is usually due to essential hypertension. In many patients blood pressure decreases substantially during gestation and pregnancies proceed uneventfully. However, such women are at increased risk for the development of superimposed preeclampsia (12), which is diagnosed when blood pressure suddenly increases in late pregnancy, often in association with the onset of proteinuria and/or hyperuricemia, thrombocytopenia, and liver function abnormalities. Some women with chronic hypertension manifest proteinuria early in pregnancy as a result of the presence of intrinsic renal disease; by far the greatest number encountered in women of childbearing age are patients with diabetic nephropathy. Most other forms of chronic hypertension are rare in gestation, but, when they occur, they can be deceptive. These include several collagen diseases, such as periarteritis and scleroderma, and pheochromocytoma, in which life-threatening hypertensive crises can occur. Cushing's syndrome may exacerbate in pregnancy and is associated with poor fetal outcome. Finally there are two causes of secondary hypertension which may ameliorate in pregnancy: In women with primary aldosteronism, increased levels of progesterone may decrease kaliuresis and lower blood pressure, while the pressor resistance to angiotensin may normalize pressure in gravidas with renal artery stenosis. In all these instances superimposed preeclampsia is difficult to diagnose.

Some pregnant women experience mild or moderate elevations of blood pressure in late pregnancy or the immediate puerperium which normalize rapidly post partum. This entity, designated *transient hypertension*, usually has a benign course and probably identifies women destined to have essential hypertension later in life.

The remainder of this chapter focuses on the diagnosis and treatment of preeclampsia and chronic essential hypertension, since these are the disorders most commonly encountered.

IV. DIAGNOSIS OF PREECLAMPSIA

Establishing the diagnosis of preeclampsia implies that the hypertensive condition is caused by pregnancy, with the potential for various manifestations, including several life-threatening syndromes. The inherent implication in this diagnosis is that when the disease is progressing, the only cure may be delivery. The explosive nature of preeclampsia and its potential for malignant consequences in both mother and child have led clinicians to err on the side of overdiagnosis. Given the possible sequelae of underdiagnosis, this approach is appropriate.

Preeclampsia occurs more often in nulliparous women, complicating about 6% of such pregnancies (12). The clinical diagnosis of preeclampsia in multiparas is frequently erroneous, a fact best illustrated in studies where diagnoses based on clinical criteria were followed up with postpartum renal biopsies (13). The abnormality noted was often that of nephrosclerosis or a primary kidney disease and not the characteristic lesion of preeclampsia.

Identification of patients at high risk for preeclampsia is important because it singles out those who require closer surveillance and identifies individuals who may be candidates for the newer preventive and therapeutic strategies. The risk factors for pure or superimposed preeclampsia are (1) nulliparity, (2) family history of preeclampsia, (3) multiple gestation, (4) chronic hypertension, (5) diabetes, (6) hydatidiform mole, (7) nonimmune hydrops fetalis, (8) extremes of reproductive age, and, possibly, (9) histories of intrauterine growth retardation or (10) early severe preeclampsia in a previous gestation.

A. Physical Signs

1. Blood Pressure

Elevations in blood pressure after midpregnancy in previously normotensive women are often the initial clue to the development of preeclampsia. Blood pressure measurements are taken at every antepartum visit; thus it is not surprising that hypertension has been the focus of much of the investigation into the pathophysiological processes and therapy of preeclampsia. More recently it has been suggested that hypertension is but one of many signs and symptoms of a multisystem illness. Some even emphasize that focusing on this sign alone has led to erroneous approaches to therapy, ones which unduly emphasize lowering the blood pressure (14).

The standard criteria for diagnosing hypertension in pregnancy are (1) systolic blood pressure increases of 30 mm Hg or greater and (2) diastolic blood pressure (Korotkoff V) increases of 15 mm Hg or greater compared to the average of values prior to 20 weeks gestation (15). When prior blood pressure values are not known, a reading of 140/90 mm Hg is considered abnormal. Thus, a level of 120/80 mm Hg may represent substantial hypertension in a woman whose previously recorded value was 90/50 mm Hg. Failure to appreciate that seemingly "normal" levels of blood pressure may be abnormal is one reason a clinician may overlook the diagnoses of preeclampsia. A modest rise in blood pressure in the second trimester may be the initial sign of the disease, and if the physician does not recognize this and schedules a revisit 3 to 4 weeks later, the patient may experience severe hypertension and/or other syndromes dangerous to both mother and fetus. Thus, any elevation in blood pressure must be evaluated, and it is prudent to overdiagnose rather than miss mild cases.

Controversy exists on how to measure blood pressure in pregnant women. The United States National High Blood Pressure Education Program (NHBPEP) Working Group recommends that Korotkoff V (disappearance) be used to designate diastolic pressure, while a World Health Organization task force suggests Korotkoff IV (muffling). Johenning and Barron (16) note the superiority of using the fifth sound, since it is the value used in nonpregnant populations and the fourth sound may overestimate diastolic pressure in 5 to 10 mm Hg.

2. Proteinuria

The definition of abnormal proteinuria is 300 mg/24 hr or above. Dipstick determinations of proteinuria may be erroneous or misleading (17), and it is advisable to confirm qualitative evidence of proteinuria with a timed urine collection (usually 24 hours, but shorter durations will suffice when close supervision is required). The magnitude of proteinuria may vary greatly from barely abnormal to frankly nephrotic levels. The diagnosis of preeclampsia in the absence of proteinuria is uncertain; however, it is important to recognize that proteinuria may be a late manifestation of this disorder. Therefore, it may be necessary to treat women as preeclamptic before proteinuria develops.

3. Edema

Edema frequently occurs during normal gestation and its presence alone is not a useful diagnostic criterion for preeclampsia; nor does its absence make preeclampsia an unlikely diagnosis. Sudden and rapid weight gain is more likely in women in whom preeclampsia develops.

B. Symptoms

Women with preeclampsia are frequently asymptomatic; thus the diagnosis is often made on discovering elevated blood pressure associated with sudden weight gain and qualitative proteinuria after a previous uneventful antepartum visit. Many women have nonspecific symptoms, such as mild headache, various aches, and fatigue. There are, however, several symptoms which can be ominous and are important to recognize, since they may signify imminent explosive disease with serious complications (Table 1).

Table 1 Ominous Signs and Symptoms in Women with Preeclampsia

Blood pressure ⩾160 mm Hg systolic or ⩾110 mm Hg diastolic
Proteinuria of new onset at a rate of ⩾2 g/24 hr or ⩾100 mg/dl in a randomly collected specimen
Increasing serum creatinine levels (especially > 177 μmol/L [2 mg/dl] unless the level was known to be elevated previously)
Platelet count < 100,000 μL or evidence of microangiopathic hemolytic anemia (e.g., schistocytes or increase in lactic acid dehydrogenase and direct bilirubin levels)
Upper abdominal pain, especially epigastric and right-upper-quadrant pain
Headache, visual disturbances, or other cerebral signs
Cardiac decompensation (e.g., pulmonary edema, usually associated with underlying heart disease or chronic hypertension)
Retinal hemorrhage, exudates, or papilledema (these signs are extremely rare in the absence of other indicators of severity and, when present, almost always indicate underlying chronic hypertension)
Fetal growth retardation

Source: Ref. 15.

C. Laboratory Tests

Laboratory tests are important in establishing the diagnosis and assessing the severity of preeclampsia. It is helpful to record baseline data in high-risk patients at an early stage of pregnancy. The standard laboratory evaluation for a woman suspected of having preeclampsia includes urinanalysis, hematocrit, and platelet count; serum creatinine, urea nitrogen, uric acid, and albumin levels; as well as liver function (Table 2). A particular constellation of laboratory abnormalities designated by the eponym HELLP syndrome (hemolysis, elevated liver function tests, low platelet count) is often seen in the woman complaining of epigastric pain. Peripheral smears also show evidence of microangiopathic hemolytic anemia, and these patients have life-threatening disease requiring emergency delivery (18).

Numerous other laboratory abnormalities have been identified in patients with preeclampsia. They have helped to identify certain features of the path-

Table 2

Test	Rationale
Hemoglobin and hematocrit	Hemoconcentration supports diagnosis of preeclampsia and is an indicator of severity. Values may be decreased, creased, however, if hemolysis accompanies the disease.
Blood smear	Signs of microangiopathic hemolytic anemia (e.g., schistocytes) favor diagnosis of preeclampsia and may be present when blood pressure is only mildly elevated.
Platelet count	Decreased levels suggest severe preeclampsia.
Urinalysis	If qualitative dipstick is 1+ or greater, a quantitative measurement of protein excretion should be done. Hypertensive gravidas with proteinuria should be considered preeclamptic (pure or superimposed) until proved otherwise.
Serum creatinine level	Abnormal or rising levels, especially when associated with oliguria, suggest severe preeclampsia.
Serum uric acid level	Increased levels aid in the differential diagnosis of preeclampsia and are an indicator of disease severity.
Serum oxaloacetic transaminase	Abnormal values suggest severe preeclampsia with hepatic involvement.
Lactic acid dehydrogenase	Elevated levels are associated with both hemolysis and hepatic involvement and suggest severe preeclampsia.
Serum albumin	Values may be decreased even in the absence of heavy proteinuria and may relate to "capillary leak" or hepatic involvement in preeclampsia.

Source: Ref. 15.

ogenesis of preeclampsia, and some have been proposed as useful predictors of the disease when measured early in pregnancy.

Indeed, early prediction of preeclampsia has long been a quest of both investigators and clinicians. For the investigator, laboratory abnormalities present before clinical manifestations of the disease provide invaluable clues to pathogenesis. For the clinician, reliable predictors allow early intervention and close surveillance. Thus far, analysis of currently available predictive tests suggests that they do not have sufficient sensitivity nor specificity to be recommended (19).

D. Differential Diagnosis

As noted, preeclampsia is rare before 20 weeks, unless trophoblast disease is present. When hypertension, proteinuria, and edema develop in the latter part of pregnancy in a previously normotensive nulliparous women, the diagnosis is fairly secure. However, there are many other scenarios, less clear-cut, in which the possibility of other disorders must be considered.

When signs and symptoms appear after midpregnancy, additional diagnostic considerations include transient hypertension and chronic hypertension, either essential or secondary, the latter including systemic illness such as lupus erythematosus. Of course, *superimposed* preeclampsia may develop with any of these conditions and treatment is individualized, based on all aspects of maternal and fetal well-being (see later discussion). The development of severe preeclampsia at midpregnancy or early in the last trimester, particularly in a multiparous woman, suggests that an underlying chronic medical condition is present.

The rapid development of renal insufficiency and thrombocytopenia in pregnant women with hypertension and proteinuria raises the possibility of thrombotic microangiopathy (either thrombotic thrombocytopenic purpura [TTP] or hemolytic uremic syndrome [HUS]). These ominous conditions have many features in common with the "HELLP" variant of preeclampsia, and differentiation among them is not always straightforward (20).

V. PATHOPHYSIOLOGICAL MECHANISMS OF PREECLAMPSIA

Preeclampsia, a multisystem disorder, is characterized by vasospasm, reduced blood flow, and ischemia in the kidney, liver, brain, and placenta. There are enhanced activation of the coagulation cascade and increased platelet aggregation. Past studies of the pathophysiological characteristics of preeclampsia focused on mechanisms of hypertension, cardiovascular hemodynamics, renal function, and coagulation. More recently, techniques in the fields of molecular and cell biology have been applied to research concerning the pathophysiological characteristics and cause of preeclampsia.

A. The Placenta

Many consider the placenta to be the major culprit in the pathophysiological mechanisms of preeclampsia, in part because delivery is the only definitive cure. Abnormalities in placentation, occurring between 10 and 20 weeks gestation, long before any clinical signs or symptoms, may be among the earliest pathological developments in this disorder (21). In normal pregnant women, the maternal spiral arteries, the blood vessels that supply the placenta, are transformed from thick walled muscular arteries into saclike flaccid vessels. This transformation permits greater volumes of blood delivery at a lower pressure and flow rate and appears to be due to invasion of maternal vessels by the trophoblast, resulting in the destruction of the elastic muscular walls and the endothelium of these vessels (22). In woman destined to have preeclampsia, trophoblastic invasion of maternal vessels is not as extensive, especially in the myometrial segments of the spiral arteries (23). The result is that these vessels remain muscular and responsive to vasoactive stimuli.

The net results of these alterations in the uteroplacental vessels are ischemic changes in the placenta and, ultimately, morphological damage and impairment of functional activity. One clinical implication of all this is that if reduced uteroplacental blood is involved in the pathogenesis preeclampsia, then antihypertensive therapy is not likely to cure the disorder, and theoretically could even aggravate it. Also, since uteroplacental perfusion is compromised in women with preeclampsia, reduction of blood pressure may jeopardize fetal well-being.

It is not known what causes the failure of trophoblast invasion of the maternal spiral arteries in women destined to have preeclampsia. Moreover, it is not clear how this process leads to maternal disease. One hypothesis, discussed further later, is that placental ischemia leads to release into the circulation of substances that mediate the multisystemic manifestations of preeclampsia.

There is also growing evidence that preeclampsia is characterized by generalized endothelial cell dysfunction, and that many of the features of the disorder, including vasospasm, increased intravascular coagulation, and reduced organ flow, are a direct consequence of endothelial dysfunction. Roberts and colleagues (24) have hypothesized that reduced placental perfusion results in release of circulating factors (e.g., mitogenic substances, lipid peroxides, and antiendothelial cell antibodies) that cause generalized endothelial cell damage in the maternal vasculature. Indeed, the observation that vascular prostacyclin production is diminished whereas thromboxane A2 generation is increased (25) are in accord with the notion that endothelial damage and platelet aggregation are involved in the pathogenesis of the disease. Additional supportive evidence for a role of altered prostaglandins in the pathophysiological processes of preeclampsia is supplied by reports of the efficacy of low-dose aspirin in preventing preeclampsia in susceptible individuals (discussed later).

Other products of endothelial cells such as EDRF (5) and endothelin (26) may be involved in the pathogenesis of preeclampsia.

The net results of these abnormalities of vascular endothelial function and prostaglandin metabolism are generalized vasospasm, increased intravascular coagulation, and decreased organ perfusion, leading to the multisystemic clinical manifestations characteristic of preeclampsia described later.

B. Blood Pressure

The hypertension of preeclampsia is characterized by marked lability, reversal of the normal circadian rhythm, and increased sensitivity to several vasoconstrictors (e.g., norepinephrine, and AII). Whereas in normal pregnancy, plasma renin activity (PRA) is elevated (compared with that in nonpregnant individuals), most authors observe that PRA and aldosterone secretion are suppressed in women with preeclampsia (27). This suggests that the hypertension is not mediated by angiotensin II, although given the increased sensitivity to pressors, AII may still play a role. It is hoped that further investigation of vascular endothelial cell function will clarify the mechanism of hypertension in preeclampsia.

C. Cardiac Function

There is controversy regarding the cardiovascular hemodynamics in preeclampsia with reports of a wide spectrum of hemodynamic profiles (1,28). Cardiac outputs have been reported to be high, normal, or low, usually with high systemic vascular resistance. This controversy has important therapeutic implications, since some recommend treating severe preeclamptics with a combination of volume expansion and vasodilator therapy (28) while others point out that such an approach may lead to pulmonary edema (29). There is wide variability in the clinical presentation of preeclampsia. Thus, each patient needs to be evaluated on an individual basis, a strategy that is usually appropriate for any seriously ill patient.

D. Plasma Volume

Plasma volume, usually measured by Evans Blue dye dilution, is reduced in women with preeclampsia, and there is evidence that such reductions may precede the development of hypertension (30).

E. Renal Function

Functionally patients demonstrate proteinuria and reduced glomerular filtration rate and renal plasma flow. There are also decreased urate clearance, hypocalciuria, and often decreased ability of the kidney to excrete sodium (31).

F. The Liver

Liver dysfunction may occur in preeclampsia, and the clinical spectrum encompasses mild elevations of liver enzymes to liver rupture (32). As noted, evidence of liver dysfunction may be an indication of severe disease and fetal jeopardy, especially when accompanied by signs of a microangiopathic hemolytic anemia (see "HELLP" Syndrome).

G. The Brain

Eclampsia, the convulsive phase of the disorder, is a major cause of death in women with this disease. The mechanisms leading to convulsions are not known; cerebral edema, vasospasm leading to severe ischemia or hemorrhage, and hypertensive encephalopathy have all been postulated (33).

VI. THERAPY OF PREECLAMPSIA

The principles of treating preeclampsia have changed little over the past three decades, despite advances in understanding its pathophysiological mechanisms. In essence, the progress made relates to early recognition, close maternal and fetal surveillance, seizure prophylaxis, judicious use of antihypertensive therapy, and timely delivery.

A. Prevention

1. Low-Dose Aspirin

Within the last 10 years the tantalizing possibility of preventing preeclampsia appeared to be within our grasp. Yet, as of 1994 there was still uncertainty as to the utility of these new preventive strategies. Preliminary data from several small clinical trials conducted in the mid-1980s suggested that low-dose aspirin (50 to 150 mg daily) administered early in gestation may prevent preeclampsia (34). It was hypothesized that such therapy reversed the imbalance between prostacyclin and thromboxane that may be responsible for many of the manifestations of this disease. More recently a few larger studies (35–38) have been completed and it appears there are several unanswered questions. For example, two groups came to different conclusions regarding the effectiveness of aspirin in preventing preeclampsia in relatively low-risk normotensive nulliparas (35,36) and in one study (36) there was an increased incidence of placental abruption in women ingesting aspirin. In another study of higher-risk patients aspirin appeared to have no effect on the incidence of preeclampsia, however, this was not a placebo-controlled trial (37). Most recently, a large multicenter trial performed in the United Kingdom failed to demonstrate a beneficial effect of aspirin in a low to moderate risk population (38). Other concerns are the time in pregnancy when therapy should be instituted and the appropriate dose. Most would agree that therapy should begin before 24 weeks, and that aspirin is not effective once clinical manifestations of preeclampsia are apparent. Regarding dose, although amounts as low as 50 mg daily may be sufficient, this issue has not been rigorously evaluated.

One large multicenter trial of aspirin in "high-risk" patients is nearing completion. While there is still no consensus on whether to treat at all, and who should be treated, some physicians are prescribing aspirin to a few select patients who appear to be at high risk for preeclampsia, including those with a history of recurrent fetal death, marked fetal growth retardation, or previous pregnancies complicated by severe preeclampsia of early onset and poor fetal outcome.

2. Calcium Supplementation

On the basis of epidemiological evidence that the incidence of preeclampsia is lower in populations with high dietary intake of calcium (39), and that high-calcium diets lower blood pressure in pregnant women, calcium supplementation (1 to 2 grams of elemental calcium in addition to dietary intake) during pregnancy has been proposed for the prevention of preeclampsia (40). Preliminary data from one large and well-performed clinical trial appeared promising but were inconclusive (41). A large multicenter trial designed to evaluate the efficacy of calcium supplementation in the prevention of preeclampsia is nearing completion.

B. Treatment of Preeclampsia

1. The Need For Hospitalization

When hypertension develops in late pregnancy, especially when the diagnosis of preeclampsia appears certain, hospitalization is usually recommended. This approach is even advisable when preeclampsia is only suspected, given the explosive nature of the disease, and once the diagnosis is made, patients are best treated in the hospitals until delivery. Occasionally, if after careful evaluation a woman appears to have very mild disease (i.e., minimally elevated blood pressure, normal renal function, minimal proteinuria, normal fetal testing), or if signs and symptoms ameliorate, she can be discharged, and her clinical course closely followed at home (often with frequent nurse visits and home fetal monitoring).

2. Delivery

Delivery is the only cure for preeclampsia, although occasionally the disease appears to develop in the first postpartum week, or transiently worsen in the immediate puerperium. The decision to deliver is extremely important for the future health and well-being of the fetus and is made by the obstetrician, but internists involved in the care of pregnant women must be cognizant of the issues involved in such decisions.

When preeclampsia develops close to term, and fetal maturity is certain, then delivery is advisable. Difficulties arise when the disease manifests at a time when the fetus is still quite immature and its survival in doubt; then one must decide whether it is safe for the mother to postpone delivery. Most physicians would terminate the pregnancy in the presence of persistent severe hypertension (diastolic blood pressure above 110 mm Hg), abnormal liver function test results, low platelet count (below 100,000/mm^3), deteriorating renal function, significant headache or visual disturbances, and right upper quadrant discomfort (Table 1). Conservative management in such cases may not be associated with improved fetal outcome and may in fact result in serious maternal morbidity (42). On the other hand, when a woman remote from term has but mild to moderate hypertension, and no signs of deteriorating renal or hepatic function or coagulopathy, temporization should be attempted, though it may be necessary to administer antihypertensive therapy to maintain blood pressure in a safe range (e.g., below 110 mm Hg diastolic; see later discussion). Such women are best treated in the hospital, where it is easier to monitor progression of the disease and intercede rapidly if complications arise. Also, hospitalization permits frequent antepartum testing, including nonstress testing, sonography, and biophysical profiling, the tests that help predict fetal jeopardy, and the decision to continue temporization can be made on a day to day basis. It must be stressed, however, that conservative treatment of early preeclampsia entails risks and is most appropriate at a tertiary care center, where aggressive monitoring of maternal and fetal status is possible (43).

3. Nonpharmacological Therapy

If a decision to postpone delivery is made, then the most important therapeutic intervention is enforcing modified bed rest. This is obviously best accomplished in a hospital setting, as most women are unable to get sufficient rest at home, especially if they have small children.

Dietary modifications have not been shown to alter the course of preeclampsia favorably. Still, in cases of edema and labile blood pressure many physicians prescribe moderate (e.g., 60 to 80 mEq/day) sodium restriction. As mentioned, it appears that adequate calcium intake may play a role in prevention; however, there is little information on the effects of calcium or other minerals once preeclampsia has developed.

4. Antihypertensive Therapy

The role of antihypertensive therapy in the management of preeclampsia is controversial, largely because of the concern that lowering maternal blood pressure might further compromise placental perfusion, while there is no evidence to suggest that it would cure or reverse preeclampsia (Table 3). At best it may help prevent premature delivery in situations where the level of blood pressure is the most worrisome manifestation of disease. Thus, reduction of pressure is performed primarily for maternal safety.

There is disagreement regarding what level of blood pressure should be treated. In the peripartum period, many authorities would begin therapy when diastolic pressure was 105 mm Hg or greater. Excessive reduction of blood pressure (e.g., below 90 mm Hg) should be prevented since it may compromise placental function.If temporization is planned, then it is advisable to start treatment when diastolic levels approach 100 mm Hg. Therapy should be individualized, however, taking into consideration the woman's early pregnancy blood pressure, the rate of rise, and the symptoms. If we are unable to control blood pressure satisfactorily with two antihypertensive agents within 24 to 48 hours, the advisability of continuing the pregnancy is questionable.

Agents with a rapid onset of action are most desirable when pressure is high and delivery appears imminent (within 24 to 48 hours). The ideal drug should act quickly, reduce pressure in a controlled manner (i.e., avoiding precipitous declines), and result in no adverse maternal or fetal effect. The drug most commonly used to manage hypertension in the peripartum period has been intravenous hydralazine (44). Treatment should always be gentle, commencing with 5-mg doses, followed by 5 to 10 mg every 20 to 30 minutes.

Of interest is a recent report (45) which, though limited in scope, noted that hydralazine used to treat women with eclampsia was associated with a greater incidence of serious ventricular arrhythmias compared to that of patients receiving labetalol (see later discussion). Also, as of this writing, there is some uncertainty regarding the continued availability of intravenous hydralazine in the United States. Thus although this drug has the longest "track record" by far in obstetric medicine, physicians may be forced to use other agents with which there is less experience.

Parenteral labetalol has been administered to women with preeclampsia with favorable results (46). This combined alpha-1- and beta-blocker is effective in treating hypertension in the peripartum period and compares favorably with hydralazine with respect to fetal effects. There is always concern that drugs with beta-blocking action may compromise the ability of the fetus

Table 3 Drug Therapy of Acute, Severe Hypertension in Pregnancy[a]

Drug	Dose/route[b]	Onset of action	Adverse effects[c]	comments
Agent of choice				
Hydralazine	5 mg i.v./i.m., then 5–10 mg every 20–40 min; or constant infusion of 0.5–10 mg/hr	i.v.: 10 min i.m.: 10–30 min	Headache, flushing, tachycardia, nausea, vomiting; possible increase in ventricular arrhythmia	Broad experience of safety and efficacy
Second-line agents				
Labetalol	20 mg i.v., then 20–80 mg every 20–30 min, up to 300 mg; or or constant infusion of 1–2 mg/min until desired effect, then stop or reduce to 0.5 mg/min	5–10 mm	Flushing, nausea, vomiting, tingling of scalp	Limited experience in pregnancy
Nifedipine	5–10 mg p.o.; repeat in 30 min if necessary, then 10–20 mg p.o. every 3–6 hr	10–15 min	Flushing, headache, tachycardia, nausea, inhibition of labor	May have synergistic interaction with $MgSO_4$; limited experience in pregnancy
Diazoxide	30–50 mg i.v. every 5–15 min	2–5 min	Inhibition of labor; hyperglycemia, fluid retention with repeated doses	Doses of 150–300 mg may cause severe hypotension; may displace phenytoin from serum protein binding sites
Relative contraindication				
Nitroprusside	0.5–10 μg/kg/min by constant i.v. infusion	Instantaneous	Cyanide toxicity, nausea, vomiting	Use only in critical care unit at low doses for briefest time feasible; may cause fetal cyanide toxicity

[a]Indicated for acute elevation of Korotkoff Phase V diastolic blood pressure to >105 mm Hg; goal is gradual reduction to 90–100 mm Hg.
[b]Abbreviations: i.v., intravenously; i.m., intramuscularly; p.o., per os (orally).
[c]All agents may cause marked hypotension, especially in severe preeclampsia.
Source: Ref. 75.

to withstand hypoxic stress, but there is preliminary evidence that suggests that uteroplacental blood flow is maintained after parenteral use of labetalol (47).

Calcium channel blockers have several features that make them attractive agents for control of hypertension in preeclampsia: a rapid onset of action; freedom from serious side effects, including hypotension; and renal vasodilatation. Unfortunately, there is limited information on the use of these agents in pregnancy (48,49). Most reports through 1993 involved the calcium channel blocker nifedipine, suggesting that this drug is quite effective in controlling blood pressure, with good fetal outcomes. There are, however, anecdotal reports that the interaction of magnesium sulfate and calcium channel blockade has led to precipitous falls in blood pressure (50). Therefore, it is advisable to await the results of additional trials before using these agents on a routine basis.

5. *Prevention and Treatment of Convulsions*

There continues to be controversy on how to prevent and/or treat eclamptic convulsions. In the United States, parenteral magnesium sulfate is routinely administered in the peripartum period to prevent convulsions (44), and this approach has been endorsed in the Consensus Report (15). Recently, Belfort and colleagues have utilized Doppler techniques to demonstrate magnesium sulfate-induced dilatation of the intracranial vasculature in preeclamptic women (51). Thus it is possible that the anticonvulsant properties of magnesium may be in part secondary to relief of vasospasm.

Outside the United States, phenytoin, phenobarbital and diazepam, or nothing is used as an alternative to magnesium sulfate. A large multicenter trial comparing magnesium sulfate, diazepam, and phenytoin in patients with eclampsia is under way and reports have appeared that calcium channel blockers with central action may provide alternative ways to prevent and treat eclampsia (52).

6. *Hemodynamic Monitoring*

In very severe or extremely complicated cases, invasive hemodynamic monitoring may be useful, particularly when respiratory difficulty or bleeding arises. We find the need for Swan Ganz catheterization relatively uncommon, as most cases can be managed with clinical acumen alone.

7. *Postpartum Issues*

Although delivery is the "cure" for preeclampsia, it is important to recognize that the disease may only become apparent in the postpartum period, particularly during the first week of the puerperium. Moreover, several of the clinical and laboratory abnormalities may worsen post partum, before they remit. This has been well documented in women with HELLP syndrome, in whom the nadir of thrombocytopenia is often most severe 48 to 72 hours post partum (53). Hypertension, too, can persist after delivery and in many patients, 2 to 3 weeks is required for hypertension to resolve completely. This is particularly important in the woman who wishes to breast feed, since antihypertensive agents are likely to enter breast milk (54), although concentrations are low.

VII. RECURRENCE OF PREECLAMPSIA AND PROGNOSIS

Elegant studies of Chesley and colleagues have demonstrated that the development of preeclampsia or eclampsia is not predictive of the later development of essential hypertension (55). The extent to which this is true seems to depend on the certainty of the diagnosis of preeclampsia. Multiparous women, who are more likely to have chronic hypertension, are more likely to have hypertension later in life (13).

With respect to future pregnancies, the long held view that preeclampsia is a disease of first pregnancy is for the most part true. However, in contrast to women who have had a previous normotensive pregnancy, women with preeclampsia as nulliparas *are* at increased risk for development of either hypertension or preeclampsia in subsequent pregnancies (56). It appears that these risks are related to the time of onset of preeclampsia during the first pregnancy, with the highest risk in those whose disease manifested remote from term, particularly in the second trimester.

VIII. CHRONIC HYPERTENSION DURING PREGNANCY

The prevalence of chronic hypertension in pregnancy is not known and differs widely in different geographic areas but is probably between 3% and 10% of all pregnancies. As noted, many or most multiparas whose elevated blood pressure is first discovered in late pregnancy have or eventually will have essential hypertension.

The vast majority (85% or above) of pregnancies in women with chronic hypertension result in healthy term infants, but there appears to be an overall increase in perinatal morbidity and mortality (57), most of which is associated with superimposed preeclampsia.

A. Clinical Evaluation of Hypertensive Patients Before Conception

Hypertensive women contemplating pregnancy should be extensively evaluated prior to conceiving. It is important to exclude secondary forms of hypertension which have a guarded pregnancy prognosis. If diagnosed, curable secondary hypertension (hormone secreting masses primarily of adrenal nature, and renovascular hypertension) should be treated before pregnancy. Patients with intrinsic renal disease should be advised about the risks of pregnancy especially if azotemia (creatinine level above 1.4 mg/dl) and hypertension are present (58). These concerns are especially applicable to women who have had renal transplantation particularly when cyclosporine (which causes hypertension) is part of the immunosuppressive regimen. Such pregnancies should preferably be undertaken after consultation with a nephrologist who has expertise in this area.

Hypertensive women considering pregnancy should be advised as follows: Most cases of mild to moderate essential hypertension are associated with a favorable outcome, but there is an increased risk of superimposed preeclampsia. Such preconception counseling permits adjustments in life-style that may be necessary during pregnancy if elevated blood pressure resists control—specifically the possibility that restricted activity (including job furlough), bed rest, or even hospitalization may be advisable. Furthermore, certain antihypertensive agents that either are contraindicated in pregnancy (e.g., angiotensin converting inhibitors) or have not been used extensively and thus whose teratogenic potential is virtually unknown (most antihypertensives) can be discontinued, and if necessary other medications believed safer for pregnancy prescribed. Finally, one should counsel women with a history of severe hypertension, especially those who require multidrug therapy, against conceiving, and such a scenario is an indication for therapeutic abortion in early pregnancy.

B. Treatment

1. Life-Style Modifications

Close medical supervision is the mainstay of management of pregnant women with chronic hypertension. It is advisable to try to control the blood pressure without medication when possible, and in patients with mild hypertension this goal is not difficult to attain since blood pressure falls in most pregnant women during the first and second trimesters. Indeed, in women with preexisting hypertension the decrement may be as great as 20 mm Hg.

Some of the strategies for nonpharmacological therapy of hypertension during pregnancy differ from those in nonpregnant individuals. Whereas weight reduction and exercise might benefit a nonpregnant individual, these measures are not advised during gestation. On the other hand, pregnancy is an ideal time to abandon smoking given the motivational incentives that accompany this condition.

2. Restriction of Activity

Bed rest, especially in the lateral recumbent position, is believed to maximize uteroplacental blood flow and is considered established therapy in women with preeclampsia or chronic hypertension. All pregnant women with elevated blood pressure, whatever the cause, should be advised to limit their activities when possible and set aside time during the day when they can be "off their feet." Women manifesting severe hypertension should be treated in a hospital setting, where rest can be enforced and medications adjusted rapidly.

3. Diet

Weight reduction should be completed prior to attempting conception and cannot be recommended during pregnancy. Hypertensive pregnant women have lower plasma volume than normotensives, and some studies suggest that the severity of hypertension correlates with the degree of plasma volume contraction (59). For this reason, sodium restriction is generally not recommended during pregnancy. If, however, a pregnant woman with chronic hypertension has been successfully treated with a low-salt diet prior to pregnancy, then it is reasonable to continue this during pregnancy, although extreme sodium restriction (below 75 mEq/day) is not recommended.

As noted previously, calcium supplementation is being evaluated for the prevention of gestational hypertension. It might be argued that suspicion of benefit is grounds for calcium supplementation, given that it is an innocuous mineral. However, pregnant women are hypercalciuric and manifest increased urinary supersaturation ratios for calcium oxalate and phosphate (60). Thus, in addition to proving benefit in relation to blood pressure reduction, current trials must demonstrate the safety of such therapy, most specifically in regard to provoking renal stone formation.

4. Home Blood Pressure Monitoring

The rationale for close observation of the pregnant hypertensive woman is that changes in clinical status (such as development of superimposed preeclampsia) can be recognized before they become severe. This is easier to accomplish if patients are instructed to take their blood pressure at home and keep a record of the readings. They can then contact medical personnel if the blood pressure rises significantly, before a scheduled visit.

C. Antihypertensive Therapy

1. Rationale for Treatment

The majority of women with chronic hypertension in pregnancy have mild to moderate elevations in blood pressure, and thus the risk of acute cardiac or cerebrovascular complications is extremely low. In the small percentage of women who have severe hypertension (and who decline to terminate), the increased risk of cerebral hemorrhage, heart failure, and myocardial infarction necessitates close monitoring and aggressive treatment at all stages of gestation.

As noted, objectives of treatment in pregnant women are to minimize the short-term risks to the mother of elevated blood pressure, while avoiding therapeutic maneuvers that compromise fetal well-being. The specific goals for the mother are to prevent the cardiovascular complications associated with severe hypertension and, if possible, to prevent preeclampsia. When maternal hypertension is severe (diastolic blood pressure 110 mm Hg or above), treatment should be instituted to prevent hypertensive vascular damage.

The indications for treatment of mild to moderate hypertension during pregnancy are less clear, in nonpregnant individuals, treatment is recommended for prevention of long-term cardiovascular consequences of elevated blood pressure. For the relatively short duration of a pregnancy these concerns are not relevant, whereas the prevention of preeclampsia and maintenance of fetal well-being are. The literature is controversial as to whether treatment of mild to moderate hypertension prevents preeclampsia or improves fetal outcome (61,62). Given the uncertainty surrounding the hazards of antihypertensive treatment during pregnancy (e.g., decreases in placental perfusion and/or adverse effects on embryo or fetus), treatment of mild to moderate hypertension must be undertaken cautiously. Excessive blood pressure reduction is to be avoided and a conservative approach is recommended. If diastolic blood pressure early in the first trimester is between 90 and 100 mm Hg, it is reasonable to await the expected physiological decrease in blood pressure before prescribing antihypertensives. If in the initial trimester the diastolic blood pressure is below 90 mm Hg and the patient is ingesting antihypertensive drugs, reduction of dose or discontinuance of the medication can be considered. The NHBPEP Working Group recommended treatment when diastolic blood pressures are consistently 100 mm Hg (Korotkoff V) or greater (15).

2. *Antihypertensive Medications*

The ideal drug is one with established antihypertensive action in gravid women and no evidence of immediate or long-term effects on fetus or neonate. There is a paucity of information concerning use of antihypertensive drugs in gestation, especially the evaluation of fetal risks. It is unfortunate that there are so few well conducted studies of safety and efficacy of antihypertensive medications in pregnant women. Most, limited in scope, are performed at the request and with the support of pharmaceutical companies (the vast majority outside the United States) and do not meet the standards for good trials. Keeping these criticisms in mind, let us explore drugs currently used to treat chronic hypertension in pregnancy (Table 4).

Table 4 Drug Therapy of Chronic Hypertension in Pregnancy[a,c]

Drug [FDA Class][c]	Daily Dose	Adverse Effects and Comments
Agent of choice		
Methyldopa [C]	500–3000 mg in 2–4 divided doses	Safety for mother and fetus (after 1st trimester) is well documented.
Second-line agents		
Hydralazine [C]	50–300 mg in 2–4 divided doses	Few controlled trials but extensive experience with few serious adverse effects documented; several reports of neonatal thrombocytopenia.
Labetalol [C]	200–1200 mg in 2–3 divided doses	Less experience than methyldopa; efficacy and short-term safety appear equal to methyldopa's
Beta-adrenergic inhibitors [C]	Dependent on specific agent used	May cause fetal bradycardia and impair fetal responses to hypoxia. Risk of intrauterine growth retardation when begun in 1st/2nd trimester.
Nifedipine [C]	30–120 mg in 1–4 divided doses depending on preparation used	Limited data; may inhibit labor; may have synergistic action with MgSO4.
Clonidine [C]	0.1–0.8 mg in 2 divided doses	Limited data.
Prazosin [C]	1–30 mg in 2–3 divided doses	Limited data.
Thiazide diuretics [D assignation in reference[282]]	Dependent on agent used	Most controlled studies in normotensive gravidas; few data in hypertensive gestation. Implicated in volume depletion, electrolyte imbalance, pancreatitis, and thrombocytopenia.

Contraindicated		
Angiotensin converting enzyme inhibitors [X][d]	Dependent on agent used	High rates of fetal loss in animals. Many cases of oligohydramnios, intrauterine growth retardation, neonatal anuric renal failure, occasionally fatal. Use only when absolutely necessary to preserve maternal well-being and other agents are unsuccessful.

[a]Note that safety during the first trimester has not been established for any antihypertensive agent.

[b]Drug therapy indicated for uncomplicated chronic hypertension when phase V diastolic BP $\geqslant$100 mm Hg. Treatment at lower levels may be indicated for patients with renal disease and/or diabetes mellitus.

[c]United States Food and Drug Administration Classification.

[d]Our classification: noted as [D] in PDR.

Source: Ref. 75.

a. Central Adrenergic Inhibitors. Methyldopa, an alpha$_2$-agonist, has been most extensively evaluated in gravidas with chronic hypertension, including two relatively large randomized trials and a long-term follow-up study of offspring of mothers exposed during pregnancy (63–65). Most published data attest to its safety, but one study in animals (66) noted depletion of neonatal cardiac catecholamines. While there have been no reports suggesting an impaired ability of the human fetus or newborn to mount an adequate cardiac response to stress, this theoretical problem warrants scrutiny. Methyldopa's proven track record in pregnancy makes it the drug of choice for the treatment of pregnant women with chronic hypertension (15).

There have been very vew reports of use of the alpha$_2$-agonist clonidine in pregnancy (67). We cannot recommend use of clonidine because of limited experience with this medication in comparison to methyldopa, a drug with a similar mechanism of action as well as an extensive record of use in gravid women.

b. Beta-Adrenoreceptor-Blockers. Beta-blockers have been used quite extensively in pregnancy (68–70). However, their safety has not been as conclusively established as has methyldopa's. These agents cross the placenta. Except perhaps for intrauterine growth retardation (IUGR), other claims of neonatal respiratory depression, bradycardia, and hypoglycemia in humans, as well as observations of altered fetal cardiovascular responses to hypoxia in animals, have not been confirmed in prospective, randomized comparisons (70). Thus, there is still reason to be cautious.

c. Combined Beta-Alpha-Adrenergic-Blockers. Labetalol compares favorably with methyldopa and is considered appropriate as a second-line agent (71,72). Of concern, however, are reports of hepatotoxicity in nonpregnant patients and a report of an increase in retroplacental clots in gravidas receiving the drug (72).

d. Calcium Channel Blockers. As noted in the Preeclampsia section, there is limited information regarding use of calcium channel blockers. As of 1994, published data are too limited to warrant their use in gravidas with chronic hypertension and thus we restrict their use (predominantly of nifedipine) to instances where hypertension is severe, other agents appear ineffective, and there is a desire to prolong the pregnancy.

e. Angiotensin Converting Enzyme Inhibitors. Angiotensin converting enzyme (ACE) inhibitors, extensively used in nongravid, young hypertensives, are contraindicated in pregnancy because of serious neonatal problems including renal failure and death (73). Current thinking is that the detrimental effects occur during second and third trimester exposure, and there are no conclusive data that ACE inhibitors are teratogenic. This is important in counseling women who conceived while ingesting ACE inhibitors. Ideally, hypertensive women contemplating pregnancy should be treated with other agents. When it is necessary to use these agents we advise our patients to discontinue them as soon as they miss their period.

f. Diuretics. The use of diuretics during gestation is controversial. One major concern, albeit theoretical, is that these agents may prevent the physiological volume expansion that accompanies normal pregnancy. In this respect there is extensive experience with prophylactic diuretics in nonhypertensive pregnant populations, without clear-cut evidence of adverse effects (74), but there is little information on saluretic use in women with chronic hypertension. Nevertheless, we concur with the recommendations of the NHBPEP Working Group Report that pregnant hypertensives may be treated with diuretics if they are taking these agents prior to pregnancy or if they have a history of salt-sensitive hypertension.

D. Secondary Hypertension

Only a small percentage of pregnant hypertensives have secondary hypertension, and the principles by which such patients are treated are similar to those outlined here and covered in Chapter 11.

IX. CONCLUSION

Successful treatment of hypertension complicating pregnancy requires cognizance of normal gestational physiological mechanisms; appreciation of the complexities of a disorder unique to pregnancy, preeclampsia; and awareness of the implications for the fetus of any contemplated therapeutic intervention. Many of the principles used when treating hypertension in nongravid populations are not relevant during pregnancy. In addition, there are many variables involved in treating gravid women; thus it is essential that therapy be individualized. It is our belief that a team of internists familiar with pregnancy and obstetricians familiar with hypertension ensures the highest chance of a successful outcome.

REFERENCES

1. Wallenburg Henk CS. Hemodynamics in hypertensive pregnancy. In: Rubin PC, ed. Handbook of Hypertension, Hypertension in Pregnancy. New York: Elsevier, 1988:66–101.
2. Walters BWJ, Thompson ME, Lee A, DeSwiet M. Blood pressure in the puerperium. Clin Sci 1986; 71:589–594.
3. Terragno NA, McGiff JC, Murray S, Terragno A. Patterns of prostaglandin production in the bovine fetal and maternal vasculature. Prostaglandins 1978; 16: 847–855.

4. Tamai T, Matsuura S, Tatsumi N, et al. Role of sex steroid hormones in relative refractoriness to angiotensin II during pregnancy. Am J Obstet Gynecol 1984; 149:117.
5. Molnar M, Hertelendy F. N-Nitro-Larginine, an inhibitor of nitric oxide synthesis, increases blood pressure in rats and reverses the pregnancy induced refractoriness to vaspressor agents. Am J Obstet Gynecol 1992; 166:1560–1567.
6. Davison JM, Dunlop M. Renal hemodynamics and tubular function in normal human pregnancy. Kidney Int 1980; 18:152–161.
7. Baylis C. Effects of early pregnancy on glomerular filtration rate and plasma volume in the rat. Renal Physiol 1980; 2:333–339.
8. August P, Sealey JE. The renin-angiotensin system in normal and hypertensive pregnancy and in ovarian function. In: Laragh JH, Brenner BM, eds. Hypertension: Pathophysiology, Diagnosis and Management. New York: Raven Press, 1990:1761–1778.
9. Abdul-Karim R, Assali NS. Pressor response to angiotensin in pregnant and nonpregnant women. Am J Obstet Gynecol 1961; 82:246–251.
10. Baker PN, Pipkin FB, Symonds EM. Longitudinal study of platelet angiotensin II binding in human pregnancy. Clin Sci 1992; 82:377–381.
11. Hughes EC, ed. Obstetric-Gynecologic Terminology. Philadelphia: FA Davis, 1972:422–423.
12. Chesley LC. Hypertensive Disorders in Pregnancy. New York: Appleton-Century-Crofts, 1978.
13. Fisher KA, Luger A, Spargo BH, et al. Hypertension in pregnancy: clinical-pathological correlations and remote prognosis. Medicine 1981; 60:267–276.
14. Roberts JM, Redman CWG. Pre-eclampsia: more than pregnancy induced hypertension. Lancet 1993; 341:1447–1451.
15. National High Blood Pressure Education Program Working Group Report on High Blood Pressure in Pregnancy. Am J Obstet Gynecol 1990; 163:1689–1712.
16. Johenning AR, Barron WM. Indirect blood pressure measurement in pregnancy. Korotkoff phase 4 versus phase 5. Am J Obstet Gynecol 1992; 167:577–580.
17. Kuo VS, Koumantiakis G, Mappl SC, Gallery EDM. Proteinuria and its assessment in normal and hypertensive pregnancy. Am J Obstet Gynecol 1992; 167: 723–728.
18. Weinstein L. Syndrome of hemolysis, elevated liver enzymes and low platelet count: a severe consequence of hypertension in pregnancy. Am J Obstet Gynecol 1982; 142:159.
19. Dekker GA, Sibai BM. Early detection of preeclampsia. Am J Obstet Gynecol 1991; 165:160–172.
20. Saltiel C, Legendre C, Grumfeld J, et al. Hemolytic uremic synetrome Syndrome in association with pregnancy. In: Kaplan BS, Trompetes RS, Moake JL, eds. Hemolytic Uremic Syndrome and Thrombotic Thromboytopnia Purpura. New York: Marcel Dekker, 1992:241–255.
21. Fox H. The placenta in pregnancy hypertension. In: Rubin PC, ed. Handbook of Hypertension. Vol. 10. Hypertension in Pregnancy. New York: Elsevier, 1988:16–37.
22. Pijnenborg R, Bland JM, Robertson WB, et al. The pattern of interstitial trophoblastic invasion of the myometrium in early pregnancy. Placenta 1981; 2:303–316.

23. Khong TY, De Wolf F, Robertson WB, et al. Inadequate maternal vascular response to placentation in pregnancies complicated by pre-eclampsia and by small-for-gestational age infants. Br J Obstet Gynaecol 1986; 93:1049.
24. Roberts JM, Taylor RN, Musci TJ, et al. Preeclampsia: an endothelial cell disorder. Am J Obstet Gynecol 1989; 161:1200–1204.
25. Friedman SA. Preeclampsia: a review of the role of prostaglandins. Obstet and Gynecol 1988; 71(1):122–137.
26. Schiff E, Gen-Baruch G, Peleg E, et al. Immunoreactive circulating endothelin-1 in normal and hypertensive pregnancies. Am J Obstet Gynecol 1992; 166:625–628.
27. August P, Lenz T, Ales KL, et al. Longitudinal study of the renin-angiotensin-aldosterone system in hypertensive pregnant women: deviations related to the development of superimposed preeclampsia. Am J Obstet Gynecol 1990; 163: 1612–1621.
28. Cotton DB, Lee W, Huhta JC, et al. Hemodynamic profile of severe pregnancy induced hypertension. Am J Obstet Gynecol 1988; 158:523–529.
29. Mabie WC, Ratts TE, Sibai BM. The central hemodynamics of severe preeclampsia. Am J Obstet Gynecol 1989; 161:1443–1448.
30. Chesley LC, Lindheimer MD. Renal hemodynamics and intravascular volume in normal and hypertensive pregnancy. In: Rubin PC, ed. Handbook of Hypertension. Vol. 10. Hypertension in Pregnancy. New York: Elsevier, 1988:38–65.
31. Lindheimer MD, Katz AI. The kidney in pregnancy. In: Brenner BM, Rector FC Jr, eds. The Kidney, 3d ed. Philadelphia: WB Saunders, 1986:1253–1295.
32. Romero R, Vizoso J, Emamian M, et al. Clinical significance of liver dysfunction in pregnancy-induced hypertension. Am J Perinat 1988; 5:146–151.
33. Donaldson JO. Neurology of Pregnancy. 2d ed. London: WB Saunders, 1989.
34. Imperiale TF, Stollenwerk-Petrulis A. A meta-analysis of low-dose aspirin for the prevention of pregnancy-induced hypertensive disease. JAMA 1991; 226: 261–265.
35. Hauth JC, Goldenberg RL, Parker CR, et al. Low-dose aspirin therapy to prevent preeclampsia. Am J Obstet Gynecol 1993; 168:1083–1093.
36. Sibai B, Caritis S, Thom E, et al. Prevention of preeclampsia with low-dose aspirin in healthy nulliparous pregnant women trial. N Engl J Med 1993; 329: 1213–1218.
37. Italian Study of Aspirin in Pregnancy. Low-dose aspirin in prevention and treatment of intrauterine growth retardation and pregnancy-induced hypertension. Lancet 1993; 341:396–400.
38. CLASP Collaborative Group. CLASP: a randomized trial of low-dose aspirin for the prevention and treatment of pre-eclampsia among 9364 pregnant women. Lancet 1994; 343:619–629.
39. Belizan JM, Villar J. The relationship between calcium intake and edema-, proteinuria-, and hypertension-gestosis: an hypothesis. Am J Clin Nutr 1980; 33: 2202–2210.
40. Belizan JM, Villar J, Repke J. The relationship between calcium intake and pregnancy-induced hypertension: up-to-date evidence. Am J Obstet Gynecol 1988; 158:898–902.

41. Belizan J, Villar J, Gonzalez L, et al. Calcium supplementation to prevent hypertensive disorders of pregnancy. N Engl J Med 1991; 325(20):1399–1405.
42. Sibai BM, Taslimi M, Abdella TN, et al. Maternal and perinatal outcome of conservative management of severe preeclampsia in midtrimester. Am J Obstet Gynecol 1985; 152(suppl 1):32–37.
43. Sibai BM, Akl S, Fairlie F, Morett M. A protocol for managing severe preeclampsia in the second trimester. Am J Obstet Gynecol 1990; 163:733–738.
44. Pritchard JA, Cunningham FG, Pritchard FA. The Parkland Memorial Hospital protocol for treatment of eclampsia: evaluation of 245 cases. Am J Obstet Gynecol 1984; 148(7):951–963.
45. Bhorat IE, Naidoo DP, Rout CC, Moodley J. Malignant ventricular arrhythmias in eclampsia: a comparison of labetolol with dihydralazine. Am J Obstet Gynecol 1993; 168:1292–1296.
46. Lunell NO, Nyllund L, Lewander R, et al. Acute effect of an antihypertensive drug, labetalol, on uteroplacental blood flow. Br J Obstet Gynaecol 1982; 89: 640–644.
47. Jouppila P, Kirkinen P, Koivula A, et al. Labetalol does not alter the placental and fetal blood flow or maternal prostanoids in pre-eclampsia. Br J Obstet Gynaecol 1986; 93:543–547.
48. Walters BNJ, Redman CWG. Treatment of severe pregnancy-associated hypertension with the calcium antagonist nifedipine. Br J Obstet Gynaecol 1984; 91: 330–336.
49. Sibai BM, Barton JR, Akl S, et al. A randomized prospective comparison of nifedipine and bed rest versus bed rest alone in the management of preeclampsia remote from term. Am J Obstet Gynecol 1992; 167:879–884.
50. Snyder SW, Cardwell MS. Neuromuscular blockade with magnesium sulfate and nifedipine. Am J Obstet Gynecol 1989; 161:35–36.
51. Belfort MA, Moise KJ Jr. Effect of magnesium sulfate on maternal brain blood flow in preclampsia: a randomized, placebo-controlled study. Am J Obstet Gynecol 1992; 167:661–666.
52. Belfort MA, Carpenter RJ, Kirshon B, et al. The use of nimodipine in a patient with eclampsia: Color flow doppler demonstration of retinal artery relaxation. Am J Obstet Gynecol 1993; 169:204–206.
53. Martin JN, Blake PG, Perry KG, et al. The natural history of HELLP syndrome: patterns of disease progression and regression. Am J Obstet Gynecol 1991; 164: 1500–1513.
54. Committee on Drugs of the American Academy of Pediatrics. The transfer of drugs and other chemicals into human breast milk. Pediatrics 1989; 84:924–936.
55. Chesley LC, Annitto JE, Cosgrove RA. The remote prognosis of eclamptic women: sixth periodic report. Am J Obstet Gynecol 1976; 124:446–459.
56. Sibai BM. Management and counseling of patients with preeclampsia remote from term. Clin Obstet Gynecol 1992; 35(2):426–436.
57. Page EW, Christianson R. The impact of mean arterial blood pressure in middle trimester upon the outcome of pregnancy. Am J Obstet Gynecol 1976; 125: 740.

58. Cunningham FG, Cox SM, Harstad TW, et al. Chronic renal disease and pregnancy outcome. Am J Obstet Gynecol 1990; 163:453–459.
59. Gallery EDM, Hunyor SN, Gyory AZ. Plasma volume contraction: a significant factor in both pregnancy-associated hypertension and chronic hypertension in pregnancy. Q J Med 1979; 48:593.
60. Maikranz P, Holley JH, Parks JH, et al. Gestational hypercalciuria causes pathological urine calcium oxalate supersaturations. Kidney Int 1989; 136:108–113.
61. Redman CWG. Controlled trials of antihypertensive drugs in pregnancy. Am J Kidney Dis 1991; XVII:149–153.
62. Blake S, Macdonald D. The prevention of the maternal manifestations of preeclampsia by intensive antihypertensive treatment. Br J Obstet Gynaecol 1990; 198:244–248.
63. Redman CWG, Beilin LJ, Bonnar J, et al. A randomized comparison of early with conservative use of antihypertensive drugs in the management of pregnancy-induced hypertension. Br J Obstet Gynaecol 1990; 97:134–141.
64. Sibai BM, Mabie WC, Shamsa F, et al. A comparison of no medication versus methyldopa or labetalol in chronic hypertension during pregnancy. Am J Obstet Gynecol 1990; 162:960–967.
65. Leather HM, Baker P, Humphreys DM, et al. A controlled trial of hypotensive agents in hypertension in pregnancy. Lancet 1968; 2:488–490.
66. Bodis J, Sulyok E, Ertl T, et al. Methyldopa in pregnancy hypertension and the newborn. Lancet 1982; 2:498–499.
67. Horvath JS, Phippard A, Korda A, et al. Clonidine hydrochloride: a safe and effective antihypertensive agent in pregnancy. Obstet Gynecol 1985; 66:634–638.
68. Rubin PC, Butters L, Clark DM, et al. Placebo-controlled trial of atenolol in treatment of pregnancy-associated hypertension. Lancet 1983; 1:431–434.
69. Butters L, Kennedy S, Rubin PC. Atenolol in essential hypertension during pregnancy. Br Med J 1990; 301:587–589.
70. Montan S, Ingemarsson I, Marsal K, et al. Randomized controlled trial of atenolol and pindolol in human pregnancy: effects on fetal hemodynamics. Br Med J 1992; 304:946–949.
71. Plouin PF, Breart G, Maillard F, et al. Comparison of antihypertensive efficacy and perinatal safety of labetalol and methyldopa in the treatment of hypertension in pregnancy: a randomized controlled trial. Br J Obstet Gynaecol 1989; 95:868–876.
72. Redman CWG. A controlled trial of the treatment of hypertension in pregnancy: labetalol compared with methyldopa. In: Riley A, Symonds EM, eds. The Investigation of Labetalol in the Management of Hypertension in Pregnancy. Amsterdam: Excerpta Medica, 1982:101–110.
73. Hanssens M, Kierse MJNC, Vankelecom F, Van Assche FA. Fetal and neonatal effects of treatment with angiotensin-converting enzyme inhibitors in pregnancy. Obstet Gynecol 1991; 78:128.
74. Collins R, Yusef S, Peto R. Overview of randomized trials of diuretics in pregnancy. Br Med J 1985; 290:17–23.
75. Barron WM. Hypertension. In: Barron WM, Lindheimer MD, eds. Medical Disorders in Pregnancy. St. Louis: Mosby, 1994.

11

Hypertension and Endocrine Disease

SHELDON G. SHEPS AND WILLIAM F. YOUNG, JR.

Mayo Medical School
and Mayo Clinic and Mayo Foundation
Rochester, Minnesota

I. INTRODUCTION

Although an uncommon form of hypertension, endocrine hypertension provides the clinician with a unique treatment opportunity in the field of hypertension, that is, to render a surgical cure or achieve a dramatic response to pharmacological therapy. Because individualization of therapy is dependent on an accurate diagnosis of the form of endocrine hypertension, each section of this chapter includes discussions on the clinical features and diagnostic approach as a prelude to individualized treatment.

II. PHEOCHROMOCYTOMA

A. Clinical Features

Pheochromocytoma is a rare tumor that can occur at any age, but the peak incidence is in the fourth through the sixth decade. Among the general population of Olmsted County, Minnesota, the incidence of pheochromocytoma is 9.5 per million population per year, whereas in Scandinavia the rate is between 0.4 and 2.1. These rates vary, largely related to acquisition of the material, both clinically and at autopsy. The incidence of pheochromocytoma among hypertensive persons has decreased greatly because essential hypertension has been diagnosed in more people in recent years as the blood pressure limit for normal values has been reduced. The diagnosis of pheochromocytoma continues to be a challenge as a substantial proportion of cases found at autopsy are still missed clinically (1).

Pheochromocytoma may be part of a polyglandular endocrine derangement or may be associated with other neuroectodermal disorders (2). There is an increased incidence in families, particularly when the index case is a child or young adult with pheochromocytoma and also when pheochromocytoma is present in both adrenal glands. Autosomal dominant inheritance occurs in patients with multiple endocrine neoplasia (MEN) type II, in association with pancreatic islet cell tumors, and in neuroectodermal disorders (such as neurofibromatosis and von Hippel–Lindau disease).

Pheochromocytomas arise from the chromaffin cells that are located in the adrenal medulla, but also in paraganglions, which may be located anywhere from the base of the brain (such as the glomus jugulare) to the testes. About 5% of occurrences are bilateral, and about 10% of the tumors are extra-adrenal and solitary. Nearly all tumors produce symptoms or signs related to the excessive production and release of catecholamines. Although a few patients are asymptomatic, most have repetitive stereotypical episodes of paroxysms due to the release of catecholamines. The episodes usually are uniform in composition. The onset of each episode is characteristically sudden, and peak severity is reached within a few minutes. The duration is less than 15 minutes in half the patients and less than an hour in most. The paroxysms either are spontaneous or are elicited by exercise, bending over, urination, defecation, pressure on the abdomen, induction of anesthesia, or injection of drugs (histamine, guanethidine, glucagon, droperidol, tyramine, metochlopramide, cytotoxic drugs, saralasin, tricyclic antidepressants, or phenothiazines). The episodes consist of headache, palpitations, pallor, and perspiration. Unusual lability of blood pressure, accelerated hypertension, and a suprarenal or midline abdominal mass are additional clues. Hypertension may appear only with an episode or may be more persistent (3) (Figure 1). In rare instances, presenting features of hypotension and polyuria are induced by a tumor that predominantly secretes epinephrine, dopa, or dopamine.

A malignant pheochromocytoma can be diagnosed only by the demonstration of tumor cells in sites where chromaffin tissue is not normally found (e.g., lymph nodes, liver, bone, muscle, or lung). Malignancy is more frequent in extra-adrenal tumors and tumors in young persons. The frequency ranges from 3% to 14%. Nuclear deoxyribonucleic acid (DNA) ploidy studies by flow cytometry have shown that patients with a normal DNA histogram follow a benign course, whereas 30% to 40% of the remainder have or develop evidence of malignant disease in follow-up studies (4).

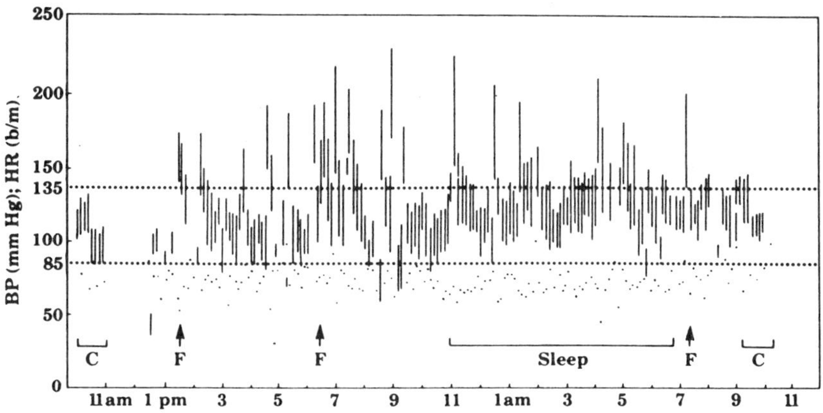

Figure 1 Blood pressure readings in a patient with phenchromocytoma, illustrating paroxysms of hypertension. There is orthostatic hypotension with positional changes, especially during calibration (C). (From Ref. 3.)

B. Diagnosis

Although the history and examination may give clues to the presence of one of the heritable syndromes and to sporadic pheochromocytoma, the diagnosis must be made on the biochemical determination of excess production of catecholamines or metabolites. In rare instances, totally asymptomatic and biochemically negative tumors may be found, but when these patients undergo operation, manipulation of these tumors almost always causes cardiovascular crises.

The values of urinary norepinephrine, epinephrine, dopamine, total metanephrines, and vanillylmandelic acid (VMA) are usually determined from urine collected for a 24-hour period, but they can be expressed as hourly rates or on a per milligram of creatinine basis in less complete specimens. Catecholamines in plasma are chemically labile, and many alterations in physiological and pathological states can affect their concentrations. One must pay careful attention to the circumstances in preparation of the patient for these collections (blood, urine). The question of which test or tests to use in screening is not easy to answer (5). Any single test chosen may have negative results on occasion, but most have positive results in all patients.

Given an excellent biochemical technique for measuring a particular substance, the decision then comes down to practice style. When an accurately collected 24-hour urine specimen can be obtained, the measurement of total metanephrine excretion is the least invasive and most economic screening test. The measurement of VMA is almost as good. If a screening test has abnormal results, they should be confirmed by tests of all three: metanephrines, VMA, and fractionated free catecholamines. In some centers, overnight collection is done on the theoretical basis that reduced sympathetic activity during sleep would more readily allow detection of an elevated autonomous hypersecretion of catecholamines.

When doing biochemical tests, it is important to recognize the physiological and other circumstances that can interfere with interpretation of the test and the specific interferences, such as the presence of methylglucamine, a component of many iodine-containing contrast mediums, that falsely lower metanephrine levels for as long as 72 hours after its parenteral use. Sotalol falsely increases urinary metanephrine levels, and labetalol hydrochloride, a drug commonly used to manage pheochromocytoma, can interfere with all of the biochemical determinations (6) (Table 1). It is rarely necessary to use pharmacological tests, but, if desired, provocative tests using glucagon and metoclopramide and a suppressive test with clonidine may be considered. The specific measurement of epinephrine and its metabolites can be of considerable value in the early diagnosis of pheochromocytoma in the adrenal medulla in MEN type II.

The combination of determination of urinary metanephrines as the screening test and confirmation by determination of urinary free catecholamines is an excellent laboratory regimen for identifying patients with pheochromocytoma. When repeated collections and other diagnostic studies yield normal findings, a valuable procedure is to have the patient collect a timed specimen in a urine container (with appropriate preservatives) after what the patient considers a "typical spell" and to analyze this specimen for catecholamines, metabolites, and creatinine.

C. Localization

Although pheochromocytoma is most commonly found in the adrenal glands and paragangliomas within the abdomen, preoperative localization by computed tomography (CT) or magnetic resonance imaging (MRI) should be attempted because of the many locations in which a functioning tumfor may be found. This should be considered after biochemical and clinical diagnostic studies. MRI will likely become the preferred technique as it becomes more universally available. It identifies the adrenal lesions as well as computed tomography, but it is better for extra-adrenal tumors. MRI does not require the administration of any glucagon or contrast media, which can provoke a catecholamine crisis unless the patient is protected with alpha- and beta-adrenergic blockade. MRI relaxation times of pheochromocytomas may be dramatically increased in comparison with those of normal adrenal tissue. CT and MRI are the only imaging techniques that visualize normal adrenal glands when the diagnosis is equivocal.

Table 1 Situations and Drugs That Interfere with Biochemical Diagnosis of Pheochromocytoma

Stimulation of endogenous catecholamines

Plasma and urine catecholamines are most sensitive, but metanephrines and VMA can be abnormal as well: emotional and physical stress, surgery, acute central nervous system disturbance (stroke, hemorrhage, tumor, encephalopathy), acute coronary ischemia, angiography, hypoglycemia, caffeine, nicotine, diazoxide, theophylline, drug withdrawal (alcohol, clonidine), vasodilator therapy (nitroglycerin, sodium nitroprusside, calcium channel blockers administered acutely)

Exogenous catecholamines

All the test results can be abnormal, but HPLC and radioenzymatic assays are more specific and sensitive for catecholamines: nose drops, sinus and cough remedies, bronchodilators, appetite suppressants

Drugs altering catecholamine metabolism

1. Reduction in plasma or urine catecholamines: $alpha_2$-agonists, chronic use of calcium channel blockers, converting enzyme inhibitors, bromocriptine
2. Decreased VMA; catecholamines and metanephrines increased: methyldopa,[a] monoamine oxidase inhibitors[b]
3. Variable changes in any test: phenothiazines,[b] tricyclic antidepressants,[b] L-dopa[b]
4. Increase in plasma or urine catecholamines: $alpha_1$-adrenergic blockers, beta-adrenergic blockers, labetalol

Specific interference

1. ↓ Metanephrine: metanephrine assay interference by the methylglucamine[c] in radiographic contrast medium
2. ↓ Urinary catecholamines: mandelamine destroys catecholamines in bladder urine
3. VMA ↓: clofibrate
   VMA ↑: nalidixic acid, anileridine
4. Labetalol: Metabolite(s) interfering with all tests
5. Increase in urine metanephrines: sotalol

[a]HPLC assays can accurately determine catecholamines and metanephrines in presence of methyldopa.
[b]Drugs with prolonged half-lives may need to be discontinued for 2 to 3 weeks before accurate determinations can be made.
[c]Methylglucamine destroys a reagent in the Pisano metanephrines assay; this is most pronounced in urine collected the same day as the contrast medium is administered but may last up to 72 hours. HPLC, high-performance liquid chromatography; VMA, vanillylmandelic acid.
Source: Ref. 5.

Scintigraphy with meta-iodobenzylguanidine (MIBG) is another technique for localizing pheochromocytomas. MIBG is concentrated in adrenergic vesicles so that images can be detected in catecholamine-producing tumors and in some normal tissues in some patients (adrenals, heart, salivary glands). In general, the normal adrenal medulla in humans is not imaged. About 10% of tumors are not detected. False-positive results are rare (1% to 2%). The advantage of scintigraphy is that is can image the entire body. Labetalol and many other compounds can interfere with the uptake of the isotope by catecholamine-containing cells (6). Positive results by scintigraphy can be used to direct subsequent MRI and CT efforts to provide precise anatomical localization of the tumor (or tumors). Positron emission tomography with compounds such as 2-[fluorine-18]-fluoro-2-deoxy-D-glucose and ^{11}C-hydroxyephedrine can localize pheochromocytomas not imaged by MIBG.

A useful strategy with sporadic cases of pheochromocytoma is to perform CT of the adrenal areas, the rest of the abdomen, and then the pelvis; if the result is negative, MIBG scintigraphy directs the next location to image with MRI. MIBG also has an important place in the evaluation of familial cases and of patients in whom the presence of metastases, multiple tumors, extra-adrenal tumors, or malignancy is being considered. Echocardiography (including transesophageal techniques) may be necessary to demonstrate intracardiac tumors, although gated MRI should disclose tumors in this location. Intramural tumors within the bladder wall require cystoscopic examination and biopsy (after appropriate adrenergic blockade) to confirm the diagnosis. These procedures are complementary when used appropriately and are not duplicative.

D. Individualized Therapy

Preparing a patient for the surgical excision of a pheochromocytoma is as critical as the operation itself. The effects of catecholamine storms on the body can be prevented by appropriate adrenergic receptor blockade. Alpha-adrenergic blockade (phenoxybenzamine, phentolamine, prazosin, doxazosin, or terazosin) is initiated until the patient is normotensive with slight orthostatic hypotension. Oral fluid and sodium loading restores the intravascular volume. Beta-adrenergic blockers are added for 3 days before operation in almost all patients; caution should be taken if cardiomegaly or cardiomyopathy exists. Alpha- and beta-adrenergic blockers used in this fashion do not interfere with diagnostic testing, and treatment can be initiated while pursuing biochemical and localization studies. The combination alpha- and beta-adrenergic blocker labetalol can be successfully used in many patients, but individual patients may not respond as well as when these drugs are administered separately in full doses. Recall that labetalol, however, interferes with the diagnostic and localization tests. In a patient who does not respond as well as expected to adrenoreceptor blockade, consideration should be given to adding converting enzyme inhibitors because renin levels are often elevated in these patients; sometimes the elevation is due to inadequate volume repletion at the same time as the adrenoreceptor blockade is being initiated. Calcium channel blockers or the rate-limiting catecholamine enzyme inhibitor metyrosine can be considered also. Preoperative preparation with glucocorticoids should be done in patients likely to have bilateral adrenalectomy, such as those with MEN type II.

Surgical excision remains the only definitive therapy. Laparoscopic adrenalectomy has been performed, but a transabdominal approach is generally necessary to allow thorough exploration of all chromaffin tissue in the abdomen and associated intra-abdominal disease, particularly cholelithiasis (occurring in almost 30% of patients with pheochromocytoma), which can be repaired at the same time. During surgery, careful attention to anesthesia, cardiovascular hemodynamics, and blood volume is imperative; the use of intravenous sodium nitroprusside to control blood pressure is routine. Other parenteral drugs can be used successfully (Table 2). The operative mortality rate at the Mayo Clinic from 1980 to 1989 was 1 in 110 patients with pheochromocytoma (0.9%). In our prior experience, the 5-year survival rate for our patients was 97% for those with benign tumors and 43% for those with malignant tumors (7).

A postoperative 24-hour urine collection for catecholamine and metabolite analyses a week or so after the operation is an essential part of management to be certain that all of the abnormalities have resolved and that there is no residual functioning tumor. It does take a few days to deplete extratumor stores of catecholamines, and a urine collection obtained too early may still be modestly abnormal. This baseline determination is important because after surgical treatment with curative intent, 5% to 10% of patients have a recurrence. DNA ploidy of the tumor should be ascertained and assigned the highest grade of several specimens. When DNA is normal, follow-up can be limited to repeating biochemical tests if symptoms recur. For those

Table 2 Agents Used for Blood Pressure Control in Pheochromocytoma

Preoperative
Alpha-blockers
Beta-blockers
Alpha-beta-blockers
Calcium channel blockers
Angiotensin converting enzyme inhibitors
Intraoperative
Nitroprusside
Nicardipine
Nitroglycerine
Phentolamine
Esmolol
Labetalol
Adenosine

with abnormal ploidy, annual biochemical studies should be done indefinitely because the malignancy rate may be as high as 30% to 40%.

When inoperable (for cure) or metastatic tumor is present, consideration can be given to debulking of tumor by surgical intervention and therapeutic embolization to reduce the tumor load and catecholamine production. Excess circulating catecholamines often can be controlled with adrenergic blocking drugs alone or in combination with the other drugs mentioned earlier. If doses of 50 Gy or more can be administered to the tumor, radiation therapy may be successful. Repeated therapeutic doses of MIBG have not produced substantial long-lasting benefit. Chemotherapy has not yielded persistent beneficial effects on catecholamine production or tumor growth, although striking transient decreases (lasting up to a year) have been reported after cyclic administration of cyclophosphamide, vincristine, and dacarbazine (8).

III. PRIMARY ALDOSTERONISM

Hypertension, hypokalemia, suppressed plasma renin activity (PRA), and increased aldosterone excretion characterize the syndrome of primary aldosteronism first described in 1954 (9,10). Prevalence estimates for primary aldosteronism vary from 0.05% to 2% of the hypertensive population (11, 12). At least six subtypes of primary aldosteronism have been identified: unilateral corticotropin-responsive aldosterone-producing adenoma (APA), bilateral adrenal hyperplasia (idiopathic hyperaldosteronism [IHA]), glucocorticoid-remediable aldosteronism (GRA), primary adrenal hyperplasia (PAH), renin-responsive APA, and aldosterone-producing adrenocortical carcinoma (Table 3). APA and IHA are found in 64% and 32% of the patients with primary aldosteronism, respectively (13). These data may be biased by the more frequent clinical recognition of the severe hypokalemia and hypertension associated with APA. When careful screening techniques are used, IHA is diagnosed more frequently than APA (12).

Table 3 Types of Primary Aldosteronism

Types	Prevalence, %
Aldosterone-producing adenoma (APA)	64 ± 10
Corticotropin-responsive (common)	
Renin-responsive (rare)	
Idiopathic hyperaldosteronism (IHA)	32 ± 10
Primary adrenal hyperplasia	<1%–2%
Aldosterone-producing adrenocortical carcinoma	1
Familial hyperaldosteronism (FH)	
Glucocorticoid-remediable aldosteronism (FH type I)	<1–2
FH type II (APA or IHA)	<1–2

PAH and renin-responsive APA are uncommon subtypes. PAH is characterized by a hyperplastic adrenal that resembles IHA morphologically, but mimics the APA response to physiological maneuvers and unilateral or subtotal adrenalectomy (14). The renin-responsive APA appears as an APA morphologically and in response to unilateral adrenalectomy, but it responds to physiological maneuvers as do the hyperplastic glands of IHA (15).

Two forms of familial hyperaldosteronism (FH) have been described: GRA (FH type I) is autosomal dominant and associated with variable degrees of hyperaldosteronism, high levels of hybrid steroids (e.g., 18-hydroxycortisol), and suppression with exogenous glucocorticoids. Fusion of the 5′-regulatory region of the 11 beta-hydroxylase gene to the coding sequences of the aldosterone synthase gene results in ACTH-dependent activation of aldosterone synthase on cortisol and cortisol precursors (16). Sixty patients in 17 kindreds have now been identified to have this chimeric gene (Lifton, personal communication). The second form of FH, FH type II, was reported by Stowasser et al. (17) and refers to the familial occurrence of APA or IHA or both in five families (13 patients).

Distinguishing the subtype of primary aldosteronism is critical to the appropriate individualization of therapy. The hypertension and hypokalemia are cured with adrenal surgery in most patients with APA and PAH, whereas pharmacological therapy is more effective for patients with IHA and GRA.

A. Clinical Features

Few symptoms accompany the syndrome of primary aldosteronism. Patients with marked hypokalemia may have muscle weakness, cramping, headaches, palpitations, polydipsia, polyuria, or nocturia. There are no specific physical findings. The degree of hypertension is usually moderate to severe and may be resistant to pharmacological intervention (18).

In addition to the hypokalemia, abnormalities detected in routine clinical laboratory tests should raise suspicion as to the presence of primary aldosteronism. For example, mild metabolic alkalosis (serum bicarbonate level above 31 mEq/L) and relative hypernatremia (serum sodium level above 142 mEq/L) are frequent findings. The effect of chronic potassium depletion on insulin secretion and action results in elevated fasting plasma glucose levels in approximately 25% of patients. Electrocardiographic changes of mild left ventricular hypertrophy and of hypokalemia, including prolonged ST segment, U waves, and T-wave inversion, may be found.

B. Diagnosis

The diagnostic approach to primary aldosteronism may be considered in three parts. First, screening for primary aldosteronism is usually triggered by the finding of spontaneous hypokalemia or easily provoked hypokalemia in the hypertensive patient. Spontaneous hypokalemia is uncommon in patients with uncomplicated hypertension and, when present, strongly suggests associated mineralocorticoid excess (19). However, normokelamia does not exclude primary aldosteronism. Several studies have shown that 7% to 38% of patients with primary aldosteronism (12,20,21) and most patients with GRA have baseline serum potassium levels greater than 3.6 mEq/L (22). Before an extensive and expensive evaluation is initiated, screening studies with serum potassium, 24-hour urinary potassium level, and paired random plasma aldosterone concentration (PAC) and PRA should be obtained (Figure 2). Approximately 30% of patients with essential hypertension and almost all patients with primary aldosteronism have subnormal upright PRA levels (23). Thus, a low PRA level is not specific for primary aldosteronism. The diagnostic significance of a low PRA value is enhanced with a simultaneously obtained PAC (24). The ratio of PAC (in nanograms/deciliter [Ng/dl]) to PRA (ng/ml/h) was less than 20 in 323 patients with

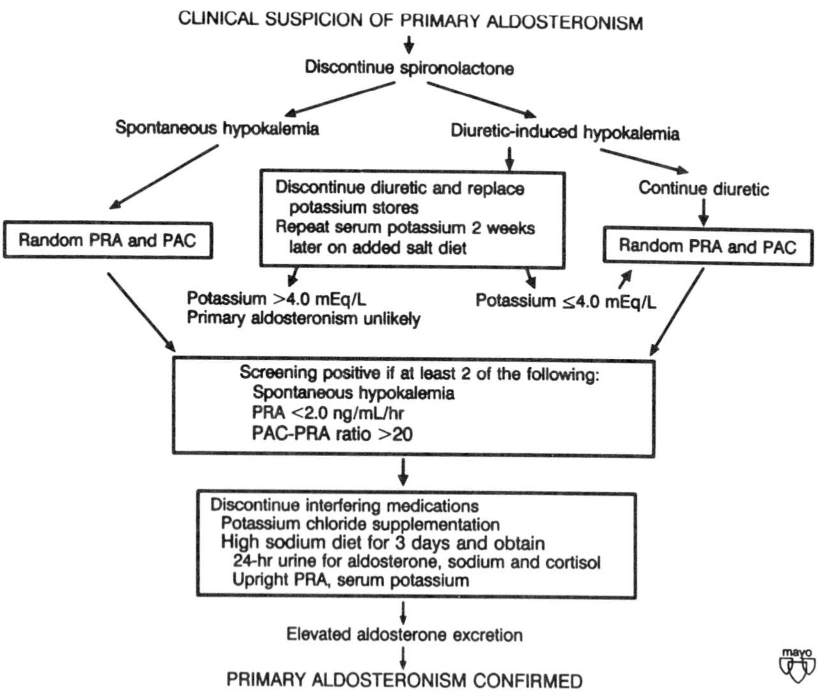

Figure 2 Screening and confirmatory studies for primary aldosteronism. PRA, plasma renin activity; PAC, plasma aldosterone concentration. (From Ref. 26.)

essential hypertension and more than 40 in 9 patients with primary aldosteronism due to APA (24). It has been suggested that a PAC/PRA ratio of more than 33 should trigger further studies to confirm primary aldosteronism (25). In a subgroup of 60 patients with primary aldosteronism diagnosed at the Mayo Clinic, the mean PAC/PRA ratio was 56 (26). However, this ratio was less than 25 in 11 patients and less than 20 in 5 patients. Patients with at least two of the following findings should be evaluated further for the possibility of primary aldosteronism: (1) spontaneous or easily provoked hypokalemia and inappropriate kaliuresis, (2) upright PRA less than 3.0 ng/ml/h, and (3) random PAC/PRA ratios of more than 20 (Figure 2).

Second, the diagnosis of primary aldosteronism must be confirmed by demonstrating nonsuppressible urine or plasma aldosterone levels and normal glucocorticoid excretion. The list of drugs and hormones capable of affecting the renin-angiotensin-aldosterone axis is extensive, and frequently, in patients with severe hypertension, a "medication-contaminated" evaluation is unavoidable. The optimal antihypertensive agents to be used during this evaluation include $alpha_1$-adrenergic receptor blockers and guanadrel (Hylorel) (13). It is impossible to interpret data obtained from patients on treatment with spironolactone (Aldactone). Therefore, spironolactone treatment should not be initiated until the evaluation is completed and final treatment decisions made. Aldosterone suppression testing can be performed with orally administered sodium chloride and measurement of urinary aldosterone level (13) or with intravenous sodium chloride loading and measurement of PAC (20). An angiotensin converting enzyme inhibitor (captopril) has also been used to demonstrate autonomous aldosterone secretion (27).

The third part of the evaluation guides the therapeutic approach by distinguishing APA and PAH from IHA and GRA (Figure 3). Unilateral adrenalectomy in patients with an APA or PAH results in normalization of both the hypertension and hypokalemia in approximately 60% to 70% of cases; in IHA and GRA, unilateral or bilateral adrenalectomy seldom corrects the hypertension (26). The studies outlined in this section should be considered only after the diagnosis of primary aldosteronism is confirmed. This differentiation may require one or more studies, of which the first is computerized adrenal imaging with CT or MRI. The diagnostic accuracy of adrenal CT scanning is approximately 90% (26). In general, the clinical picture of patients with APA differs from that of patients with IHA—patients with APA have more severe hypertension, more profound hypokalemia (less than 3.0 mEq/L), higher plasma (above 25 ng/dl) and urinary (above 30 μg/24 hr) aldosterone levels, and younger age (below 50 years). Patients fitting these descriptors are considered to have a "high probability of APA" (Figure 3). However, these factors are not absolute predictors of unilateral versus bilateral adrenal abnormality. The patient with a "high probability of APA"

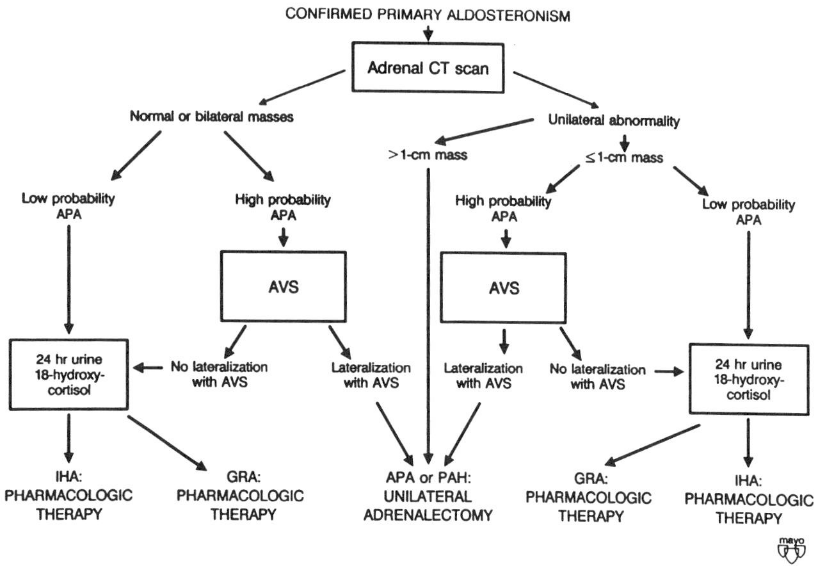

Figure 3 Subtype evaluation of primary aldosteronism. The details are discussed in the text. CT, computed tomography; APA, aldosterone-producing adenoma; IHA, idiopathic hyperaldosteronism; PAH, primary adrenal hyperplasia; GRA, glucocorticoid-remediable aldosteronism; AVS, adrenal venous sampling. (From Ref. 26.)

who has a unilateral adrenal nodule larger than 1 cm should be considered for unilateral adrenalectomy. However, even in this group there is a risk of operating on a nonfunctioning nodule. The concern regarding apparent adrenal microadenomas (1 cm or less) is that they may represent areas of hyperplasia, and unilateral adrenalectomy would be inappropriate (28). The most frequent error may be incorrectly labeling a small APA as IHA on the basis of CT findings of bilateral multinodularity or normal-appearing adrenals (29).

Selective adrenal venous sampling for aldosterone helps resolve these diagnostic dilemmas. One of the first tests used to distinguish APA from IHA (30) continues to be the most accurate, but it is an invasive and difficult technique. The cumulative failure rate for catheterization of the right adrenal vein is 26% (13), and the performance of this test should be limited to referral centers.

Patients with documented primary aldosteronism, normal adrenal computerized imaging, or no lateralization of aldosterone on adrenal venous sampling should be evaluated for the possibility of GRA (Figure 3). Typically these patients are diagnosed in their second to third decades and have a positive family history of hypokalemia-associated hypertension. Screening for GRA is accomplished with measurement of 24-hour urine 18-hydroxycortisol excretion (22) or a direct genetic blood test to detect the chimeric gene (16). The 24-hour urinary excretion of 18-hydroxycortisol in patients with GRA is typically above 3000 nmol (22).

C. Individualized therapy

The treatment goal is to prevent morbidity and mortality associated with hypertension and hypokalemia. The appropriate treatment of primary aldosteronism is highly dependent on the cause. Although hypertension is frequently cured with unilateral adrenalectomy in patients with APA and PAH, the average cure rate for IHA is only 19% with unilateral or bilateral adrenalectomy (13). Patients with IHA and GRA should be treated medically.

1. Surgical Treatment of APA and PAH

The treatment of choice for patients with APA and PAH is unilateral total adrenalectomy (31). The blood pressure response to spironolactone before surgery is a predictor of the blood pressure response to unilateral adrenalectomy in patients with APA (13). To decrease the surgical risk, hypokalemia should be corrected with spironolactone (Aldactone) before operation. Accurate preoperative localization allows for a unilateral posterior retroperitoneal surgical approach, which is associated with short postoperative hospitalization and minimal morbidity and mortality rates (32). With unilateral adrenalectomy, stress steroid coverage is unnecessary.

Typically, the hypertension does not resolve immediately after operation but rather does so over 1 to 6 months. Although nearly 100% of patients have improved blood pressure control postoperatively, average long-term cure rates with unilateral adrenalectomy for APA are 60% to 70% (26). Persistence of hypertension may be related to resetting of baroreceptors, established hemodynamic changes, structural changes of the blood vessels, altered sensitivity of the vessels to pressor substances, renal functional or structural changes, and coincident primary hypertension. Chronic medical therapy should be given to patients who have persistent hypertension postoperatively, or who are poor surgical candidates; women with hypertension/hypokalemia controlled with low-dose spironolactone; or those who refuse surgical treatment.

2. Pharmacological Treatment of IHA

Nondrug therapy including a sodium-restricted diet (less than 100 mEq sodium/day), maintenance of ideal body weight, tobacco avoidance, and regular aerobic exercise contributes significantly to the success of pharmacological treatment. Potassium supplementation, in the form of medication or as a diet rich in potassium, is ineffective in correcting the hypokalemia associated with primary aldosteronism. Frequently, hypertension and hypokalemia can be controlled with a first-step agent, such as spironolactone or amiloride. If hypertension persists despite dose titration, then a second-step agent (e.g., calcium channel antagonist, angiotensin converting enzyme inhibitor, or a thiazide diuretic) is added to the pharmacological program (Table 4).

3. First-Step Agents (Potassium-Sparing Agents)

a. Spironolactone. Competitive antagonism to aldosterone is the basis of the major form of medical intervention for primary aldosteronism. Spironolactone (Aldactone) is the first-line agent for women. The dosage is 100 mg/day initially and is increased to 400 mg/day if necessary for blood pressure control. Hypokalemia responds promptly; hypertension may take as long as 4 to 8 weeks to be corrected. Frequently, after several months of therapy, this dosage can be decreased to as little as 50 mg/day; dosage titration is based on blood pressure response and serum potassium level. Potassium supplementation should not be given concurrently with spironolactone because of the potential for development of hyperkalemia. Unfortunately, spironolactone also blocks testosterone biosynthesis and peripheral androgen action; this blocking results in significant side effects, including impotence, decreased libido, gynecomastia, and menstrual irregularities. Spironolactone has been shown to increase the half-life of digoxin, and for patients taking this drug the dosage may need to be adjusted when treatment with spironolactone is started. Concomitant therapy with salicylates should be avoided because they interfere with the tubular secretion of an active metabolite and decrease the effectiveness of spironolactone.

b. Amiloride. Amiloride (Midamor) is the drug of choice for men and for patients intolerant of spironolactone. It is not an aldosterone antagonist. Amiloride is an organic base that blocks sodium channels in a mineralocorticoid-independent portion of the distal renal tubule, thus increasing sodium and chloride excretion and decreasing potassium and hydrogen ion excretion. The dosage is 5 mg twice daily (10 mg/day) initially with meals and is increased up to 30 mg/day if necessary for control of hypokalemia (33). Potassium supplementation should not be given concurrently with amiloride because of the potential development of hyperkalemia. Side effects include headaches, fatigue, impotence, and gastrointestinal complaints.

c. Triamterene. Triamterene (Dyrenium) is a pteridine compound with some structural resemblance to folic acid. It directly affects tubular transport and, independently of aldosterone, causes increased sodium and chloride

Table 4 Orally Administered Drugs Used to Treat Hypertension and Hypokalemia in Patients with Primary Aldosteronism

Generic name (trade name)	Dosage mg/day[a] Initial	Maximum	Side effects
First-step agents (potassium-sparing agents)			
Spironolactone (Aldactone)	100	400[b]	Gastrointestinal (GI) discomfort, impotence, decreased libido, menstrual irregularities, gynecomastia
Amiloride (Midamor)	10[b]	30[b]	Headaches, fatigue, impotence, GI symptoms
Triamterene (Dyrenium)	200[b]	300[b]	GI symptoms, leg cramps, dizziness
Second-step agents			
Thiazide diuretic			
Hydrochlorothiazide (Esidrix)	12.5	50	Hypokalemia
Calcium channel antagonist			
Nifedipine (Procardia, Adalat)	30[c]	120[c]	Flushing, edema, constipation, dizziness, GI discomfort, headache, weakness
Nifedipine (Procardia XL)	30	120	
Angiotensin converting enzyme inhibitor			
Enalapril (Vasotec)	5	40[b]	Headache, dizziness, fatigue, GI symptoms, cough; acute renal failure in patients with bilateral renal artery stenosis
Lisinopril (Prinivil, Zestril)	5	30	Cough; acute renal failure in patients with bilateral renal artery stenosis
Aldosterone-producing adrenal malignancies			
Adrenolytic agent			
Mitotane (Lysodren)	1000[c]	10,000[c]	Anorexia, nausea, diarrhea, lethargy, confusion, dizziness, rash
Adrenal enzyme inhibitor			
Ketoconazole (Nizoral)	600	1200	Hepatotoxicity, impotence, GI symptoms, rash, asthenia syndrome

[a]Given once daily unless otherwise indicated.
[b]Given as two doses daily.
[c]Given in three doses daily.

excretion. Potassium excretion is decreased as a result of inhibition of secretion at the distal nephron. The initial dosage is 100 mg twice daily (200 mg/day) after meals. The dosage can be increased up to 300 mg/day if necessary for control of hypokalemia. Side effects include nausea, emesis, leg cramps, and dizziness. A possible interaction resulting in acute renal failure has been reported in patients who also are taking indomethacin. Therefore, use of nonsteroidal anti-inflammatory agents should be avoided during treatment. This drug is used only if spironolactone and amiloride were not tolerated.

If one potassium-sparing agent is not effective or causes significant side effects, then a different one should be used. However, two of these agents should not be given concurrently. Furthermore, a second-step antihypertensive agent frequently is needed for patients with IHA.

d. Second-Step Agents. The hypertension of IHA often is inadequately controlled with a potassium-sparing agent alone. Nifedipine (Procardia, Adalat) is effective for decreasing plasma aldosterone levels and returning plasma potassium concentration and blood pressure to normal in some patients with primary aldosteronism (34). Angiotensin converting enzyme inhibitors also are effective in patients with IHA, returning blood pressure to normal, decreasing aldosterone secretion rates, and improving potassium balance (35).

Hypervolemia is a major reason for resistance to drug therapy, and low doses (e.g., 12.5 to 50 mg of hydrochlorothiazide daily) of a thiazide or related sulfonamide diuretic are effective agents to be used in combination with the potassium-sparing diuretic (18). Unfortunately, these agents often lead to further hypokalemia. Therefore, serum potassium levels should be monitored. Guidelines for the use of these antihypertensive agents are briefly summarized in Table 4.

e. Glucocorticoid-Remediable Aldosteronism. In the rare patients with type I FH, chronic treatment with physiological doses of a glucocorticoid normalizes the blood pressure and corrects the hypokalemia. However, treatment with spironolactone in these patients is just as effective and precludes the potential disruption of the pituitary-adrenal axis (36).

f. Aldosterone-Producing Adrenal Malignancy. This malignant tumor should be suspected in patients with aldosterone-producing tumors that are more than 3 cm in diameter (most APAs are less than 3 cm in diameter). It is very difficult to make this diagnosis on microscopic examination. The only absolute criterion is the presence of local invasion or metastatic lesions. Surgical excision is the treatment of choice. Mitotane (o,p′-DDD) or cisplatin is used in patients with persistent tumor. Associated excessive glucocorticoid and mineralocorticoid overproduction may be controlled with ketoconazole (Nizoral) (Table 4).

IV. OTHER FORMS OF MINERALOCORTICOID EXCESS

In addition to those listed in Table 3, other syndromes of excess mineralocorticoid in the setting of low PRA have been described.

A. Hyperdeoxycorticosteronism

1. Congenital Adrenal Hyperplasia

Congenital adrenal hyperplasia (CAH) is caused by enzymatic defects in adrenal steroidogenesis that result in deficient cortisol secretion. The lack of cortisol feedback inhibition on the hypothalamus and pituitary results in an ACTH-driven buildup of cortisol precursors at the sites proximal to the enzymatic deficiency. The most common form of CAH, 21-hydroxylase deficiency, is not associated with hypertension. Two uncommon forms of CAH, 11-beta-hydroxylase deficiency and 17-alpha-hydroxylase deficiency, result in hypersecretion of the mineralocorticoid 11-deoxycorticosterone (DOC). The increased circulating levels of DOC result in hypertension, hypokalemia, low PRA, and low levels of aldosterone. These defects are inherited in an autosomal recessive manner and typically diagnosed in childhood. However, partial enzymatic defects have been shown to be the cause of hypertension in adults (37).

2. 11-Beta-Hydroxylase Deficiency

Approximately 5% of all cases of CAH are due to 11-beta-hydroxylase deficiency, and the prevalence in whites is 1 in 100,000 (38). In addition to high levels of DOC and 11-deoxycortisol, the substrate mass effect results in increased levels of adrenal androgens. Patients present in childhood with hypertension, hypokalemia, virilization in females, and pseudoprecocious puberty in males. The diagnosis is confirmed with the finding of markedly increased levels of DOC, 11-deoxycortisol, and adrenal androgens. Treatment with glucocorticoid replacement normalizes the steroid abnormalities and hypertension. Glucocorticoid replacement options in adults include dexamethasone 0.5 to 0.75 mg daily, prednisone 5 mg a.m. and 2.5 mg p.m., or hydrocortisone 20 mg a.m. and 10 mg p.m.

3. 17-Alpha-Hydroxylase Deficiency

17-Alpha-hydroxylase deficiency is very rare; approximately 120 cases have been reported (39). This defect results in decreased cortisol and sex hormone production. Genetic 46,XY males present with either pseudohermaphroditism or as phenotypic females, and 46,XX females exhibit primary amenorrhea. Therefore, this form of CAH may not come to medical attention until puberty. The steroid biochemical findings include low concentrations of plasma adrenal androgens, plasma 17-alpha-hydroxyprogesterone, aldosterone, cortisol, and PRA, and increased plasma concentrations of DOC, corticosterone, and 18-hydroxycorticosterone. As with 11-beta-hydroxylase deficiency, treatment with glucocorticoid replacement normalizes the steroid abnormalities and hypertension. Sex steroids also need to be replaced.

4. DOC-Producing Tumor

DOC-producing adrenal tumors are usually large and malignant, but one case of a benign DOC-secreting adrenal tumor has been reported (40) with no evidence of tumor recurrence 12 years after the original report (Dr. Saruta, personal communication). Some of these tumors secrete androgens and estrogens in addition to DOC and thus may cause virilization in women and feminization in men. This diagnosis is confirmed by a high plasma DOC or urinary tetrahydrodeoxycorticosterone value and a large adrenal tumor on CT scan. Optimal treatment is complete surgical resection.

5. Primary Cortisol Resistance

Elevated cortisol secretion and plasma cortisol concentrations without evidence of Cushing's syndrome are found in patients with this rare familial syndrome of primary cortisol resistance (41). The presenting signs and symptoms are variable and include hypokalemic alkalosis, hypertension, increased plasma DOC concentrations, and increased adrenal androgen secretion. Several defects in glucocorticoid receptors and the steroid-receptor complex are probably responsible for this syndrome. Treatment options for the mineralocorticoid-dependent hypertension are blockade of the mineralocorticoid receptor with spironolactone and suppression of ACTH secretion with dexamethasone (42).

B. Apparent Mineralocorticoid Excess Syndromes

Cortisol is a potent mineralocorticoid. The kidney metabolizes cortisol (Kendall's compound "F") to cortisone (compound "E," metabolically inactive) via 11-beta-hydroxysteroid dehydrogenase (11-beta-OHSD). Deficiency of this enzyme results in a high intrarenal concentration of cortisol, hypertension, hypokalemia, suppressed PRA, and low aldosterone levels (43). The diagnosis of 11-beta-OHSD deficiency is made by documenting an increased ratio of urinary metabolites of cortisol (tetrahydrocortisol [THF] + 5-alpha-tetrahydrocortisol [allo-THF]) to those of cortisone (tetrahydrocortisone [THE]). The ratio of (THF + alloTHF)/THE is approximately 1:1 in normal subjects; in patients with 11-beta-OHSD deficiency this ratio is above 7:1. Two types of defects in the renal metabolism of cortisol have been described. Type 1 apparent mineralocorticoid excess (AME) syndrome refers to deficiency in the 11-beta-OHSD enzyme. The type II form of AME is secondary to a deficiency in the A-ring reduction metabolic pathway (44).

Treatment options include blockade of the mineralocorticoid receptor with spironolactone or suppression of endogenous cortisol secretion with dexamethasone. The congenital forms are rare autosomal recessive disorders and have been documented in 20 patients. The acquired forms are more common and include licorice-induced hypertension and Cushing's syndrome.

1. Licorice-Induced Hypertension—Type I AME Syndrome

Licorice-induced hypokalemic hypertension, which is reversible with spironolactone administration, was documented more than 30 years ago (45), but the underlying pathophysiological mechanism was only recently discovered (43). Natural licorice is derived from the root of the plant Glycyrrhiza glabra. Confectionery licorice contains approximately 0.3% glycyrrhizic acid, which, after ingestion, is converted to glycyrrhetinic acid, a potent inhibitor of 11-beta-OHSD. Analyses of urinary F:E ratios in patients with licorice-induced hypertension have documented a reversible acquired 11-beta-OHSD deficiency (46). Doses of 50 to 100 g of crude glycyrrhiza (150 to 300 mg glycyrrhizic acid) per day in true confectionery licorice are necessary to produce the syndrome (45). All patients with hypertension and hypokalemia should be questioned about possible licorice ingestion. Inhibition of 11-beta-OHSD can be documented by measurement of 24-hour urinary F:E ratio and metabolite ratios.

2. Cushing's Syndrome—Type II AME Syndrome

a. Clinical Features. Hypertension is present in approximately 75% to 80% of patients with Cushing's syndrome (47). The mechanisms of hypertension include increased production of DOC, increased vascular reactivity to catecholamines, and overload of cortisol inactivation with stimulation of the mineralocorticoid receptor. Deficient cortisol ring A reduction due to overload of metabolizing enzymes results in a type II variant of AME in patients with severe hypercortisolism (48).

In addition to hypertension, the clinical manifestations of excessive cortisol production include central weight gain, oligomenorrhea, hirsutism, facial plethora and rounding, depression, poor wound healing, easy bruising, red/purple striae, and proximal muscle weakness.

b. Diagnosis. Cushing's syndrome is caused by hypersecretion of corticotropin (ACTH) (ACTH-dependent Cushing's syndrome) or by primary adrenal hypersecretion of glucocorticoids (ACTH-independent Cushing's syndrome [Table 5]). The diagnostic evaluation of Cushing's syndrome typically proceeds as outlined in Figure 4. First, hypercortisolism must be suspected as a result of the known manifestations of the disorder and then confirmed with measurements of serum and 24-hour urine cortisol concentrations.

Table 5 Causes of Cushing's Syndrome

Types	Prevalance, %
ACTH-dependent	
Pituitary	
Corticotrope adenoma	72
Corticotrope multinodular hyperplasia	<1
Ectopic	
Ectopic ACTH-secreting tumor	12
Ectopic CRH-secreting tumor	<1
Ectopic ACTH- and CRH-secreting tumor	<1
ACTH-independent	
Unilateral adrenal disease	
Adenoma	7
Carcinoma	5
Bilateral adrenal disease	
Macronodular hyperplasia	1
Primary pigmented nodular adrenal disease	1

ACTH, adrenocorticotropic hormone; CRH, corticotropin-releasing hormone.

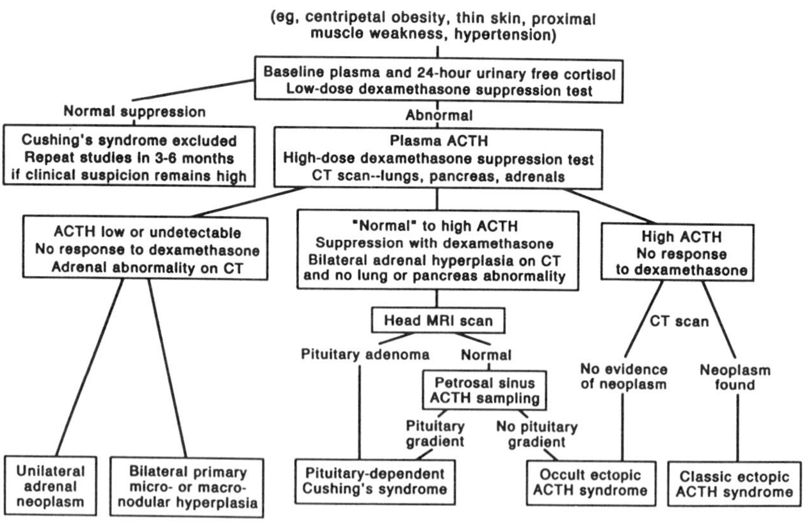

Figure 4 Evaluation of Cushing's syndrome. The details are discussed in the text. ACTH, adrenocorticotropic hormone; CT, computed tomography; MRI, magnetic resonance imaging.

Autonomous hypercortisolism (Cushing's syndrome) is confirmed with the low-dose dexamethasone suppression test (dexamethasone 0.5 mg orally every 6 hours for 48 hours); 24-hour urinary cortisol excretion of 20 μg or above confirms the diagnosis. Then the plasma ACTH concentration classifies the subtype of hypercortisolism as ACTH-dependent ("normal" to high levels of ACTH) or ACTH-independent (undetectable ACTH) (Figure 4).

In patients with ACTH-dependent hypercortisolism the high-dose dexamethasone suppression test (dexamethasone 2 mg orally every 6 hours for 48 hours) helps differentiate pituitary from ectopic ACTH hypersecretion; a 24-hour urinary cortisol excretion that decreases 50% or more from baseline values is consistent with pituitary-dependent disease. However, some types of ectopic ACTH-secreting tumors (e.g., bronchial carcinoid) may also be suppressed by high-dose dexamethasone administration (49). When a pituitary tumor is not found on computerized pituitary imaging, further evaluation with computerized lung imaging and inferior petrosal sinus sampling for ACTH and with ovine corticotropin-releasing hormone stimulation is indicated (50).

In patients with ACTH-independent hypercortisolism, the high-dose dexamethasone suppression test shows no suppression in urinary cortisol excretion. In these patients computerized imaging of the adrenal glands usually indicates the type of adrenal disease (Table 5).

c. Individualized Therapy. Transsphenoidal pituitary adenomectomy is the treatment of choice for patients with pituitary-dependent disease. The long-term surgical cure rate for ACTH-secreting microadenomas is approximately 80%. If pituitary surgery is not curative, bilateral adrenalectomy and pituitary irradiation are adjunctive treatment options. Surgical extirpation of an adrenal adenoma or carcinoma or the source of ectopic ACTH production is the treatment of choice for patients with primary adrenocortical disease or ectopic ACTH production. Bilateral adrenalectomy is the preferred treatment for patients with ACTH-independent bilateral macronodular or micronodular hyperplasia. Pharmacological therapy is reserved for patients not cured with the surgical approach. Ketoconazole and mitotane (o,p′-DDD) are two examples of agents used to block glucocorticoid production.

The hypertension associated with Cushing's syndrome should be treated until a surgical cure is obtained. Spironolactone, at dosages used to treat primary aldosteronism, is effective in reversing the hypokalemia associated with the type II AME syndrome. Second-step agents include thiazide diuretics, beta-adrenergic receptor blockers, and calcium channel antagonists. The hypertension associated with the hypercortisolism usually resolves over several weeks after the surgical cure, and antihypertensive agents can be tapered and withdrawn. Approximately 26% of patients have persistent hypertension despite cure of the hypercortisolism (51).

V. OTHER ENDOCRINE CAUSES OF HYPERTENSION

A. Thyroid Dysfunction

Dysfunction of the thyroid gland may be the sole cause of hypertension or contribute significantly to underlying essential hypertension. Thyroid-directed treatment in the hypertensive patient may normalize the blood pressure or facilitate the treatment of hypertension. The types of thyroid disease associated with hypertension include hyperthyroidism, hypothyroidism, and medullary thyroid carcinoma (associated with pheochromocytoma in the MEN type IIA and IIB syndromes).

1. Clinical Features

Hyperthyroidism occurs when excessive amounts of circulating thyroid hormones interact with thyroid hormone receptors on peripheral tissues. This results in increased metabolic activity and increased sensitivity to circulating catecholamines. Thyrotoxic patients usually have high cardiac output and increased systolic blood pressure.

Hypothyroidism results from deficiency of thyroid hormones, which causes many metabolic processes to slow. Patients with hypothyroidism have a high prevalence of hypertension, primarily diastolic (52). Hypothyroidism is characterized by low cardiac output, high peripheral vascular resistance, and increased level of sympathetic activity.

2. Diagnosis

The clinical suspicion of thyroid gland dysfunction is confirmed with laboratory tests. Increased levels of blood thyroid hormones (thyroxine and triiodothyronine) and low serum levels of thyroid-stimulating hormone (TSH) are the hallmarks of hyperthyroidism. The serum TSH level is a very sensitive indicator of the effect of circulating thyroid hormones on one target tissue, the pituitary. The diagnosis of hypothyroidism is based on low serum levels of thyroid hormone and increased serum levels of TSH. The TSH-based laboratory approach to the diagnosis of thyroid dysfunction is outlined in Figure 5.

3. Individualized Treatment

The accurate diagnosis of the type and form of thyroid dysfunction is critical to directing the appropriate therapy. For example, hyperthyroidism due to Graves' disease is most effectively treated with ^{131}I, whereas hyperthy-

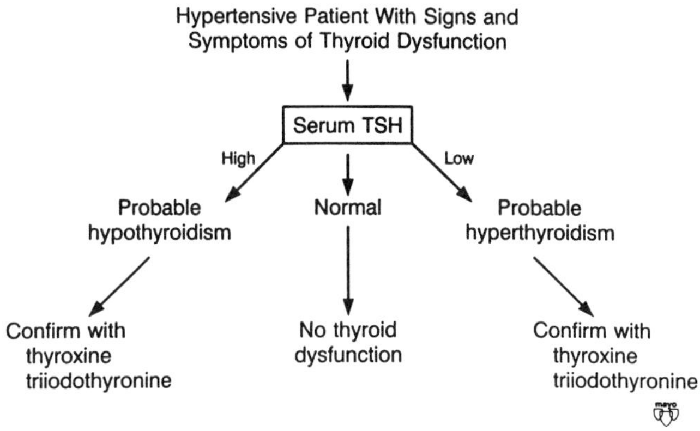

Figure 5 A thyroid-stimulating hormone- (TSH)-based algorithm for the laboratory investigation of thyroid function. The TSH assay should be "sensitive," with a lower limit of detection $\leqslant 0.05$ mIU/L. If pituitary insufficiency is suspected, the diagnosis of hypothyroidism should be made on the basis of serum concentrations of total and free thyroxine.

roidism caused by a toxic multinodular goiter should be treated surgically. Hypothyroidism is effectively treated with synthetic levothyroxine. The reader is referred to recent reviews for the specific details of the nuances of treatment approaches (53). During the wait for the thyroid-directed therapy to be effective, the hypertension may be treated. The systolic hypertension of hyperthyroidism responds to treatment with beta-adrenergic blockade. Vasodilators and diuretics are effective agents to treat the diastolic hypertension associated with hypothyroidism.

B. Hyperparathyroidism

Hypercalcemia is associated with an increased incidence of hypertension (54). Primary hyperparathyroidism (an autonomous overproduction of PTH) is a common cause of hypercalcemia. The prevalence of hypertension in patients with primary hyperparathyroidism is increased twofold (54). In most of cases the disease is caused by a benign solitary parathyroid adenoma. However, the hyperparathyroidism, when associated with MEN syndromes, is usually due to hyperplasia of all four parathyroid glands.

Most patients with primary hyperparathyroidism are asymptomatic. The side effects of chronic hypercalcemia may be the focus of the presentation: polyuria and polydipsia, constipation, osteoporosis, renal lithiasis, peptic ulcer disease, and hypertension. The history and physical examination rarely give any specific indications of primary hyperparathyroidism. The hallmarks of this disorder are hypercalcemia, hypophosphatemia, and increased serum concentrations of PTH. The first step in the diagnosis is to document hypercalcemia on two separate occasions. In the patient with hypercalcemia, the measurement of serum PTH is the most specific way of making the diagnosis of primary hyperparathyroidism. If the serum concentration of PTH is not increased, the clinical data should be reviewed and nonparathyroid causes of hypercalcemia investigated. Causes of hypercalcemia with a low serum PTH concentration include pheochromocytoma, hyperthyroidism, cancer (including multiple myeloma), vitamin D intoxication, and sarcoidosis.

Most of the pharmacological agents used to treat primary hypertension may be applied, except that thiazide diuretics may aggravate the hypercalcemia and should be avoided. After successful surgical removal of the parathyroid adenoma, the hypertension resolves in approximately 50% of patients (55).

C. Acromegaly

Growth hormone excess results in sodium retention and an increased incidence of hypertension in patients with acromegaly (56). Acromegaly is characterized by acral and soft tissue overgrowth, progressive dental malocclusion, degenerative arthritis, low-pitched sonorous voice, excessive sweating

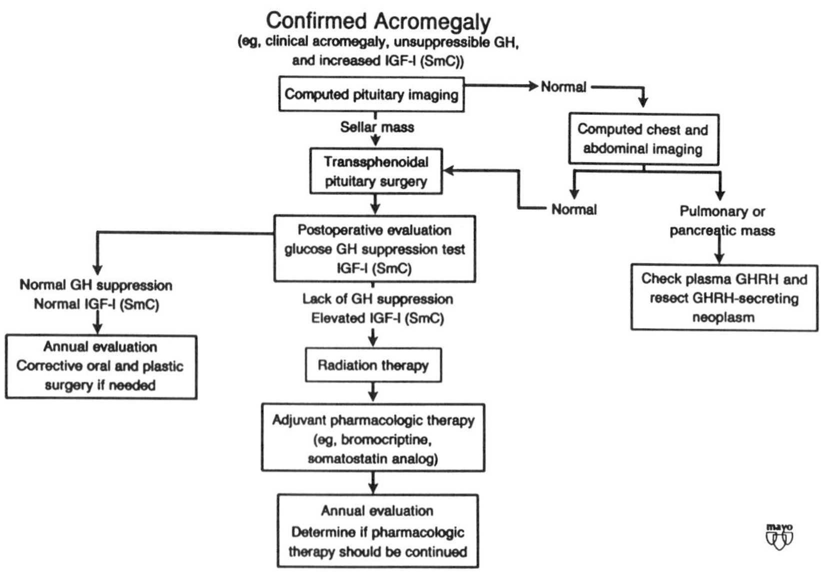

Figure 6 Algorithm for the treatment of acromegaly. GH, growth hormone, GHRH, growth hormone-releasing hormone. (From Ref. 57.)

and oily skin, hypertension, and cardiac dysfunction. The diagnosis of acromegaly depends on two criteria: a growth hormone level that is not suppressed to less than 2 μg/L after an oral glucose load (75 to 100 g) and an increased serum concentration of somatomedin C (insulinlike growth factor I). Pituitary imaging and treatment options are summarized in Figure 6 (57). The initial agent to treat the associated hypertension should be a thiazide diuretic.

VI. CONCLUSION

As noted, the therapy of the hypertension that commonly accompanies various endocrine disorders depends upon an accurate differential diagnosis. With that in hand, definitive therapy of both the hypertension and the underlying endocrinopathy are usually possible.

REFERENCES

1. Sutton M, Sheps SG, Lie JI. Prevalance of clinically unsuspected pheochromocytoma: review of a 50-year autopsy series. Mayo Clin Proc 1981; 56:354–360.
2. Sheps SG, Jiang N-S, Klee GG, van Heerden JA. Recent developments in the diagnosis and treatment of pheochromocytoma. Mayo Clin Proc 1990; 65:88–95.
3. National High Blood Pressure Education Program Working Group Report on Ambulatory Blood Pressure Monitoring. Arch Intern Med 1990; 150:2270–2280.
4. Nativ O, Grant CS, Sheps SG, et al. The clinical significance of nuclear DNA ploidy pattern in 184 patients with pheochromocytomas. Cancer 1992; 69:2683–2687.
5. Sheps SG, Jiang N-S, Klee GG. Diagnostic evaluation of pheochromocytoma. Endocrinol Metab Clin North Am 1988; 17:397–414.
6. Khafagi FA, Shapiro B, Fig LM, et al. Labetalol reduces iodine-131 MIBG uptake by pheochromocytoma and normal tissues. J Nuc Med 1989; 30:481–489.
7. van Heerden JA. Pheochromocytoma. In Cameron JO ed. Current Surgical Therapy, 4th ed. St. Louis: BC Decker, 1992.
8. Averbuck SD, Steakley CS, Young RC, et al. Malignant pheochromocytoma: effective treatment with a combination of cyclophosphamide, vincristine, and dacarbazine. Ann Intern Med 1988; 109:267–273.
9. Conn JW: Presidential address. Part I. Painting background. Part II. Primary aldosteronism, a new clinical syndrome. J Lab Clin Med 1955; 45:3–17.
10. Mader IJ, Iseri LT. Spontaneous hypopotassemia, hypomagnesemia, alkalosis and tetany due to hypersecretion of corticosterone-like mineralocorticoid. Am J Med 1955; 19:976–988.
11. Berglund G, Andersson O, Wilhelmsen L. Prevalence of primary and secondary hypertension: studies in a random population sample. Br Med J 1976; 2:554–556.
12. Streeten DHP, Tomycz N, Anderson GH Jr: Reliability of screening methods for the diagnosis of primary aldosteronism. Am J Med 1979; 67:403–413.
13. Young WF Jr, Klee GG: Primary aldosteronism: diagnostic evaluation. Endocrinol Metab Clin North Am 1988; 17:367–395.

14. Irony I, Kater CE, Biglieri EG, Shackleton CHL. Correctable subsets of primary aldosteronism: primary adrenal hyperplasia and renin responsive adenoma. Am J Hyperten 1990; 3:576–582.
15. Tunny TJ, Gordon RD, Klemm SA, Cohn D. Histological and biochemical distinctiveness of atypical aldosterone-producing adenomas responsive to upright posture and angiotensin. Clin Endocrinol 1991; 34:363–369.
16. Lifton RP, Dluhy RG, Powers M, et al. A chimaeric 11β-hydroxylase/aldosterone synthase gene causes glucocorticoid-remediable aldosteronism and human hypertension. Nature 1992; 355:262–265.
17. Stowasser M, Gordon RD, Tunny TJ, et al. Familial hyperaldosteronism type II: five families with a new variety of primary aldosteronism. Clin Exp Pharmacol Physiol 1992; 19:319–322.
18. Bravo EL, Fouad-Tarazi FM, Tarazi RC, et al. Clinical implications of primary aldosteronism with resistent hypertension. Hypertension 1988; 11(suppl I):I207–I211.
19. Fishman LM, Kuchel O, Liddle GW, et al. Incidence of primary aldosteronism uncomplicated "essential" hypertension: a prospective study with elevated aldosterone secretion and suppressed plasma renin activity used as diagnostic criteria. JAMA 1968; 205:497–502.
20. Weinberger MH, Grim CE, Hollifield JW, et al. Primary aldosteronism: diagnosis, localization, and treatment. Ann Intern Med 1979; 90:386–395.
21. Bravo EL, Tarazi RC, Dustan HP, et al. The changing clinical spectrum of primary aldosteronism. Am J Med 1983; 74:641–451.
22. Rich GM, Ulick S, Cook S, et al. Glucocorticoid-remediable aldosteronism in a large kindred: clinical spectrum and diagnosis using a characteristic biochemical phenotype. Ann Intern Med 1992; 116:813–820.
23. Jose A, Kaplan NM. Plasma renin activity in the diagnosis of primary aldosteronism: failure to distinguish primary aldosteronism from essential hypertension. Arch Intern Med 1969; 123:141–146.
24. Hiramatsu K, Yamada T, Yukimura Y, et al. A screening test to identify aldosterone-producing adenoma by measuring plasma renin activity: results in hypertension patients. Arch Intern Med 1981; 141:1589–1593.
25. McKenna TJ, Sequeira SJ, Heffernan A, et al. Diagnosis under random conditions of all disorders of renin-angiotensin-aldosterone axis, including primary hyperaldosteronism. J Clin Endocrinol Metab 1991; 73:952–957.
26. Young WF Jr, Hogan MJ, Klee GG, et al. Primary aldosteronism: diagnosis and treatment. Mayo Clin Proc 1990; 65:96–110.
27. Hambling C, Jung RT, Gunn A, et al. Re-evaluation of the captopril test for the diagnosis of primary hyperaldosteronism. Clin Endocrinol 1992; 36:499–503.
28. Radin DR, Manoogian C, Nadler JL. Diagnosis of primary hyperaldosteronism: importance of correlating CT findings with endocrinologic studies. Am J Roentgenology 1992; 158:553–557.
29. Doppman JL, Gill JR Jr, Miller DL, et al. Distinction between hyperaldosteronism due to bilateral hyperplasia and unilateral aldosteronoma: reliability of CT. Radiology 1992; 184:677–682.

30. Melby JC, Spark RF, Dale SL, et al. Diagnosis and localization of aldosterone-producing adenomas by adrenal-vein catheterization. N Engl J Med 1967; 277: 1050–1056.
31. Ferriss JB, Brown JJ, Fraser R, et al. Results of adrenal surgery in patients with hypertension, aldosterone excess, and low plasma renin concentration. Br Med J 1975; 1:135–138.
32. Grant CS, Carpenter P, van Heerden JA, Hamberger B. Primary aldosteronism: clinical management. Arch Surg 1984; 119:585–590.
33. Kremer D, Boddy K, Brown JJ, et al. Amiloride in the treatment of primary hyperaldosteronism and essential hypertension. Clin Endocrinol (Oxf) 1977; 7: 151–157.
34. Nadler JL, Hsueh W, Horton R. Therapeutic effect of calcium channel blockade in primary aldosteronism. J Clin Endocrinol Metab 1985 60:896–899.
35. Griffing GT, Melby JC. The therapeutic effect of a new angiotensin-converting enzyme inhibitor, enalapril maleate, in idiopathic hyperaldosteronism. J Clin Hypertens 1985; 3:265–276.
36. Ganguly A, Grim CE, Bergstein J, et al. Genetic and pathophysiological studies of a new kindred with glucocorticoid-suppressible hyperaldosteronism manifest in three generations. J Clin Endocrinol Metab 1981; 53:1040–1046.
37. Guthrie GP, Wilson EA, Quillen DL, Jawad MJ. Adrenal androgen excess and defective 11β-hydroxylation in women with idiopathic hirsutism. Arch Intern Med 1982; 142:729–735.
38. White PC, New MI, Dupont B. Congenital adrenal hyperplasia. N Engl J Med 1987; 316:1519–1524.
39. Biglieri EG, Kater CE. 17α-Hydroxylation deficiency. Endocrinol Metab Clin North Am 1991; 20:257–268.
40. Kondo K, Saruta T, Saito I, et al. Benign desoxycorticosterone-producing adrenal tumor. JAMA 1976; 236:1042.
41. Brandon DD, Markwick AJ, Chrousos GP, Loriaux DL. Glucocorticoid resistance in humans and non-human primates. Cancer Res 1989; 49(suppl):2203s–2213s.
42. Javier EC, Reardon GE, Malchoff CD. Glucocorticoid resistance and its clinical presentations. Endocrinologist 1991; 1:141–148.
43. Stewart PM, Wallace AM, Valentino R, et al. Mineralocorticoid activity of liquorice: 11-beta-hydroxysteroid dehydrogenase deficiency comes of age. Lancet 1987; 2:821–824.
44. Ulick S, Tedde R, Mantero F. Pathogenesis of the type 2 variant of the syndrome of apparent mineralocorticoid excess. J Clin Endocrinol Metab 1990; 70:200–206.
45. Salassa RM, Mattox VR, Rosevear JW. Inhibition of the "mineralocorticoid" activity of licorice by spironolactone. J Clin Endocrinol Metab 1962; 22:1156–1159.
46. Farese RV Jr, Biglieri EG, Shackleton CHL, et al. Licorice-induced hypermineralocorticoidism. N Engl J Med 1991; 325:1223–1227.
47. Walker BR, Edwards CRW. Cushing's syndrome. In: James VHT, ed. The Adrenal Gland. 2d ed. New York: Raven Press, 1992:289–318.

48. Ulick S, Wang JZ, Blumenfeld JD, Pickering TG. Cortisol inactivation overload: a mechanism of mineralocorticoid hypertension in the ectopic adrenocorticotropin syndrome. J Clin Endocrinol Metab 1992; 74:963–967.
49. Leinung MC, Young WF Jr, Whitaker MD, et al. Diagnosis of corticotropin-producing bronchial carcinoid tumors causing Cushing's syndrome. Mayo Clin Proc 1990; 65:1314–1321.
50. McNally PG, Howlett TA. Investigation of Cushing's syndrome by inferior petrosal sinus sampling. Trends Endocrinol Metab 1993; 4:117–112.
51. O'Neal LW, Kissane JM, Hartroft PM. The kidney in endocrine hypertension: Cushing's syndrome, pheochromocytoma, and aldosteronism. Arch Surg 1970; 100:498–505.
52. Streeten DHP, Anderson GH Jr, Howland T, et al. Effects of thyroid function on blood pressure: recognition of hypothyroid hypertension. Hypertension 1988; 11:78–83.
53. Shapiro LE, Surks MI. Managing hypothyroidism. Endocrinologist 1991; 1: 343–347.
54. Salahudeen AK, Thomas TH, Sellars L, et al. Hypertension and renal dysfunction in primary hyperparathyroidism: effect of parathyroidectomy. Clin Sci 1989; 76:289–296.
55. Diamond TW, Botha JR, Wing J, et al. Parathyroid hypertension: a reversible disorder. Arch Intern Med 1986; 146:1709–1712.
56. Thuesen L, Christensen SE, Weeke J, et al. A hyperkinetic heart in uncomplicated active acromegaly: explanation of hypertension in acromegalic patients? Acta Med Scand 1988; 223:337–343.
57. Young WF Jr. Acromegaly. In: Rakel RE, ed. Conn's Current Therapy 1990. Philadelphia: WB Saunders, 1990:557–559.

12

Hypertensive Crises

C. VENKATA S. RAM

University of Texas Southwestern Medical Center at Dallas
Dallas, Texas

Despite the high prevalence of hypertension, hypertensive crises occur only infrequently in clinical practice, developing in no more than 1% to 2% of hypertensive patients (1). Hypertensive crises may develop in patients with chronic hypertension but may also occur in patients with hypertension that is newly discovered or of short duration.

Although any form of hypertension may lead to the development of hypertensive crises, the chief determinant of the complication is the level of blood pressure rather than its cause. Another factor contributing to the development of hypertensive crisis is the abruptness with which the blood pressure rises. In previously normotensive individuals, acute elevations in arterial pressure may cause target organ damage to a greater extent at any given level of blood pressure than in those with chronic hypertension. This scenario seems to be especially important, moreso than the absolute level of blood pressure, under certain clinical situations (e.g., onset of hypertension as in children with acute glomerulonephritis, toxemia of pregnancy, and drug-induced hypertension). In the management of a patient with hypertensive crisis, prompt therapy should take precedence over diagnostic studies. Acute acomplications of hypertensive crisis are largely reversible, but the degree of reversibility depends on how soon appropriate treatment is rendered. In some situations (e.g., aortic dissection or acute left ventricular failure) immediate reduction of blood pressure is indicated, not because of its absolute level but because certain coexisting complications may make even moderate hypertension dangerous.

Hypertensive crises can be conveniently categorized into emergencies and urgencies (Tables 1 and 2). There is no arbitrary level of blood pressure separating hypertensive emergencies and urgencies, although, in the former, the blood pressure levels generally tend to exceed 200/130 mm Hg. Hypertensive emergencies carry poor prognosis unless the blood pressure is reduced quickly, whereas hypertensive urgencies pose less immediate danger, but may become emergencies if the blood pressure is not vigorously controlled. In typical hypertensive emergencies, the blood pressure should be reduced in a few hours, whereas in hypertensive urgencies blood pressure reduction can be accomplished in several hours or days.

I. ACCELERATED AND MALIGNANT HYPERTENSION

A. Clinical Manifestations

Salient clinical features of accelerated/malignant hypertension include headache, malaise, weight loss, and visual disturbances ranging from blurring to blindness. Drowsiness and altered mental status are commonly observed.

Table 1 Examples of Hypertensive Emergencies

Accelerated/malignant hypertension[a]
Hypertensive encephalopathy
Acute left ventricular failure
Acute aortic dissection
? Intracranial hemorrhage
Pheochromocytoma crisis
MAO inhibitor + tyramine interaction
Eclampsia
Substance-/drug-induced acute hypertension

[a]Can also be considered as an urgency.

Table 2 Examples of Hypertensive Urgencies

Accelerated/malignant hypertension[a]
Severe hypertension associated with coronary artery disease
Severe hypertension in the kidney transplant patient
Preoperative hypertension
Hypertension associated with burns

[a]Can also be considered as an emergency.

Congestive heart failure can be a presenting feature of malignant hypertension as a direct consequence of left ventricular dysfunction or of volume retention resulting from associated renal insufficiency. Azotemia and proteinuria are common and renal function deteriorates rapidly without proper therapy. Even with appropriate treatment, renal function may decline at times as a result of reduced renal perfusion. Anemia is common; the degree may give a clue as to the proximate cause: severe anemia suggests underlying chronic renal disease, whereas mild anemia may reflect microangiopathic hemolysis.

B. Management

Patients with accelerated/malignant hypertension should be treated in the hospital since the goal is not simply to lower the blood pressure but to monitor, stabilize, and reverse the damage to target organs and to exclude reversible causes of hypertension. Preferably, the patients should be treated in an intensive care unit. However, in the absence of significant target organ failure, patients can be managed on the wards.

Sodium restriction is not necessary during early stages of treatment unless there is evidence of fluid overload. Similarly, the need for immediate diuretic therapy must be individualized. Diuretic therapy may be needed subsequently to potentiate the hypotensive effects of certain vasodilators such as nitroprusside. Diuretics should not be used unnecessarily since volume depletion in malignant hypertension can further aggravate the pathophysiological mechanisms.

Sodium nitroprusside is a suitable drug for immediate reduction of severe hypertension. The details of its use will be discussed later. Prompt reduction in blood pressure can similarly be accomplished by bolus injections or slow infusion of diazoxide or labetalol.

While parenteral therapy is widely used in the initial treatment of malignant hypertension, various oral therapies can also be successfully used. Captopril, minoxidil, clonidine, prazosin, labetalol, and nifedipine have all been used for initial treatment of malignant hypertension. The choice of oral versus parenteral therapy depends on the monitoring facilities, condition of the patient, and coexisting complications. Once the blood pressure is brought to safe levels, long-term therapy must be initiated with appropriate oral agent(s) based on the renal, cardiac, and neurological status of the patient.

II. HYPERTENSIVE ENCEPHALOPATHY

Hypertensive encephalopathy should be quickly recognized and effectively treated since it carries a poor prognosis if untreated, but is rapidly reversible with proper treatment (2). The clinical manifestations of hypertensive encephalopathy are precipitated not only by severity of blood pressure elevation but also by the abrupt onset of hypertension.

A. Clinical Features

Clinical manifestations of hypertensive encephalopathy include severe generalized headache; restlessness; neurological dysfunction consisting of confusion, somnolence, and stupor; and, if untreated, progressive worsening of the sensorium culminating in coma and death. Other clinical features may include projectile vomiting, visual disturbances ranging from blurring to frank blindness, and transient focal neurological deficits. Sometimes (especially in children) generalized or focal seizures may dominate the clinical picture. Although papilledema is present in most patients, its absence should not exclude the diagnosis of hypertensive encephalopathy.

Hypertensive encephalopathy must be distinguished from other acute neurological complications of hypertension such as cerebral infarction or hemorrhage and uremic encephalopathy (2) (Table 3). The only definitive criterion to confirm the diagnosis of hypertensive encephalopathy is a prompt response of the patient's condition to antihypertensive therapy. The syndrome usually resolves within 1 to 12 hours with appropriate control of hypertension.

B. Management

Once the diagnosis of hypertensive encephalopathy is suspected, the blood pressure should be lowered rapidly, yet the diastolic blood pressure should remain at or slightly above 100 mm Hg. Rapid reduction in the blood pressure produces prompt relief of symptoms of hypertensive encephalopathy and parenteral drugs are preferred to prevent permanent neurological damage.

III. ACUTE AORTIC DISSECTION

The increased occurrence of dissecting aortic aneurysms in patients with hypertension and the usual presence of hypertension in patients with dissecting aneurysm of the aorta are well established (3). The primary event in aortic dissection is rupture of the intima with subsequent exposure of the media to the intraluminal pressure of the aorta, which separates the layers of the aorta, causing a classic "double-barrel" aorta.

A. Clinical Features

The usual patient with a dissection of the aorta, especially one involving the ascending aorta, is an elderly male with a chronic history of hypertension

Table 3 Differential Features of Hypertensive Encephalopathy and Cerebrovascular Accidents

	Evolution	Headache	Consciousness	Signs
Hypertensive encephalopathy	Subacute (12–18 hr)	Severe Generalized Recent onset	Initially clear but progresses to coma	Nausea and vomiting Visual disturbance Seizures Transient neurological deficits
Cerebral infarction	Rapid (few min to 6 hr)	None or mild	Inattentive Coma very rare	Fixed neurological deficits
Cerebral embolus	Sudden	None or mild	Mild lethargy	Changing signs
Cerebral hemorrhage	Rapid	Sudden Severe Occipital	Rapid progression to coma	Dense deficits
Subarachnoid hemorrhage	Rapid	Sudden Severe Local to general	Normal or altered, depending on the site and secondary involvement	Fever Stiff neck Aphasia Cranial nerve palsies

who has severe and persistent chest pain. The symptoms of acute dissection are listed in Table 4.

Of all the symptoms, severe pain is the most important manifestation. It is easily confused with the pain of acute myocardial infarction. The pain of dissection is abrupt in onset and is quite severe from the beginning. Other symptoms of aortic dissection depend on the location and progression of the dissection. Physical findings that can be seen in acute aortic dissection can be manifold, depending on the extent and location of the dissecting process.

Table 4 Clinical Features of Acute Aortic Dissection

Severe pain in the chest, intrascapular region, neck, midback, sacral area
Syncope
Confusional state or headache
Blindness
Hemoptysis
Dyspnea
Nausea and vomiting
Melena or hematemesis
Oliguria, anuria, or hematuria
Paralysis

The clinical diagnosis of aortic dissection is based upon a high index of suspicion and the presenting features. Once the diagnosis is suspected, immediate medical therapy should be implemented pending the diagnostic tests. A chest X-ray may show a recent widening of the mediastinum but unless compared with the previous films, it is not a useful study.

Two-dimensional echocardiography, transesophageal echocardiography, and magnetic resonance imaging (MRI) have all been utilized to diagnose aortic dissection (4). Digital and/or conventional angiography provides more thorough information concerning the anatomy of dissection and the course taken by the dissecting hematoma.

B. Initial Management

Once the diagnosis of acute aortic dissection is apparent, the following steps should be undertaken. If the patient is hypertensive, blood pressure should be reduced to near normal levels. When instituting antihypertensive therapy, one should keep in mind that the force and velocity of ventricular contraction (dp/dt) and the pulsatile flow are important determinants of the shearing force acting on the aortic wall (5). Attempts should be made to decrease the dp/dt with a suitable agent; therefore, the objective of appropriate antihypertensive therapy is to reduce the velocity of myocardial shortening, which can be done with drugs which exert negative inotropic effects. An ideal agent would be trimethaphan, which has a balanced hemodynamic action and is rapidly effective. Since this drug is a ganglion blocking agent, it decreases the neural transmission at the myocardial contractility sites and therefore decreases the pulsative flow and blunts the sharpness of the pulse wave generated by the heart. The other options would include labetalol, a combined alpha- and beta-blocking drug, or the ultra-short-acting beta-blocker esmolol (6). The goal of antihypertensive therapy is to lower the blood pressure to the lowest level tolerated by the patient without causing cerebral, myocardial, or renal hypoperfusion.

C. Definitive Therapy

The choice between continuing medical therapy and surgical intervention depends on the different clinical behavior of proximal and distal dissections in the early phase of the disease. Surgery is the definitive treatment of choice for proximal dissection because of the potentially devastating consequences of the progression of the hematoma and frequent association of this type with pulse deficits, aortic regurgitation, pericardial tamponade and neurological dysfunction, and so on.

For the patients with uncomplicated distal dissection, continuation of chronic medical therapy offers a slight advantage over surgical therapy. The advantage of medical therapy is largely due to the fact that patients with distal dissection tend to have advanced atherosclerotic or cardiac disease. Surgery should be undertaken in these patients if there is evidence of rupture or vital organ compromise or inability to contain the hematoma with appropriate medical therapy.

IV. MISCELLANEOUS CONDITIONS

Hypertension is often present in patients with coronary artery disease or congestive heart failure which may present as crises. These are covered in Chapter 7. Other causes include the following, which are also covered elsewhere:

Pheochromocytoma (Chapter 11)
Drug toxicity (Chapter 13)
Eclampsia (Chapter 10)

A hyperadrenergic state mimicking pheochromocytoma crisis has been reported after abrupt discontinuation of the antihypertensive drug clonidine (7). When clonidine is abruptly discontinued (especially high doses) or even sometimes rapidly tapered, a syndrome has been noted consisting of nausea, palpitations, anxiety, sweating, nervousness, and headache—along with marked elevation of the blood pressure. In some patients the blood pressure rises beyond the pretreatment level. The probable mechanism of the clonidine withdrawal syndrome is a sudden activation of sympathetic activity.

Symptoms of clonidine withdrawal can be relieved by reinstitution of clonidine. If there is marked elevation of blood pressure and the patient is experiencing symptoms—such as palpitations, chest discomfort, or epigastric discomfort—intravenous administration of phentolamine or labetalol is recommended.

A. Hypertensive Crisis Associated with Drug and Food Reactions: Monoamine Oxidase Inhibitors

Patients receiving monoamine oxidase (MAO) inhibitors are at risk of development of hypertensive crisis if they should also take drugs such as ephedrine or amphetamines, or foods containing high quantities of tyramine. In the presence of an inhibitor of MAO, tyramine and indirectly acting sympathetic amines escape oxidative degradation, enter the systemic circulation, and potentiate the actions of catecholamines. Sympathomimetic amines such as those contained in nonprescription cold remedies can also provoke this response. Immediate treatment is similar to that of pheochromocytoma crisis (8).

B. Hypertensive Crisis Due to Systemic Vasculitis

Abrupt onset of severe hypertension has been known to occur as a complication of necrotizing vasculitis (9). Possible mechanisms include a direct increase in peripheral vascular resistance as a result of the vasculitis, or via activation of the renin-angiotensin system from renal ischemia.

C. Postoperative Hypertension

Severe hypertension may occur in some patients in the postoperative period, especially after open heart operations and carotid artery surgery. The cause of severe postoperative hypertension is multifactorial: withdrawal of antihypertensive drugs, pain, volume overload, and sympathetic activation. Patients with cerebrovascular and coronary artery disease are at particular risk of development of postoperative hypertension. Therapy should be individualized, and in some situations immediate lowering of the blood pressure is warranted.

V. MANAGEMENT OF HYPERTENSIVE CRISES

The need to hospitalize the patient and the choice of therapeutic options, including the use of parenteral versus oral therapy, depend on the clinical evaluation of the patient. Patients with hypertensive emergencies should be hospitalized; those with hypertensive urgencies may not require admission. The therapeutic principle underlying the management of hypertensive crisis is not only to lower the blood pressure quickly but to prevent, arrest, and reverse the target organ dysfunction and damage. Therefore, close supervision of the patient while the blood pressure is being lowered is mandatory. There are no firm guidelines as to the degree of desired blood pressure reduction, but a reasonable goal for most hypertensive emergencies is to lower the diastolic blood pressure to 100 mm Hg (or to reduce the mean arterial pressure by 25%) over a period of minutes to hours. The following sections provide a review of the parenteral drugs useful in the management of hypertensive emergencies and urgencies (Table 5).

A. Nitroprusside

Sodium nitroprusside is one of the most potent blood pressure lowering drugs and possesses the advantageous properties of rapid onset and offset of action. The hypotensive response occurs within seconds after infusion is started and is dissipated almost as rapidly when the infusion is discontinued. The actions of nitroprusside are almost exclusively confined to the vascular smooth muscle, where it relaxes both the arteries and the veins. During nitroprusside administration, systemic arterial and venous pressures are reduced.

Table 5 Parenteral Drugs Useful in the Immediate Control of Severe Hypertension

Drug	Route and dosage	Onset	Offset	Comments
Nitroprusside	i.v. Infusion, 0.3 μg/kg/min to 8 μg/kg/min	Seconds	3–5 min	Thiocyanate toxicity may occur with prolonged (>48 hr) or high-dose infusion (>15 μg/kg/min), particularly in renal insufficiency
Nicardipine	i.v., 5–15 mg/hr	5–15 min	30–40 min	May cause reflex tachycardia
Labetalol	i.v., 20 mg q 10 min (can increase to 80 mg doses)	5 min or less	3–6 hr	Prompt response; can be followed with same drug taken orally
Trimethaphan	i.v. Infusion pump, 0.5–5 mg/min	1–5 min	10 min	Drug of choice for treatment of aortic dissection
Diazoxide	i.v., 50–150 mg q 5 min or as infusion of 7.5–30 mg/min	1–5 min	4–25 hr	Should not be used for patients with angina pectoris, myocardial infarction, dissecting aneurysm
Enalaprilat	i.v., 1.25 mg q 6 hr	15 min	4–6 hr	May be particularly advantageous in patients with pulmonary edema

Although the exact mechanism by which nitroprusside dilates the vasculature has not been firmly established, it may interfere with the intracellular activation of calcium, thereby inhibiting the release of calcium from storage sites, or it may facilitate the extrusion of intracellular calcium or enhance sequestration of intracellular calcium.

The cardiac output response to nitroprusside is quite variable and depends largely on the preexisting hemodynamic status of the patient. In hypertensive patients not in congestive heart failure, cardiac output usually falls; in those with low output states the cardiac ejection fraction consistently increases.

Because of nitroprusside's rapid onset of action and potency, infusion must be closely monitored by means of an infusion pump or a microdrip regulator and intra-arterial blood pressure recording. In 1991, the FDA revised the labeling of nitroprusside to underscore the dangers of hypotension and other side effects (10). The initial infusion rate should be no higher than 0.3 μg/kg/min, and this can be increased every 5 minutes until the desired blood pressure level is obtained. Once the desired effect of nitroprusside is achieved, the infusion usually can be maintained with minimal adjustment, but the blood pressure should be continuously monitored. Parenteral treatment of hypertensive crisis generally is needed only for 12 to 48 hours and the drug should be discontinued as soon as alternate modes of therapy have proved effective. Because of its short duration of action, the effects of stopping the therapy will be seen within a few minutes. If indicated, treatment can be resumed promptly. Hypotension is the most common but avoidable side effect of nitroprusside therapy.

The immediate metabolic product of nitroprusside is cyanide, which is liberated by the direct combination of nitroprusside with the sulfhydryl groups in red cells and tissues. The circulating cyanide then is rapidly converted in the liver to thiocyanate by the enzyme rhodanase or transsulfarase, which in turn is removed almost exclusively by the kidney with a half-life of approximately 1 week.

Cyanide toxicity from nitroprusside, although extremely rare, has been reported. Prophylactic infusion of hydroxocobalamin (vitamin B_{12a}) at 25 mg/hr has been shown to decrease the cyanide concentration and tissue hypoxia resulting from nitroprusside infusion during surgery (11). Hydroxocobalamin has one cyanide radical less than cyanocobalamin and, therefore, allows cyanide to combine and form cyanocobalamin, which is then excreted in the urine. When cyanide toxicity is suspected on the basis of hypoxemia and metabolic acidosis, nitroprusside infusion should be discontinued and 3% solution of sodium nitrite (4 to 6 mg) be given by slow i.v. infusion over 2 to 4 minutes, followed by an infusion of sodium thiosulfate (50 ml of a 25% solution).

Thiocyanate toxicity secondary to nitroprusside is uncommon and occurs only with high doses and in the presence of renal failure. Symptoms of thiocyanate toxicity include fatigue, nausea, anorexia, skin rashes, headaches, disorientation, and psychotic behavior. They tend to occur at plasma levels of 5 to 10 mg/dl, and levels greater than 20 mg/dl are dangerous. Therefore, during high-dose infusions of nitroprusside—and especially when renal function is impaired—determinations of plasma thiocyanate levels are recommended; treatment should be interrupted when the thiocyanate level is close to 10 mg/dl. Treatment of thiocyanate toxicity demands discontinuation of the drug and perhaps institution of dialysis.

It has been suggested that nitroprusside may enhance myocardial ischemia by preferentially dilating the coronary vessels in the nonischemic myocardium, an effect known as "coronary steal." In a comparative study, nitroprusside and nitroglycerin produced similar hemodynamic effects but the former increased the electrocardiographic ST segment elevations (12). In patients with coronary artery disease, nitroprusside, in contrast to nitroglycerin, was shown to increase ischemic injury via effecting the redistribution of blood flow away from ischemic zones (13). In contrast to the preceding findings is the observation that nitroprusside improves myocardial perfusion in experimental coronary obstruction (14). What are the clinical implications of these findings? Clinicians using nitroprusside must be aware that it has the potential to worsen myocardial ischemia in susceptible patients. Animal studies have demonstrated that high doses of nitroprusside may reduce cerebral blood flow (15). A similar effect was seen in humans (16). We are not sure about the clinical implications of these observations.

B. Intravenous Labetalol

Labetalol, a combined alpha- and beta-adrenergic blocking drug, can be used parenterally or orally for the treatment of hypertensive emergencies. Intravenous labetalol administered either as a continuous infusion or in bolus injections reduces the blood pressure promptly through its rapid onset of action (17). Controlled smooth reduction in blood pressure may be obtained by continuous infusion of labetalol at the rate of 0.5 to 2 mg/min. As with nitroprusside, close monitoring of the patient is required during the infusion of labetalol therapy. Rapid (but not abrupt) lowering of blood pressure can also be accomplished with bolus injections of labetalol (18). Bolus injections of 20 to 40 mg can be given every 10 to 15 minutes until the desired blood pressure level is obtained or until a cumulative labetalol dose of 300 mg is reached. Minibolus injections are safer than the large bolus injections. Labetalol should not be used in patients who may have contraindications to the use of beta-blockers.

C. Nicardipine Infusion

Nicardipine is a dihydropyridine calcium antagonist, recently approved by the FDA, which has been shown to exert a prompt hypotensive effect when given intravenously in patients with severe hypertension (19). Nicardipine infusion (5.0 mg/hr) can be titrated up gradually to obtain the desired therapeutic effect. Once a stable blood pressure level is reached, most patients do not require dosage alterations. Thus, nicardipine pharmacodynamics resemble those of nitroprusside in terms of the onset, duration, and offset of action. Because of its mechanism of action (calcium channel blockade), nicardipine may be beneficial in preserving tissue perfusion. This property may be particularly advantageous in patients with ischemic disorders, such as coronary, cerebrovascular, and peripheral vascular disease. From our clinical experience with the use of nicardipine (20), we believe that it may turn out to be a useful therapeutic option in the management of severe hypertension with or without target organ damage. This mode of therapy is particularly attractive since the patients can be switched to the oral formulation of the drug.

D. Trimethaphan

Trimethaphan camsylate is a ganglion blocking agent. The hypotensive effect of trimethaphan is accompanied by a reduction in left ventricular ejection rate and cardiac output. These attributes make it a drug of choice for the medical treatment of acute aortic dissection. Trimethaphan has a rapid onset of action, and its effects dissipate within a few minutes of discontinuation of the drug. The head of the bed should be elevated to augment the antihypertensive effect of this agent. Like nitroprusside, trimethaphan should be administered as a continuous intravenous drip, and constant monitoring is necessary, preferably in the intensive care unit. The usual starting dose of the drug should be 1 mg/min titrated to obtain the desired blood pressure level. After prolonged infusion, tachyphylaxis may result from intravascular volume expansion, which can be partially overcome by effective diuretic therapy.

The major disadvantage of trimethaphan is that it causes parasympathetic inhibition resulting in paralytic ileus, urinary retention, and mydriasis. These effects are likely to occur when the drug is administered for more than a day or two.

E. Diazoxide

Diazoxide has a direct relaxant effect on the vascular smooth muscle, causing a rapid fall in arterial blood pressure. The hypotensive effect of diazoxide is associated with striking increases in heart rate and cardiac output. Diazoxide has no direct effect on the myocardium, but reflex increases in the cardiac output and heart rate may pose a problem to patients with intrinsic cardiac disease. Expansion of plasma volume and edema formation occur during diazoxide therapy, partly because of its direct tubular antinatriuretic action. Because of the difficulty in achieving a smooth, controllable fall in blood pressure and the various side effects, the use of diazoxide has been sharply curtailed.

F. Phentolamine

Phentolamine, an alpha-receptor blocking agent, is specifically indicated for treating hypertensive crises associated with increased circulating catecholamines (e.g., pheochromocytoma crisis, certain cases of clonidine withdrawal syndrome, and crises resulting from MAO inhibitor and drug-food interaction). The hypotensive effect of a single intravenous bolus injection is short-lived, less than 15 minutes.

G. Nitroglycerin

The dominant effect of nitroglycerin is venodilatation, resulting in reduction of venous return (preload) to the heart. It is a weak systemic arterial dilator with a greater effect on large arteries than on smaller arteries. Low doses cause venodilatation; higher doses are required to produce a fall in systemic blood pressure (21). Because of nitroglycerin's pharmacological actions, infusion may be particularly beneficial in patients with coronary artery disease with or without hypertension. Although there are no controlled studies, nitroglycerin therapy can be considered in the management of severe hypertension associated with coronary artery disease. The usual initial dosage of nitroglycerin is 5 to 15 μg/min and is titrated upward to a desired therapeutic endpoint. It has a rapid onset (within 2 to 5 minutes) and offset of action.

H. Fenoldopam

Fenoldopam is an experimental vasodilator that acts by activating dopamine-1 (DA_1) receptors in the vascular bed. Although its effects on the renal vasculature are potent, resistance in other vascular beds is also reduced. Fenoldopam infusion has been shown to be effective in the immediate management of severe hypertension (22). It may cause significant tachycardia. The advantages of fenoldopam, if any, remain to be determined and further investigations are currently in progress.

I. Intravenous Enalaprilat

Enalaprilat, an angiotension converting enzyme (ACE) inhibitor, is available in parenteral form for rapid lowering of blood pressure in patients with severe hypertension (23). The onset of action after the intravenous injection usually occurs within 15 minutes with maximum effect taking place within 1 to 4 hours. The duration of hemodynamic effects is dose dependent, but in most patients it is approximately 6 hours. Loop diuretics potentiate the hypotensive response of i.v. enalaprilat. The dose for treating severe hypertension is likely given over a 5-minute period every 6 hours. Higher doses have not been demonstrated to produce additional therapeutic effects. The starting dose should be lower (0.625 mg) for patients on diuretic therapy.

J. Transition from Parenteral to Oral Therapy

After the immediate management of a hypertensive emergency or urgency with parenteral therapy, oral agents should be initiated at the earliest opportunity. Generally, oral therapy can be begun while tapering off the parenteral drug. If possible, oral drugs should be started with a low dose which can be increased gradually depending on the clinical response. It is important to detect and prevent postural hypotension during transition to oral therapy.

K. Role of Concomitant Diuretic Therapy

Diuretics per se have a limited role in the management of hypertensive emergencies. However, they potentiate the therapeutic response to nondiuretic agents. When the blood pressure does not respond satisfactorily to an adequate dose of the primary agent, adding a diuretic (furosemide) may be helpful. Certainly in volume overloaded states such as heart failure, concomitant administration of a loop diuretic is indicated for optimal results. Diuretics should not be used routinely in the management of hypertensive crises as prior volume depletion may be present.

VI. IMMEDIATE MANAGEMENT OF SEVERE HYPERTENSION WITH ORALLY EFFECTIVE DRUGS

Clinical experience has suggested that antihypertensive drugs given orally in either single or multiple doses lower the blood pressure immediately in patients with severe hypertension (Table 6). Oral administration of a variety of antihypertensive drugs has been utilized in patients with or without concomitant target organ damage. Obviously, this approach is most suitable for patients with hypertensive urgencies, not emergencies.

Table 6 Acute Oral Therapy for the Immediate Control of Severe Hypertension

Drug	Route and dosage	Onset	Offset	Comments
Nifedipine	10–20 mg po or sublingual	5–15 min	3–5 hr	Generally good response; short duration of action for optimal dosage not standard
Clonidine	0.2 mg po initially, then 0.1 mg/hr, up to 0.8 mg total	0.5–2 hr	6–8 hr	Prominant sedation
Captopril	6.5–25 mg po	15 min	4–6 hr	Generally good, sometimes excessive response
Minoxidil	5–10 mg po	30–60 min	12–16 hr	Tachycardia, fluid retention

A. Nifedipine

Nifedipine, a calcium channel blocker, given orally or sublingually, has been shown to reduce the blood pressure rapidly and to be useful in the management of hypertensive crises (24). Immediate reduction in the blood pressure can be accomplished with sublingual (punctured capsule, or nifedipine liquid drawn out of the capsule with a syringe) or oral administration of the capsules. The drug is also effective when the capsule is bitten and then swallowed. The advantages of nifedipine are rapid onset of action and lack of central nervous system (CNS) depression. It may cause reflex tachycardia. Since the duration of action of nifedipine is short, patients who receive this drug for hypertensive emergencies should be monitored for several hours to consider readministration of the drug. Nifedipine is a useful choice for the management of hypertensive urgencies. The hypotensive effects of sublingual nifedipine manifest within 10 minutes and the nadir is seen at about 30 minutes.

Although the sublingual route has been widely used, nifedipine capsules swallowed intact produce similar antihypertensive effects. From a pharmacokinetic viewpoint, different modalities of administration result in variable blood levels of the drug. In fact, in one study, sublingual nifedipine produced negligible blood levels in contrast to the oral mode of administration (25). Abrupt fall in the blood pressure induced by nifedipine administration can cause certain adverse effects—symptomatic hypotension, tachycardia, and ischemic events. Therefore, the clinical need to use nifedipine capsules to lower the blood pressure urgently should be carefully assessed.

B. Clonidine

Clonidine therapy has been shown to produce an immediate antihypertensive effect with repetitive dosing (26). Typically, clonidine loading is accomplished in the emergency room by administering clonidine orally 0.1 mg every hour until the desired goal is obtained. After the availability of nifedipine, clonidine loading has been used infrequently and is on the decline. Clonidine and nifedipine are equally effective in the treatment of hypertensive urgencies. Unlike clonidine, nifedipine does not cause sedation.

Zeller et al. (27) evaluated the blood pressure responses to (1) clonidine loading (given hourly), (2) initial dose of clonidine followed by placebo given hourly, and (3) maintenance therapy without loading. There was no difference in the therapeutic response to clonidine given hourly compared to a single dose. At 24 hours and at 1 week, there were no differences in control of blood pressure between the groups. These data suggest that acute oral antihypertensive drug loading to treat severe hypertension offers no advantages. On the contrary, such therapy can cause hemodynamic and other complications such as prominent sedation.

C. Angiotensin Converting Enzyme Inhibitors

Captopril, an ACE inhibitor, has been found to be effective in the immediate treatment of severe hypertension and hypertensive crises (28). Captopril lowers the blood pressure promptly without causing tachycardia and thus offers a distinct hemodynamic advantage over direct arteriolar dilators. However, the maximal effect from orally administered captopril may not be attained for as long as 2 hours. On the other hand, there are reports documenting the effectiveness of sublingual captopril in the treatment of hypertensive crisis (29). Since experience with sublingual captopril is rather limited, further data have to be generated to define its role in the acute management of hypertensive crisis. High renin states such as malignant hypertension associated with scleroderma renal crisis are particularly responsive to captopril. Volume depleted patients merit closer surveillance as converting enzyme inhibition in these individuals may cause profound hypotension and azotemia. Comparative studies have demonstrated that captopril and nifedipine are equally effective in immediate treatment of severe hypertension (30). In general, the onset of action of nifedipine is more rapid than that of captopril (by approximately 10 minutes), an insignificant factor, in my opinion.

D. Minoxidil

Minoxidil is a powerful direct vasodilator and has been successfully used in the treatment of refractory or severe hypertension. Because of its relatively rapid onset of action and sustained duration, this drug has been used for the treatment of hypertension crises. Minoxidil in doses ranging from 2.5 to 10 mg can be given every 4 to 6 hours initially in the treatment of severe hypertension. It works best when given along with a diuretic, and an adrenergic blocker is necessary to counteract the reflex tachycardia.

E. Oral Labetalol

Labetalol can be administered orally (100 to 300 mg) in the treatment of hypertensive urgencies (31). Because of its dual adrenergic blockade, the fall in blood pressure is not accompanied by reflex tachycardia, which can be beneficial especially in patients with coronary artery disease.

VII. COMPLICATIONS OF THERAPY

Rapid control of hypertension is not without hazards. Unwarranted fall in blood pressure may cause hypoperfusion to the heart, brain, or kidney, resulting in ischemic sequelae.

A. Renal Function

Accelerated/malignant hypertension and hypertensive encephalopathy are more commonly seen in patients with a background of renal insufficiency. Effective control of hypertension under such circumstances may result in transient deterioration of renal function, and temporary dialysis may sometimes be necessary. Long-term treatment of severe hypertension, however, is likely to stabilize or even improve renal function (32).

B. Cerebral Function and Effects of Acute Antihypertensive Therapy

As explained in more detail in Chapter 8, cerebral blood flow (CBF) is normally maintained with a safe margin despite wide variations in systemic blood pressure. However, CBF may be disrupted in certain hypertensive crises (e.g., hypertensive encephalopathy), and antihypertensive therapy may adversely influence cerebral circulation. Experimental data obtained from hypertensive rats suggest that different antihypertensive drugs may have different effects on cerebral blood flow (33). For example, diazoxide maintains fairly constant CBF until systemic blood pressure falls to a very low level; hydralazine causes disruption of CBF independent of change in systemic blood pressure; converting enzyme inhibitors and calcium antagonists appear to have a favorable impact on CBF. The relevance of these observations for humans remains to be determined.

C. Other Problems

The complications of antihypertensive therapy usually result from hypotension and sometimes from the nature of therapy—such as diazoxide's causing cardiac ischemia and nitroprusside's causing thiocyanate toxicity. These complications can be prevented by careful evaluation of the patient and by choice of an appropriate antihypertensive agent. In this respect, drugs with a short duration of action offer an advantage because unwanted hypotension can be quickly reversed by adjusting the dose or stopping the drug.

In patients recovering from acute cerebrovascular accident or hypertensive encephalopathy, centrally acting agents such as methyldopa or clonidine should not be used because of their sedative effects. One common error in managing hypertensive crises is premature introduction of oral drugs. Another is failure to monitor the standing blood pressure in a patient who has been receiving potent antihypertensive agents in the supine position.

VIII. RESISTANT HYPERTENSION

Much more common than hypertensive crises is resistance to therapy, usually defined as a diastolic blood pressure above 95 mm Hg despite use of three medications. There are numerous reasons for a poor response to therapy (Table 7), with the most likely being volume overload due to either excessive sodium intake or inadequate administration of diuretic (34). In one series of 91 patients whose pressure remained above 140/90 despite use of three antihypertensive agents, the mechanisms were suboptimal drug regimen (mainly inadequate diuretic) in 43%, intolerance to medications in 22%, noncompliance in 10%, and secondary hypertension in 11% (35). In a disadvantaged minority population, uncontrolled hypertension is most closely related to limited access to care, noncompliance with therapy, and alcohol-related problems (36).

Before starting extensive testing for secondary causes and altering drug therapy, blood pressure should be checked outside the office setting, since as many as half of "resistant" patients turn out to have controlled hypertension (37).

In addition to adequate diuretics to control hypertension that is truly resistant, therapy may need to include an ACE inhibitor and a calcium blocker, with minoxidil reserved for those who remain resistant to adequate therapy.

IX. SUMMARY

The most critical decision in the management of hypertensive emergencies is to assess the patient's clinical state and to ascertain whether the patient's condition truly needs emergency management. A patient with a true hypertensive crisis ideally should be treated in an intensive care unit. The choice of oral versus parenteral drug depends on the urgency of the situation, as well as the patient's general condition. The level to which the blood pressure should be lowered varies with the type of hypertensive crisis and should be individualized. The choice of parenteral drug is dictated by the clinical manifestations and concomitant medical problems associated with hypertensive crisis. There is no predestined level for the goal therapy. Complications of therapy, mainly hypotension and ischemic brain damage, can occur in patients given multiple potent antihypertensive drugs in large doses without adequate monitoring. Such complications can be minimized by gentle lowering of blood pressure, careful surveillance, and individualization of therapy. A relatively asymptomatic patient who has severe hypertension, that is, diastolic blood pressure of 130 to 140 mm Hg, need not be treated with parenteral drugs. These patients should be managed on an individual basis, and the usual course would be to intensify or alter the previous antihypertensive therapy. All too often, asymptomatic patients or those without an acute problem are unnecessarily subjected to immediate therapy. A significant immediate change in the patient's blood pressure may be gratifying to the physician

Table 7 Causes of Lack of Responsiveness to Therapy

Nonadherence to therapy
- Cost of medication
- Instructions not clear and/or not given to the patient in writing
- Inadequate or no patient education
- Lack of involvement of the patient in the treatment plan
- Side effects of medication
- Organic brain syndrome (e.g., memory deficit)
- Inconvenient dosing

Drug-related causes
- Doses too low
- Inappropriate combinations (e.g., two centrally acting adrenergic inhibitors)
- Rapid inactivation (e.g., hydralazine)
- Drug interactions
  - Nonsteroidal anti-inflammatory drugs
  - Oral contraceptives
  - Sympathomimetics
  - Antidepressants
  - Adrenal steroids
  - Nasal decongestants
  - Licorice-containing substances (e.g., chewing tobacco)
  - Cocaine
  - Cyclosporine
  - Erythropoietin

Associated conditions
- Increasing obesity
- Alcohol intake more than 1 oz of ethanol a day

Secondary hypertension
- Renal insufficiency
- Renovascular hypertension
- Pheochromocytoma
- Primary aldosteronism

Volume overload
- Inadequate diuretic therapy
- Excess sodium intake
- Fluid retention from reduction blood pressure
- Progressive renal damage

Pseudohypertension

but is not indicated for most patients with asymptomatic severe hypertension. Indiscriminate use of therapeutic options such as nifedipine and furosemide should be strongly discouraged.

Once the hypertensive crisis has resolved and the patient's condition is stable, we should look into possible factors that may have contributed to the dangerous elevation of blood pressure such as nonadherence to prescribed therapy or presence and/or progression of a secondary form of hypertension such as a renal artery stenosis. It is crucial to recognize not only what is a hypertensive crisis but also what is not.

REFERENCES

1. Kincaid-Smith P. Malignant hypertension. Cardiovasc Rev Rep 1980; 1:42–50.
2. Ram CVS. Hypertensive encephalopathy: recognition and management. Arch Intern Med 1978; 138:1851–1853.
3. Hirst AE, Johns VJ, Kime SW. Dissecting aneurysm of aorta: Review of 505 cases. Medicine 1958; 37:217.
4. Chan K-L. Impact of transesophageal echocardiography on the treatment of patients with aortic dissection. Chest 1992; 101:406–410.
5. Ram CVS, Kaplan NM. Hypertensive emergencies. In: Shoemaker WC, Thompson WL, Holbrook PR, eds. Textbook of Critical Care. Philadelphia: WB Saunders, 1984.
6. Hogan PJ. Medical management of dissecting thoracic aneurysms. Texas Heart Inst J 1990; 17:281–288.
7. Hansson L, Hunyor SN, Julius S, Hoober SW. Blood pressure crisis following withdrawal of clonidine. Am Heart J 1973; 85:605–610.
8. Lippman SB, Nash K. Monoamine oxidase inhibitor update: potential adverse food and drug interactions. Drug Safety 1990; 5:195–204.
9. O'Connell MT, Kubrusly DB, Fournier AM. Systemic necrotizing vasculitis seen initially as hypertensive crisis. Arch Intern Med 1985; 145:265–267.
10. Nightingale SL. New labeling for sodium nitroprusside emphasizes risk of cyanide toxicity. JAMA 1991; 265:847.
11. Cottrell JE, Casthely P, Brodie JD, et al. Prevention of nitroprusside induced cyanide toxicity with hydroxocobalamin. N Engl J Med 1978; 298:808–811.
12. Chiariello M, Gold HK, Lienbach RC, et al. Comparison between the effects of nitroprusside and nitroglycerin on ischemic injury during the acute myocardial infarction. Circulation 1976; 54:766.
13. Mann T, Cohn PF, Holman BL, et al. Effect of nitroprusside on regional myocardial blood flow in coronary disease: results in 25 patients and comparison with nitroglycerin. Circulation 1978; 57:732.
14. Gopal MA, Neill WA, Oxendine JM. Effect of nitroprusside on myocardial blood flow in acute regional coronary ischemia in conscious dogs with and without ventricular distension. Cardiovasc Res 1983; 17:267.

15. Candia GJ, Heros RC, Lavyne MH, et al. Effect of intravenous sodium nitroprusside on cerebral blood flow and intracranial pressure. Neurosurgy 1978; 3:50–53.
16. Brown FD, Hanlon K, Crockard HA, Mullan S. Effect of sodium nitroprusside on cerebral blood flow in conscious human beings. Surg Neurol 1977; 7: 67–70.
17. Wilson DJ, Wallin JD, Vlachakis ND, et al. Intravenous labetalol in the treatment of severe hypertension and hypertensive emergencies. Am J Med 1983; 75(suppl):95.
18. Vidt DG. Intravenous labetalol in the emergency treatment of hypertension. J Clin Hypertens 1985; 2:179.
19. Ram CVS, Boldrick RW, Heller J, et al. Rapid control of severe hypertension with intravenous infusion of nicardipine: a new therapeutic approach. J Clin Pharmacol 1989; 29:835.
20. Wallin JD, Fletcher E, Ram CV, et al. Intravenous nicardipine for the treatment of severe hypertension. Arch Intern Med 1989; 149:2662–2669.
21. Herling IM. Intravenous nitroglycerin: clinical pharmacology and therapeutic considerations. Am Heart J 1984; 108:141–149.
22. Elliott WJ, Weber RR, Nelson KS, et al. Renal and hemodynamic effects of intravenous fenoldopam versus nitroprusside in severe hypertension. Circulation 1990; 81:970–977.
23. DiPette DJ, Ferraro JC, Evans RR, Martin M. Enalaprilat, an intravenous angiotensin-converting enzyme inhibitor, in hypertensive crises. Clin Pharmacol Ther 1985; 38:199–204.
24. Bertel O, Conen D, Radu E, et al. Nifedipine in hypertensive emergencies. Br Med J 1983; 286:19–21.
25. Harten J, Burggraaf K, Danhof M, et al. Negligible sublingual absorption of nifedipine. Lancet 1987; 2:1363–1365.
26. Anderson RJ, Hart GR, Crumpler CP, et al. Oral clonidine loading in hypertensive urgencies. JAMA 1981; 246:848–850.
27. Zeller KR, Von Kuhnert L, Matthews C. Rapid reduction of severe asymptomatic hypertension: a prospective, controlled trial. Arch Intern Med 1989; 149: 2186–2189.
28. Biollaz J, Waeber B, Brunner HR. Hypertensive crisis treated with orally administered captopril. Eur J Clin Pharmacol 1983; 25:145–149.
29. Tschollar W, Belz GG. Sublingual captopril in hypertensive crisis. Lancet 1985; 1:34–35.
30. Angeli P, Chiesa M, Caregaro L, et al. Comparison of sublingual captopril and nifedipine in immediate treatment of hypertensive emergencies. Arch Intern Med 1991; 151:678–682.
31. Gonzalezs ER, Peterson MA, Racht EM, et al. Dose-response evaluation of oral labetalol in patients presenting to the emergency department with accelerated hypertension. Ann Emerg Med 1991; 20:333–338.
32. Mitchell HC, Graham RM, Pettinger WA. Renal function during long-term treatment of hypertension with minoxidil. Ann Intern Med 1980; 93:676–681.

33. Barry DI. Cerebrovascular aspects of antihypertensive treatment. Am J Cardiol 1989; 63:14C–18C.
34. Graves JW, Bloomfield RL, Buckalew VM Jr. Plasma volume in resistant hypertension: guide to pathophysiology and therapy. Am J Med Sci 1989; 298:361–365.
35. Yakovlevitch M, Black HR. Resistant hypertension in a tertiary care clinic. Arch Intern Med 1991; 151:1786–1792.
36. Shea S, Misra D, Ehrlich MH, et al. Predisposing factors for severe, uncontrolled hypertension in an inner-city minority population. N Engl J Med 1992; 327:776–781.
37. Mejia AD, Egan BM, Schork NJ, Zweifler AJ. Artifacts in measurements of blood pressure and lack of target organ involvement in the assessment of patients with treatment-resistant hypertension. Ann Intern Med 1990; 112:270–277.

13

Drug-Induced Hypertension

JOHN J. CURTIS
University of Alabama at Birmingham
Birmingham, Alabama

In reporting adverse effects, investigators seldom incriminate drugs as causes of hypertension in humans. However, there are drugs which have well-described hypertensive effects (see Table 1). Most of these agents do not pose widespread clinical problems but are of considerable interest in that they increase our knowledge of mechanisms involved in elevating blood pressure. On the other hand, corticosteroids and cyclosporine are widely used agents that frequently cause hypertension in humans and that demand more attention in therapeutic considerations.

I. LICORICE

As also described in the preceding chapter, licorice (glycyrrhetinic acid) has captured the attention of investigators because it can cause a mineralocorticoidlike hypertension in humans (1). In humans, the enzyme 11-beta-hydroxysteroid dehydrogenase (11-beta-OHSD) interconverts cortisol and cortisone (2). Glycyrrhetinic acid is a potent inhibitor of 11-beta-OHSD. This inhibition causes cortisol to remain a potent mineralocorticoid and produce hypertension that can mimic aldosterone excess. The clinical impact of this drug-induced hypertension is not great—most cases result in case reports to medical journals.

Table 1 Drugs that Induce Hypertension in Humans

Drug	Clinical impact	Mediated
Glcyrrhentinic acid	Minor	Endocrine system
Phenylephrine	Minor	Nervous system
Oral contraceptive agents	Debated—may have beneficial effects	Endocrine system
Corticosteroids	Major	Endocrine system
Cyclosporine	Major	Uncertain

II. ORAL CONTRACEPTIVES

Early in the clinical use of first-generation steroid contraceptives physicians reported that they induced hypertension in some women (3). Modern oral contraceptive pills seem to have fewer adverse effects and may even provide some cardiovascular protection (4). Because of the balance between possible adverse effects and protective effects of hormone replacement therapy, the use of oral contraceptive agents is becoming more rational with recommendations to individuals based on their risk factors and other medical risks such as smoking.

III. SYMPATHOMIMETICS

Phenylephrine, a potent alpha-receptor used mainly as a nasal decongestant, has been reported to cause elevated blood pressure in humans as have other alpha-receptor stimulators (5,6). While these cases are often dramatic, they are rare and usually occur in the setting of massive dosages.

IV. CORTICOSTEROIDS

Indeed, most of those agents that elevate blood pressure are naturally occurring substances. Corticosteroids and cyclosporine are two drugs that commonly induce hypertension in humans. Corticosteroids are given in larger than natural doses for therapeutic reasons. On the other hand, cyclosporine is a macrolide antibiotic that has no counterpart in naturally occurring human enzymes, proteins, or sugars. Cyclosporine, FK-506, and Rapamycin are all potent immunosuppressive agents (macrolide antibiotics) that seem to have similar adverse effects. Only cyclosporine is currently approved by the Federal Drug Administration (FDA) and in general clinical use in the United States. It clearly can produce hypertension.

Hypertension is one of the most characteristic features of Cushing's syndrome (excess production of cortisol). It is also a nearly universal feature of Conn's syndrome (excess production of aldosterone). Thus, both the glucocorticoid and the mineralocorticoid products of the adrenal cortex can cause elevation of blood pressure. It is not surprising then that administration of either ACTH or cortisol has been reported to induce hypertension in humans.

Synthetic glucocorticoids (methylprednisolone, prednisolone, etc.) were designed to have low mineralocorticoid activity in the hope that hypertension induction would be reduced, but the attempt has been only partly successful.

Hall et al. (7) reported that they were unable to produce hypertension in dogs using synthetic glucorticoids regardless of dose or duration of therapy. not only was hypertension not produced, but the dogs developed hypotension with chronic renal vasodilatation, increased excretion of sodium, and volume depletion. Whitworth et al. (8) in studies of humans were able to produce hypertension in a reproducible and reliable fashion. This group suggests that neither mineralocorticoid activity nor an increase in plasma volume is essential for synthetic steroids to induce an increase in blood pressure (8).

Clinical observations in renal transplantation have consistently documented reduction of hypertension when synthetic steroids are withdrawn from the patient's immunosuppressive regimen (9,10). In both systemic lupus and rheumatoid arthritis patients exposed to chronic steroid therapy, most but not all (11) studies (12,13) have also implicated steroids as a cause of hypertension.

Treatment of corticosteroid-induced hypertension is usually directed at reduction of the dose of steroids or uses of alternate day steroid therapy (10, 14). Since the mechanism whereby corticosteroids cause pressure elevation is unclear, pharmacological intervention has been somewhat empirical. Most agents that are used in treatment of essential hypertension are also used in the hypertension that is induced by steroid therapy. No single agent seems to stand out as most effective. Diuretic agents have not been demonstrated to be more or less effective than angiotensin-converting enzyme inhibitors.

V. CYCLOSPORINE

Cyclosporine is a macrolide antibiotic that has gained widespread use in organ transplantation programs since it was approved by the FDA in 1983. This immunosuppressant agent is credited with improving renal allograft survival rates by 15% to 20%. Its introduction made both liver and heart transplantation possible. However, the adverse effects of nephrotoxicity and hypertension did not become apparent until the agent was in general use.

Indeed the first randomized trials in humans were conducted in Canada (15) and Europe (16) and did not suggest that hypertension would be a problem. It should be noted that these trials were designed to determine whether the drug was a more effective immunosuppressive agent than standard therapy (azathioprine and prednisone) and were not truly designed to look at hypertension. Nonetheless both trials mentioned hypertension as a possible adverse effect and neither found the incidence to be more dramatic than standard therapy.

Jarowenko was among the first to point out that cyclosporine-treated transplantation patients had a significantly higher rate of hypertension than observed with standard therapy (17). Studies in which patients were taken off cyclosporine and returned to standard therapy also demonstrated that cyclosporine could induce hypertension (18,19). The incidence of hypertension in renal transplantation recipients was high (above 50%) before cyclosporine was employed (20). In cardiac and liver programs, however, there was not a high background rate of hypertension. Such transplant groups reported a dramatic change in the rates of hypertension seen when they switched to cyclosporine (21–23). Indeed, when cyclosporine is used in circumstances that don't involve organ transplantation, it induces hypertension in the majority of patients (24–26). Thus, while hypertension was not noted before FDA approval of cyclosporine, there is no question that in humans cyclosporine can induce hypertension. In animals, cyclosporine-induced hypertension has been less easy to produce. Indeed, the situation is similar to that noted for steroids. Some animal models become hypotensive on cyclosporine (27).

In both humans and animals, however, clearly cyclosporine causes a marked increase in renal vascular resistance (28,29). Increased renal vascular resistance is one of the earliest and most universal findings in most forms of hypertension. Thus, from a renal hemodynamic standpoint, it would be surprising if cyclosporine did not cause hypertension. Flechner et al. noted that cyclosporine in humans caused an increase in serum creatinine level (a finding not known before FDA approval)—but that unlike that by most nephrotoxic agents the renal impairment caused by cyclosporine was reversible (30). Because of this reversible nature of cyclosporine "toxicity," many investigators suspected that cyclosporine, unlike other agents that damage renal tubules, has its major effect on the renal vessels. Today it is widely accepted that cyclosporine has a major effect on the renal afferent arteriole (31–33).

Sodium retention with marked proximal reabsorption of sodium (34), urea (35), and uric acid (36,37) has been demonstrated among hypertensive patients receiving cyclosporine. These abnormalities all can be explained by afferent arteriolar vasoconstriction. Another mechanism that could also lead to sodium retention and a volume expanded type of hypertension is stimulation of the sympathetic nervous system. This, too, appears to occur with cyclosporine therapy in humans (38,39). In humans, but not in animal models (40,41), cyclosporine appears to have little if any effect on the renin-angiotensin system (42).

Thus, unlike the situation with prednisone, several aspects of the mechanism of cyclosporine-induced hypertension are understood—namely, that the hypertension induced by cyclosporine results from afferent arteriolar vasoconstriction and probably concurrent sympathetic nervous system stimulation. This leads to sodium retention in the proximal renal tubule. The hypertension is a volume expansion type of hypertension that (in humans) does not appear to involve the renin-angiotensin system.

Not known, however, are the means whereby cyclosporine causes afferent arteriolar vasoconstriction. A number of mediators have been suggested (43–46), and it is possible that cyclosporine acts directly on the blood vessel cells without the need for a mediator system. At any rate, an understanding of the steps required for cyclosporine to cause vasoconstriction would be highly valuable to address both the hypertension and the nephrotoxicity of this drug.

Treatment of the hypertension associated with cyclosporine then might logically be aimed at reduction of volume expansion with the use of diuretic agents and antihypertensive agents that are renal vasodilators. Diuretic agents can aggravate some of the problems linked to prednisone and cyclosporine—gout and hyperlipidemia. They tend to produce hypokalemia that counters cyclosporine's tendency to produce hyperkalemia. Afferent arteriolar vasoconstriction induced by cyclosporine tends to produce a "prerenal"-like increase in the blood urea nitrogen (BUN)/serum creatinine ratio that can be markedly aggravated by the volume depletion (47) caused by diuretic therapy. Thus diuretic agents can have both beneficial and detrimental effects when given in combination with cyclosporine. On balance, however, it may be difficult to control blood pressure in a volume expanded state without the use of diuretic agents, and careful medical management can achieve a euvolic state with their use.

The two groups of renal vasodilators that have been most discussed in relation to cyclosporine-induced hypertension are calcium channel blockers (CCBs) and angiotensin-converting enzyme inhibitors (ACEIs). Besides being renal vasodilators, these agents (especially CCBs) are said to have less sodium retaining effects than other antihypertensive agents that cause vasodilatation. Indeed, it has been suggested that CCBs are natriuretic (48–50).

An antihypertensive agent that can produce both antriuretic effects and vasodilatation would seem especially suited for cyclosporine-induced hypertension. CCBs seem an even more ideal choice in that the site of most effective renal vasodilatation appears to be the afferent arteriole (51,52), the very site that is alleged to be cyclosporine's target for vasoconstriction. For these reasons CCBs have gained widespread use in organ transplantation centers.

Clinical trials, however, to document the benefits that seem to follow from the use of CCBs have had mixed results. In short-term trials, a number of investigators have demonstrated that cyclosporine-treated patients show a marked decrease in renal vascular resistance with CCBs (53,54). In a longer-term study, however, Mourad et al. were unable to demonstrate any advantage of CCBs over ACEIs in cyclosporine-associated hypertension (55). Along with improvement in renal vascular resistance (at least in the short term), investigators have suggested that the prolonged acute tubular necrosis (ATN) seen with cyclosporine can be modified (56). Acute effects of CCBs on increasing renal blood flow in which in vivo fluorescence microscopy of kidney subcapsular blood flow was visualized have been reported by Rooth et al. (57).

It should be noted that CCBs add to the tendency of cyclosporine to cause gingival hyperplasia (58). It is also important to note that they can alter cyclosporine blood levels by interference with the metabolic breakdown of cyclosporine in the liver. Only the dihydropyridines, nifedipine and isradipine, have been shown not to affect cyclosporine blood levels. Some physicians find this drug interaction to be an advantage because of the high cost of cyclosporine. Thus use of a CCB that will increase blood levels of cyclosporine can markedly cut the cost of immunosuppression (59). The potential disadvantage to this approach is that the complications from drug adjustment by those who may be unaware that cyclosporine levels are being supported by a drug interaction can be catastrophic.

ACEIs are effective antihypertensive agents even when (as in cyclosporine-induced hypertension in humans) the renin-angiotensin system does not appear to be stimulated (60). Kidney transplantation patients with cyclosporine-associated hypertension have been shown to be responsive to ACEI therapy (61). Caution must be exercised, however, if one suspects transplant renal artery stenosis to be the cause of the hypertension, since in this setting ACEIs can induce acute renal failure (62).

Since cyclosporine causes afferent arteriolar vasoconstriction, patients on cyclosporine might be expected to have a hemodynamic response to ACEI that is similar to (yet much less dramatic than) that with renal artery stenosis. Curtis et al. report a mild decrease (not clinically significant) in glomerular filtration rate (GFR) when cyclosporine and captopril were used together (63). Bunke and Ganzel demonstrated that GFR increased by nearly 15 ml/min in heart transplantation patients who were switched from ACEIs to CCBs at the same time that blood pressure control improved (64). The long-term therapy study of Mourad et al. demonstrated a slightly higher serum creatinine level in the ACEI-treated patients than in the CCB-treated group, although this did not achieve statistical significance (55). It should be noted that ACEI therapy is especially effective in the treatment of posttransplantation polycythemia (which often is associated with mild hypertension) (65).

While ACEI therapy in the precyclosporine era was especially effective in posttransplantation hypertension, since cyclosporine therapy has become nearly universal most physicians have turned to CCBs. It should be remembered, however, that ACEIs can be effective even when plasma renin activity is not elevated. Moreover, in the setting of polycythemia and hypertension, ACEIs may be the drugs of choice. Despite the preceding data concerning a mild decrease in GFR, the major clinical concern is the use of ACEI in the setting of transplantation renal artery stenosis. This concern may be managed by checking renal function soon after (less than 24 hours) starting ACEI therapy. If serum creatinine level remains relatively stable, then the agents can be used, often with good results.

In addition to use of diuretics and vasodilators, cyclosporine-induced hypertension, like corticosteroid-induced hypertension, will respond to dosage reduction or discontinuation. Fortunately, the hypertension associated with these two drugs is rarely severe enough to force drug discontinuation (and its risk of provoking rejection) (66,67).

While not tested as extensively in the kidney transplantation population, the nonpharmacological interventions of weight control, sodium restriction, and alcohol restriction should reduce pressure in drug-induced hypertension (as they clearly do in essential hypertension).

In conclusion, the two major drugs that induce hypertension in humans (but surprisingly not easily in animals) are corticosteroids and cyclosporine. More seems to be known about the mechanism of cyclosporine-induced hypertension than about the mechanism of corticosteroid hypertension. In the latter, reduction of dose is accepted as highly effective in reducing blood pressure. In the former, both volume reduction and renal vasodilatation seem appropriate and CCB therapy is currently considered most effective.

REFERENCES

1. Colloredo G, Bertone V, Peci P, et al. Pseudoaldosteronism caused by licorice: review of the literature and description of 4 clinical cases. Minerva Med 1987; 78(2):93–101.
2. Whorwood CB, Sheppard MC, Stewart PM. Licorice inhibits 11 beta-hydroxysteroid dehydrogenase messenger ribonucleic acid levels and potentiates glucocorticoid hormone action. Endocrinology 1993; 132(6):2287–2292.
3. Connell EB. Oral contraceptives: the current risk-benefit ratio. J Reprod Med 1984; 20(suppl 7):513–523.
4. Sondheimer SJ. Update on the metabolic effects of steroidal contraceptives. Endocrinol Metab Clin North Am 1991; 20(4):911–923.

5. Heyman SN, Mevorach D, Ghanem J. Hypertensive crisis from chronic intoxication with nasal decongestant and cough medications. DICP 1991; 25(10): 1068–1070.
6. Lai YK. Adverse effect of intraoperative phenylephrine 10%: case report. Br J Ophthalmol 1980; 73(6):468–469.
7. Hall JE, Morse CL, Smith MJJ, et al. Control of arterial pressure and renal function during glucocorticoid excess in dogs. Hypertension 1980; 2(2):139–148.
8. Whitworth JA, Gordon D, Andrews J, Scoggins BA. The hypertensive effect of synthetic glucocorticoids in man: role of sodium and volume. J Hypertens 1989; 7(7):537–549.
9. Ghio L, Tarantino A, Edefonti A, Mocciaro A, et al. Advantages of cyclosporine as sole immunosuppressive agent in children with transplanted kidneys. Transplantation 1992; 54(5):834–838.
10. Hricik DE, Lautman J, Bartucci MR, et al. Variable effects of steroid withdrawal on blood pressure reduction in cyclosporine-treated renal transplant recipients. Transplantation 1992; 53(6):1232–1235.
11. Jackson SH, Beevers DG, Myers K. Does long-term low-dose corticosteroid therapy cause hypertension? Clin Sci 1981; 61(suppl 7):381s–383s.
12. Nashel DJ. Is atherosclerosis a complication of long-term corticosteroid treatment? Am J Med 1986; 80(5):925–929.
13. Badui E, Garcia RD, Robles E, et al. Cardiovascular manifestations in systemic lupus erythematosus: prospective study of 100 patients. Angiology 1985; 36(7): 431–441.
14. Min DI, Monaco AP. Complications associated with immunosuppressive therapy and their management. Pharmacotherapy 1991; 11(5):119S–125S.
15. A randomized clinical trial of cyclosporine in cadaveric renal transplantation. New Engl J Med 1983; 309(14):809–815.
16. Cyclosporin in cadaveric renal transplantation: one-year follow-up of multicentre trial. Lancet 1983; 2(8357):986–989.
17. Jarowenko MV, Flechner SM, Van BCT, et al. Influence of cyclosporine on posttransplant blood pressure response. Am J Kidney Dis 1987; 10(2):98–103.
18. Chapman JR, Marcen R, Arias M, et al. Hypertension after renal transplantation: a comparison of cyclosporine and conventional immunosuppression. Transplantation 1987; 43(6):860–864.
19. Curtis J, Luke R, Dubovsky E, Diethelm A, et al. Cyclosporine in therapeutic doses increases renal allograft vascular resistance. Lancet 1986; 2:477–479.
20. Bachy C, Alexandre G, van Ypersele de Strihou C. Hypertension after renal transplantation. Br Med J 1976; 2(6047):1287–1289.
21. Bellet M, Cabrol C, Sassano P, et al. Systemic hypertension after cardiac transplantation: effect of cyclosporine on the renin-angiotensin-aldosterone system. Am J Cardiol 1985; 56:927–931.
22. Starling R, Cody R. Cardiac transplant hypertension. Am J Cardiol 1990; 65(1): 106–111.
23. Lawless S, Ellis D, Thompson A, et al. Mechanism of hypertension during and after orthotopic liver transplantation in children. J Pediatr 1989; 115(3):372–379.

24. Griffiths CE, Voorhes JJ. Cyclosporine A in the treatment of psoriasis: a clinical and mechanistic perspective. J Invest Dermatol 1990; 95(5):53S–55S.
25. Deray G, Benhmida M, Le HP, et al. Renal function and blood pressure in patients receiving long-term, low-dose cyclosporine therapy for idiopathic autoimmune uveitis. Ann Intern Med 1992; 117(7):578–583.
26. Fry L. Psoriasis: immunopathology and long-term treatment with cyclosporin. J Autoimmunol 1992; 5(suppl A):277–283.
27. Parkhurst GW, Moon BH, Xia RL, et al. Cyclosporine-induced hypotension. Transplantation 1989; 48(5):756–759.
28. Kiberd B. Cyclosporine-induced renal dysfunction in human renal allograft recipients. Transplantation 1989; 48(6):965–969.
29. Rossi NF, Churchill PC, McDonald FD, Ellis VR. Mechanism of cyclosporine A-induced renal vasoconstriction in the rat. J Pharmacol Exp Ther 1989; 250(3): 896–901.
30. Flechner SM, Payne WD, Van BC, et al. The effect of cyclosporine on early graft function in human renal transplantation. Transplantation 1983; 36(3): 268–272.
31. English J, Evan A, Houghton D, Bennett W. Cyclosporine-induced acute renal dysfunction in the rat: evidence of arteriolar vasoconstriction with preservation of tubular function. Transplantation 1987; 44(1):135–141.
32. Remuzzi G, Bertani T. Renal vascular and thrombotic effects of cyclosporine. Am J Kidney Dis 1989; 13(4):261–272.
33. Mihatsch M, Theil G, Spichtin H. Morphological findings in kidney-transplants after treatment with cyclosporine. Transplant Proc 1983; 15:2821–2835.
34. Curtis J, Luke R, Jones P, Diethelm AG. Transplant hypertension with cyclosporine is sodium sensitive and less responsive to captopril than with azathioprine (abstr). Am J Kidney Dis 1986; 8:A4.
35. Laskow DA, Curtis JJ, Luke RG, et al. Cyclosporine-induced changes in glomerular filtration rate and urea excretion. Am J Med 1990; 88(5):497–502.
36. Tiller D, Hall B, Horvarth J, et al. Gout and hyperuricaemia in patients on cyclosporine and diuretics. Lancet 1985; 1(8426):453.
37. Carpenter B, Thomas R, West C. The incidence of gout in renal transplant recipients. Am J Kidney Dis 1987; 10(5):369–371.
38. Scherrer U, Vissing S, Morgan B, et al. Cyclosporine-induced sympathetic activation and hypertension after heart transplantation. N Engl J Med 1990; 323(11): 693–699.
39. Moss N, Powell S, Falk R. Intravenous cyclosporine activates afferent and efferent renal nerves and causes sodium retention in innervated kidneys in rats. Proc Natl Acad Sci 1985; 82:8222–8226.
40. Perico N, Zoja C, Benigni A, et al. Effect of short-term cyclosporine administration in rats on renin-angiotensin and thromboxane A2: possible relevance to the reduction in glomerular filtration rate. J Pharmacol Exp Ther 1986; 239(1): 229–235.
41. Lustig S, Stern N, Eggena P, et al. Effect of cyclosporin on blood pressure and renin-aldosterone axis in rats. Am J Physiol 1987; 253(6 Pt 2):1596–1600.

42. Bantle J, Boudreau R, Ferris T. Suppression of plasma renin activity by cyclosporine. Am J Med 1987; 83:59–64.
43. Brooks DP, Drutz DJ, Ruffolo RRJ. Prevention and complete reversal of cyclosporine A-induced renal vasoconstriction and nephrotoxicity in the rat by fenoldopam. J Pharmacol Exp Ther 1990; 254(2):375–379.
44. Mason J. The pathophysiology of Sandimmune (cyclosporine) in man and animals. Pediatr Nephrol 1990; 4(5):554–574.
45. Coffman T, Carr D, Yarger W, Klotman P. Evidence that renal prostaglandin and thromboxane production is stimulated in chronic cyclosporine nephrotoxicity. Transplantation 1986; 43:282–285.
46. Kon V, Sugiura M, Inagami T, et al. Role of endothelin in cyclosporine-induced glomerular dysfunction. Kidney Int 1990; 37(6):1487–1491.
47. Laskow DA, Curtis J, Luke R, et al. Cyclosporine impairs the renal response to volume depletion. Transplant Proc 1988; 20(3)(suppl 3):568–571.
48. Kaplan N. Calcium entry blockers in the treatment of hypertension: current status and future prospects. JAMA 1989; 262(6):817–823.
49. Sterzel R. Renal actions of calcium antagonists. J Cardiovasc Pharmacol 1987; 10(suppl 10):17–22.
50. Zanchetti A, Leonetti G. Natiuretic effects of calcium antagonists. Clinical implications. Drugs 1990; 2:15–21.
51. Carmines P, Navar L. Disparate effects of Ca channel blockade on afferent and efferent arteriolar responses to ANG II. Am J Physiol 1989; 256(6 Pt 2):1015–1120.
52. Epstein M. Calcium antagonists and renal protection: current status and future perspectives. Arch Intern Med 1992; 152(8):1573–1584.
53. McNally PG, Walls J, Feehally J. The effect of nifedipine on renal function in normotensive cyclosporin-A-treated renal allograft recipients. Nephrol Dial Transplant 1990; 5(11):962–968.
54. Curtis JJ, Laskow DA, Jones PA, et al. Captopril-induced fall in glomerular filtration rate in cyclosporine-treated hypertensive patients. J Am Soc Nephrol 1993; 3(9):1570–1574.
55. Mourad G, Ribstein J, Mimran A. Converting-enzyme inhibitor versus calcium antagonist in cyclosporine-treated renal transplants. Kidney Int 1993; 43(2): 419–425.
56. Dawidson I, Rooth P, Fry WR, et al. Prevention of acute cyclosporine-induced renal blood flow inhibition and improved immunosuppression with verapamil. Transplantation 1989; 48(4):575–580.
57. Rooth P, Dawidson I, Clothier N, Diller K. In vivo fluorescence microscopy of kidney subcapsular blood flow in mice: effects of cyclosporine, (NVA2)-cyclosporine, and isradipine, a new calcium antagonist. Transplantation 1988; 46(4): 566–569.
58. Seymour RA. Calcium channel blockers and gingival overgrowth. Br Dent J 1991; 170(10):376–379.
59. Chrysostomou A, Walker RG, Russ GR, et al. Diltiazem in renal allograft recipients receiving cyclosporine. Transplantation 1993; 55(2):300–304.

60. Todd PA, Goa KL. Enalapril: a reappraisal of its pharmacology and therapeutic use in hypertension. Drugs 1992; 43(3):346–381.
61. Hricik DE. Antihypertensive and renal effects of enalapril in post-transplant hypertension. Clin Nephrol 1987; 27(5):250–259.
62. Dubovsky E, Curtis J, Luke R, et al. Captopril as a predictor of curable hypertension in renal transplant recipients. Contrib Nephrol 1987; 56:117–123.
63. Curtis JJ, Laskow DA, Jones PA, et al. Captopril-induced fall in glomerular filtration rate in cyclosporine-treated hypertensive patients. J Am Soc Nephrol 1993; 3(9):1570–1574.
64. Bunke M, Ganzel B. Effect of calcium channel antagonists on renal function in hypertensive heart transplant recipients. J Heart Lung Transplant 1992; 11(6): 1194–1199.
65. Gaston RS, Julian BA, Diethelm AG, Curtis JJ. Effects of enalapril on erythrocytosis after renal transplantation. Ann Intern Med 1991; 115(12):954–955.
66. Sanders CE, Curtis JJ, Julian BA, et al. Tapering or discontinuing cyclosporine for financial reasons—a single-center experience. Am J Kidney Dis 1993; 21(1): 9–15.
67. Sinclair NR. Low-dose steroid therapy in cyclosporine-treated renal transplant recipients with well-functioning grafts: The Canadian Multicentre Transplant Study Group. Can Med Assoc J 1992; 147(5):645–657.

14

Improving Patient Compliance in the Management of Hypertension

R. BRIAN HAYNES
McMaster University
Hamilton, Ontario, Canada

I. INTRODUCTION

Hypertension is one of the first chronic disorders for which successful medical treatments were developed. These treatments lower the risk of high blood pressure at a price. Because they do not cure the disorder, patients must follow the treatments for as long as the disorder persists, often for the rest of their lives. Although hypertension is asymptomatic in its early stages, the treatments can cause symptomatic adverse effects and also are often expensive for the patient and inconvenient. Furthermore, the prescription for hypertensive patients often includes life-style changes, including weight reduction, stopping smoking, reducing the amount of salt in the diet, reducing alcohol consumption, and increasing exercise. While all of these nondrug treatments have merit, each and every one of them places a heavy behavioral demand on the patient—an additional compliance burden. Although sometimes we might wonder why patients do not follow our prescriptions, there is not much mystery here. Fortunately, there are now many validated methods of helping patients to follow their treatment regimens, the subject of this chapter.

II. THE NATURE OF NONCOMPLIANCE

A. Definition

Compliance has been defined as the extent to which a person's behavior (in terms of taking medication, following a diet, modifying habits, or attending clinics) coincides with medical or health advice (2). Some people object to the term "compliance" because they believe it implies subservience of the patient or constitutes blaming the patient for noncompliance. Some prefer "adherence" to "compliance," but it is splitting hairs to claim that "sticking to" the regimen is less pejorative than "sticking with" it. In any event, "Patient Compliance" is the Medical Subject Heading used by the National Library of Medicine to index the considerable scientific literature on this topic in MEDLINE, and this is certainly the most common term in use. Given that this is so, I will use the term "compliance" in this chapter without apology but with the explanation that it is used nonjudgmentally, unless otherwise specified. Even so, one must recognize that in specific situations it may well be appropriate to assign blame: the physician may fail to provide adequate instruction, the patient may have other priorities, or circumstances may conspire to cause the problem. Thus, when an underlying cause can be found, it should be labeled as the problem rather than using the nonspecific term "noncompliance." Unfortunately, in many cases the clinician will be unable to sort out exactly what the problem is, and the generic term will need to be applied. Fortunately, knowing the underlying problem is not always necessary for improving compliance, just as knowing the underlying cause of hypertension is not necessary for managing it.

B. Types of Noncompliance and Their Magnitude

There are many forms of noncompliance that can undermine the effectiveness of antihypertensive care (3). After community screening for high blood pressure, from 35% (4) to 49% (5) of those whose blood pressure is elevated may fail to follow through with a referral for follow-up assessment. Once assessed and prescribed therapy, over a third of patients may drop out of care entirely and are particularly likely to do so in the few months after their initial diagnosis (6,7). Once in care, patients frequently do not take all of their medication – the average consumption rate is reported as about 50% (8,9) – but the distribution is U-shaped as approximately a third of patients take virtually no medication, a third take roughly half their medication, and a third take most or all (and sometimes more than all) of their prescribed medication. Compliance with instructions to lose weight or stop smoking is still lower, with long-term rates of less than 10% for substantial weight loss (10) and smoking cessation (11).

The rates of noncompliance in most reports evoke despair as they imply that very few patients receive much benefit from antihypertensive therapy. However, most of the studies from which the figures are derived were relatively short-term and were executed relatively early in our attempts to perfect antihypertensive care. Studies with longer follow-up periods have found that most of those who leave care eventually return, and most patients in care get enough treatment to bring their blood pressure under control (12). One way of thinking about this is that the short-term disadvantages of following antihypertensive therapy substantially outweigh the short-term benefits and patients require persistent reminders of the long-term benefits to swing this unfavorable balance in a positive direction.

C. Key Determinants of Compliance

Literally hundreds of studies have attempted to "crack the compliance nut," discovering the causes of low compliance and the determinants of high compliance (1). If understanding the causes of hypertension is complicated, it is not difficult to imagine that understanding compliance is more so. Studies of sociodemographic factors, such as age, gender, socioeconomic status, intelligence, and marital status have not provided consistent findings, and neither have any consistent psychological features of noncompliance been discovered. Indeed, we are virtually all noncompliant with medical treatments at one time or another. Thus, there is no stereotypical noncomplier (this has obvious implications for detecting noncompliance; see Measurement of Compliance). There are two exceptions to this generalism: difficult social circumstances, such as marital discord, social isolation (13,14), and unemployment, adversely affect compliance, and patients with psychotic disorders, particularly those with paranoid features, tend to be less compliant (1).

The key factors that deter compliance that we can often affect include the time between screening and follow-up appointments (15–17), the amount of waiting time at clinic visits (18,19), the complexity of the regimen (20–24), adverse effects of therapy (14,25), and the cost of therapy (18,20,24). These factors affect individual patients differently, so that the physician needs to become aware of each patient's situation, with particular attention to barriers to compliance that can be modified.

III. MEASUREMENT OF COMPLIANCE (Table 1)

A. In Practice

To be efficient in managing patient compliance in usual clinical practice, it is important to be able to detect noncompliance when it occurs. Unfortun-

Table 1 Methods of Measuring Compliance

In clinical practice
Attendance at appointments
Response to antihypertensive medications
Patient self-report
In research
Pill counts at home visits
Monitoring of prescription refills
Drug assays in body fluids
Tracers
"Memory" pill containers

ately, physicians are notoriously poor judges of the compliance of their patients and it is essential to use methods of measuring compliance that have been validated (26). As it happens, most accurate measures of compliance are not very easy to apply and most easy measures are not accurate. Fortunately, however, most important compliance problems can be detected by three simple maneuvers, used in sequence:

1. Watch for patients who fail to attend appointments. Nonattendance is evidence of the most severe form of noncompliance: dropping out of treatment. Also, patients who are irregular attenders are less likely to be following their prescribed regimen (27–30).
2. Watch for nonresponders. Blood pressure does not correlate very well with medication consumption in individual patients (31). However, for patients whose blood pressure fails to respond to increments in medication, noncompliance is the most frequent explanation. This method can be augmented for some medications by observing their effects on other body processes, for example, slowing of heart rate with beta-blockers or lowering of serum potassium level and elevating of uric acid level for diuretics. However, these effects are no better correlated with medication consumption than blood pressure itself (31).
3. Ask nonresponders about their compliance. A recent meta-analysis of studies of measures of compliance has shown that the simple clinical measure of asking the patient has a sensitivity of 55% with a specificity of 87% (32). That is, about half of noncompliers will confirm this on direct questioning, and few patients who are taking most of their medication indicate that they are not. A nonthreatening approach is best, such as "Many people have difficulty taking all the medications we prescribe. During the past week, have you missed *any* tablets?" In my experience, many patients will indicate that they have taken virtually all their medication but "may have missed one or two pills on Saturday

night" when they were outside the home. Qualifying statements such as these are associated with an average compliance rate of less than 50% (31)!

B. In Research

Other ways of assessing compliance are impractical in most clinical settings but are possible—and often necessary—in research settings. Careful pill counts can be useful on one occasion, but these require a home visit, a very careful inventory of the pills, an accounting of when the pills were dispensed and whether pills from a previous prescription were added to the container, and questioning of the patient about whether he or she shares pills with others or has some of the supply in other locations, such as the car, office, or cottage (31). Some initial deception is required in setting up the visit (e.g., indicating that the main purpose of the visit is to measure the blood pressure in the home) or the result is no more likely to be accurate than asking the patient directly. Also, after the first occasion, the patient will know what's up and may modify their pill count to reflect what they feel they want the assessor to know. The deception raises ethical issues that are discussed further later, but the ethical concerns can often be dealt with satisfactorily by asking the patient at the time of the visit if his or her pills can be counted and making it clear what the reason for the count is and that it is entirely up to them. Counting pills that patients take to clinic visits gives rates of 90% to 100%, making a mockery of the procedure, although it is remarkable how many drug trials blithely report such figures.

Monitoring pharmacy records for refills of medication is a useful variant of counting pills in settings where there is a single-source pharmacy for patients (33–35). The validity of monitoring depends on the assumption that what is taken from the pharmacy actually ends up passing through the lips of the patient in the intended way, as is not always the case. Nevertheless, it can provide an inexpensive indirect method of monitoring compliance if trouble is taken to correlate pharmacy records with prescriptions, including changes in dosing and medications.

Drug assays are available for some beta-blockers (36,37), but these can be expensive and the measurements can be misleading if the medication has a short serum half-life as the patient may have taken the medication only shortly before the time of determination or may have missed only that dose. Urinary measurements, for example of diuretics, provide no more information than simply asking the patient (31). A variant on these methods is to add a tracer to the medication, such as riboflavin (38) or a homeopathic dose of digoxin (39), and measure this, but there are obvious logistical and regulatory problems of doing so. An additional disadvantage to these direct methods of compliance measurement is that they can be applied only to specific medications, compared with pill counts, prescription monitoring, memory-cap pill containers, and self-reports which apply to any medication the patient is prescribed.

Finally, there are a number of special pill containers with computerized memory chips (40) in their caps that can provide valuable information about the timing of dosing and gaps in dosing, as long as the patient removes and replaces the lid with each dosing.

IV. THE ETHICS OF ATTEMPTING TO IMPROVE COMPLIANCE

There are several circumstances in which encouraging high compliance is of dubious merit and it is important to consider each patient's situation before intervening to improve compliance (Table 2). First, the diagnosis of hypertension must be clearly established before compliance becomes an issue. Particularly for mild or labile elevations of blood pressure, multiple assessments of blood pressure must be made to determine whether the average is elevated (41).

Second, lowering the blood pressure must be of clear value for the patient before attempting to improve compliance. In the largest trial of antihypertensive therapy to date, the British Medical Research Council trial, women with mild blood pressure elevations who had no evidence of target organ damage did not show any benefit from therapy (42,43). In these circumstances, the practitioner may prescribe treatment on the basis of his or her own clinical judgment (41), but the patient must at least be permitted to take it or leave it. As an additional concern, a small proportion of patients seem very sensitive to the adverse effects of medications and the benefits of antihypertensive treatment of them may not outweigh the harm.

Third, the method of improving compliance must be of established effectiveness (44). If for no reason other than efficiency, the maneuvers used to increase compliance should have been documented to work in properly designed studies. Unfortunately, many practitioners feel that they have done their job in promoting compliance when they have instructed the patient carefully on the need for, and details of, the regimen (45). Many studies have

Table 2 Ethical Issues in Using Compliance-Enhancing Strategies

The diagnosis of hypertension must be established.
The benefits of lowering the blood pressure must outweigh the adverse effects for the individual patient.
The method of improving compliance must be of known efficacy.
The patient must be willing.

shown that "education" alone does not improve long-term compliance and, while clear instructions are necessary to promote compliance, they are not sufficient for long-term regimens such as those required for hypertension (46).

Finally, the patient must be a willing partner in the process of improving compliance. The patient obviously has a right to refuse treatment and this right must be respected. Attempts to coerce or intimidate the patient to comply (for example, by emphasizing that noncompliance will cause a stroke or heart attack) have not been shown to work any better than positive reinforcement and supportive reminders, but they do cause some patients with high anxiety levels to withdraw from care. Thus, such tactics might be considered unethical and potentially dangerous.

V. IMPROVING COMPLIANCE

Compared with the relatively straightforward research that has established the efficacy of antihypertensive medications, research into methods of improving compliance is frankly messy. Most of the interventions that have been tested to improve compliance are not easily packaged or standardized (the term "disembodied technology" might be used to describe them), and the theoretical underpinnings of these strategies are not always apparent. We will discuss these interventions at two levels, first reviewing the randomized controlled trials of attempts to improve compliance among hypertensive patients, and then describing a theory-based practical formulation of the empirical studies.

A. Empirical Research

There have been many studies of attempts to improve patient compliance with medical therapies, and adherence to antihypertensive therapy has been the most common subject of the well-executed long-term trials (46). Several of these studies have shown no benefits to compliance or blood pressure of interventions as diverse as self-monitoring of blood pressure (47,48), home visits (47), worksite care (49), programmed teaching (49), counseling by a nurse (48) or health educator (50), peer group discussions (48), tangible rewards (48), or unit dose-reminder packaging (51).

Fortunately, there are even more studies, summarized in Table 3, showing that compliance with antihypertensive therapy can be improved by a number of interventions, often including those that were not successful in the studies just cited. This is not as mysterious as it might seem: no single maneuver works very well, but the combination of complementary strategies is often beneficial and all the studies of successful strategies included two or more

Table 3 Randomized Trials of Successful Interventions to Improve Compliance with Antihypertensive Therapy

Authors	Intervention	Effect on Compliance	Effect on Blood pressure
Haynes et al.	Self-monitoring, cueing, frequent visits, rewards	+21%	Improved
Logan et al.	Worksite nurse, self-monitoring, cueing, recalls, frequent visits, rewards	+19%	Improved
Bass et al.	Cueing, recalls, frequent visits	+ 8%	Improved
Takala et al.	Written instruction, monitoring cards, recalls	+15%	Improved
Levine et al.	Counseling, social support, group discussions	Increased	Improved
Nessman et al.	Self-monitoring, group discussion, self-management	+19%	Improved
Swain et al.	Instruction, contingency contracts	+28%	Improved

maneuvers. We will return to the theoretical underpinnings and a practical formulation after a description of the effective strategies.

In 1976, Haynes and colleagues (52) reported that compliance could be improved and blood pressure lowered among uncontrolled, noncompliant hypertensives by a complex intervention with a non–health professional research assistant helping patients at their worksite to plan taking their medication in concert with usual daily activities ("cueing" or "tailoring"); teaching them to monitor their own blood pressure and compliance at home; and rewarding patients for higher compliance and blood pressure improvements by praising their efforts, allowing them to earn credits toward purchasing their blood pressure monitoring equipment, and reducing the frequency of their follow-up visits. The research assistant was not allowed to change medications but could notify the patient's physician if compliance appeared to be high without blood pressure being controlled. This "kitchen sink" approach resulted in a statistically significant, absolute 21% increase in compliance compared with that of control patients who received usual care for their physicians. Blood pressures improved significantly within the intervention group but the difference compared with the control group was not significant.

Logan and colleagues (53) used the same compliance procedures, also administered at the worksite, but in this study they were administered by nurses who also made changes in medications in consultation with the study physician. Control patients were simply referred to their family physicians for continuing care. Again there was a significant improvement in compliance in comparison with that of control patients, but this time there was also a statistically significant improvement in blood pressure control in favor of the intervention group patients. Although this intervention was quite elaborate, a full economic analysis showed that it was cost-effective in comparison with usual community care by primary care physicians (54).

The study of Bass and colleagues (55) changed the venue to family physicians' offices, with practice nurses working in an extended role with the physician, screening patients for hypertension and helping hypertensive patients to achieve high compliance through instruction, cueing, recalling of patients who missed appointments, and seeing some patients on extra visits. There was a modest improvement in compliance among intervention group patients compared with patients in control practices, and a small, statistically significant difference in systolic but not diastolic blood pressure at the end of the 4-year follow-up observation in the trial.

Several other investigations have used similarly elaborate approaches, with additional innovations, including social support and group discussions for hypertensive patients (50,56) and contingency contracts in which patients agreed to do specific tasks (e.g., showing up at clinic on time) for simple rewards (e.g., being seen on time!) (57). Of interest, in the latter study, few patients contracted to take their pills more often. Nevertheless, the dropout rate was substantially reduced and blood pressures were lowered. One of these studies (50) also showed a reduced mortality rate among patients receiving the compliance enhancement program, compared with that of controls, when the patients were followed over a 5-year period (58).

Almost all trials of what proved to be successful compliance strategies used very complicated interventions, too complex to use in most practice settings, but the studies of failed compliance strategies showed that simple, single strategies are ineffective (47–51). Is there a middle ground? A Finnish study by Takala and colleagues (59) was the first to demonstrate the success of a complex but practical approach. Patients in a community health center were given simple written information and instructions about their high blood pressure and its treatment, treatment cards on which their blood pressures and medications were recorded and amended at follow-up visits, and telephone recalls if they missed appointments. The dropout rate over 1 year was reduced from 19% in the control group to 4% in the intervention group, and significantly more intervention group patients had improvements in blood pressure. Keeping patients in care is of paramount importance and recalling nonattenders is likely the most important single intervention, although the weight of evidence would suggest that recalls would have limited effectiveness if they were the only compliance maneuver.

The descriptions of compliance interventions in reports of individual studies can leave the reader in a state of confusion about what works and what does not, particularly as the studies have come from researchers of a number of different scientific disciplines, including psychology, sociology, health education, and clinical epidemiology, each with its own jargon. Some theories of compliance behavior can clarify this situation and lead to practical generalizations.

B. Theories of Compliance and Their Practical Application

As described by Leventhal and Cameron (60), theories from psychology can provide a basis for classifying compliance strategies and understanding why certain strategies work while others do not. A full discussion of the current theories is beyond the scope of this chapter, but a simple framework classifies compliance interventions into three broad categories: cognitive, behavioral, and social support (46). Cognitive factors include what the patient knows about the disease and its treatment. Behavioral factors include the reminders and rewards a patient receives to comply with appointments and prescribed therapy. Social support is a more nebulous concept but includes the emotional support and encouragement that patients receive from their family, friends, and health professionals to help them cope with their disorder and its treatment. It is important to bear in mind that no single intervention has been shown to maintain long-term compliance; one must combine strategies from two or more of these three categories to achieve success.

1. Practical Cognitive Strategies

The cognitive aspect of most importance to compliance is what the patient understands about the details of following the regimen. The schedule of pill taking, what to do if pills are missed or delayed, what common side effects may occur, what serious side effects should be watched for, and what to do when the first prescription is running out are far more important than information about the nature of the disease and the mechanics of how the treatment works. (This is not to say that information about the disease and its treatment should not be made available to patients if they wish it, but that such information will not help improve long-term compliance and may compete with the vital information the patient needs to follow the regimen.) Information should be provided in the form of clear, simple instructions about the schedule of medication and its duration. To ensure that the necessary information has been understood, key instructions should be provided both verbally and in written form, asking the patient to verify that he or she understands the instructions. Common misconceptions should be anticipated and avoided, including that the medication can be stopped when the blood pressure is controlled, that different medications cannot be taken together at the same time of day, and that feeling tense or relaxed is a guide to when to take the medication.

At the heart of simple instructions is a simple regimen. Medications that can be given once a day are best (61–63). For patients who require more than one medication, all should be prescribed to be taken at the same time if this is consistent with therapeutic activity. (Patients often make their own regimens unnecessarily complicated by spreading their pills over the day.) If clinically sensible, combination medications may help. Mixing nondrug and drug treatments may be appropriate therapeutically but can be confusing for the patient. Despite the enthusiasm for their use shown by authors of preceding chapters, nondrug treatments are also harder for patients to follow and probably should be reserved for highly motivated patients or introduced after blood pressure is brought under control as a possible means of reducing medication (1).

2. Behavioral Strategies

Behavioral interventions are the most important ingredients of any compliance improvement program (46), the two main forms are cues (reminders) and rewards (reinforcements). Reminders of various sorts are important to keep the patient on track. Reminders about upcoming appointments can reduce nonattendance, and if patients miss appointments, they should be contacted as soon as possible (64,65). Medication should be prescribed in concert with constant features of the patient's daily schedule so that events such as brushing one's teeth act as cues to take a pill that has been prescribed at that time of day (66). Pill organizers (available at all pharmacies) also help to remind patients to take their pills and enable them to see whether they have done so.

To reward compliance, the practitioner's recognition of, and praise for, the patient's efforts to comply at each visit provide potent reinforcement. The importance of compliance should be stressed at each visit (this need take only a few seconds). Some patients need to be seen more frequently than others to ensure adequate compliance. On follow-up evaluation, if a patient's blood pressure control seems to have slipped, rather than attempting to adjust medication, the practitioner should ask the patient to return in a week and to be sure to take every pill during the week. If the blood pressure is down at the next visit, the relationship between compliance and blood pressure response to medication should be reinforced and the length of time between visits increased. If the blood pressure is still elevated and the patient indicates full compliance, then an adjustment in medication may be appropriate.

Often in practice it will not be clear whether the patient has taken the medication or not. A reasonable substitute is to base rewards on the blood pressure. The patient should be given feedback about the blood pressure, with praise if he or she has done well or encouragement to do better if the blood pressure is not controlled. Having patients monitor their own blood pressure at home may provide a useful basis for such discussions. Home monitoring has been shown to help improve compliance and lower blood pressure when combined with reinforcement from the physician (66) but does not improve compliance or blood pressure if the patient does this without subsequent discussion and reinforcement from the health care provider (47). Finally, the patient can be rewarded for high compliance and good blood pressure control by a negotiated decrease in visit frequency.

3. Social Support

Fostering social support for the patient constitutes the third route through which compliance can be enhanced (50). The patient's family and friends can help or hinder compliance. Having a chronic disorder such as hypertension is a worrisome nuisance that most people would prefer to ignore. Worse, it can also drain family resources and reduce a person's self-esteem. Frequently patients' families are far from useful allies in helping them to cope with their treatments. The family may treat the patient as if he or she is ill or fragile or may convey the notion that the disorder is the patient's "fault" because he or she is not coping properly with stress.

A word from the physician to one or more members of the family may help them become "part of the solution." Unfortunately, our understanding of family dynamics in general and of the dynamics of a specific patient's family in particular is very limited, and involving the patient's family may have unpredictable effects. At least, the patient should be consulted before there is any attempt to involve his or her family in managing the patient's medical problems. With the patient's permission, then, the family can be asked to help by reminding the patient to take the medication at times he or she is likely to forget, by providing positive reinforcement for following the treatment, by taking and recording the patient's blood pressure at home, and by helping the patient to remember and attend appointments.

C. Research Implications and Directions

Research involving antihypertensive treatments that are self-administered must include compliance measurement, and, if the research question is one of the efficacy of the treatment, methods of enhancing patient compliance must be included in the follow-up of patients in all groups being compared. Patients must not be "lost to follow-up" if at all possible, and analyses of data based on "compliers" are inherently flawed because noncompliers differ from compliers in important ways that go beyond merely failing to take the medication (67).

Research into strategies to measure and enhance patient compliance with long-term regimens flourished in the 1970s and early 1980s, partly stimulated by documentation of the benefits of antihypertensive therapy and the demonstration that noncompliance reduced the benefits for most patients to a modest fraction of that possible. Much useful information was generated by these studies, but they fell short of providing easily administered, highly effective monitoring and intervention strategies. Since the early 1980s, little new information has been found and the research effort has lagged (68). With the recent advent of so many new, effective treatments for chronic medical disorders, there are substantial need and opportunity for innovation and new research into compliance. This may require interdisciplinary teams, including psychologists, sociologists, and medical scientists, to gain new understandings of the problems so that better ways of dealing with them can be developed. Alternatively, obviating the problems of compliance may await basic research into hypertension leading to treatments that cure or treatment formulations that have ultraprolonged actions, reducing the opportunities for noncompliance.

VI. DISCUSSION

When antihypertensive therapy is prescribed, assisting the patient with compliance must be part of the treatment plan. Most compliance problems can be detected by watching for nonattendance or failure to respond to treatment or by asking those who do not respond about their compliance in a nonthreatening but direct way. In research, more accurate measurements are required and include home-visit pill counts, prescription refill monitoring, memory-cap pill containers, and drug or tracer levels in body fluids. Inadequate measurement and management of compliance in research can produce misleading results.

None of the strategies for improving compliance is very effective on its own. A simple package that will work includes keeping the regimen as simple as possible; giving clear instructions, with periodic checks to ensure understanding; calling the patient when an appointment is missed; discussing at each visit any problems the patient is having with the regimen; and congratulating patients for what they have been able to accomplish even if this is not perfect.

ACKNOWLEDGMENT

Dr. Haynes has a career scientist award from the National Health Research and Development Program of the Department of Health of Canada. G. A. Haynes assisted with the preparation of the manuscript.

REFERENCES

1. Haynes RB. Determinants of compliance: the disease and the mechanics of treatment. In: Haynes RB, Taylor DW, Sackett DL ed. Compliance in Health Care. Baltimore: Johns Hopkins University Press, 1979.

2. Haynes RB, Taylor DW, Sackett DL, eds. Compliance in Health Care. Baltimore: Johns Hopkins University Press, 1979.
3. Sackett DL, Snow JC. The magnitude of compliance and noncompliance. In: Haynes RB, Taylor DW, Sackett DL eds. Compliance in Health Care. Baltimore: Johns Hopkins University Press, 1979:11-22.
4. Carey R, Reid R, Ayers C, et al. The Charlottesville blood pressure survey: value of repeated blood pressure measurements. JAMA 1976; 236:847-851.
5. Wilbur JA, Barrow JG. Hypertension: a community problem. Am J Med 1972; 52:653-663.
6. Hedstrand H, Aberg H. Treatment of hypertension in middle-aged men. Acta Med Scand 1976; 199:281-288.
7. Langfeld SB. Hypertension: deficient care of the medically served. Ann Intern Med 1973; 78:19-23.
8. Haynes RB, Sackett DL, Gibson ES, et al. Improvement of medication compliance in uncontrolled hypertension. Lancet 1976; 1:1265-1268.
9. Sackett DL, Haynes RB, Gibson ES, et al. Randomized clinical trial of strategies of improving medication compliance in primary hypertension. Lancet 1975; 1:1205-1207.
10. Garb JR, Stunkard AJ. Effectiveness of a self-help group in obesity control: a further assessment. Arch Intern Med 1974; 134:716-720.
11. Wilson DM, Taylor DW, Gilbert JR, et al. A randomized trial of a family physician intervention for smoking cessation. JAMA 1988; 260:1570-1574.
12. Birkett NJ, Evans CE, Haynes RB, et al. Hypertension control in two Canadian communities: evidence for better treatment and overlabelling. J Hypertens 1986; 4:369-374.
13. Baekeland F, Lundwall L, Shanahan TJ. Correlates of patient attrition in the outpatient treatment of alcoholism. J Nerv Ment Dis 1973; 157:99-107.
14. Nelson A, Gold B, Hutchinson R, Benezra E. Drug default among schizophrenic patients. Am J Hosp Pharm 1975; 32:1237-1242.
15. Finnerty FA, Mattie EC. Hypertension in the inner city. I. Analysis of clinic dropouts. Circulation 1973; 47:73-75.
16. Gates SJ, Colborn DK. Lowering appointment failures in a neighbourhood health centre. Med Care 1976; 14:263-267.
17. Hoenig F, Ragg N. The non-attending psychiatric outpatient: an administrative problem. Med Care 1966; 4:96-100.
18. Alpert JJ. Broken appointments. Pediatrics 1964; 34:127-132.
19. Geersten HR, Gray RM, Ward JR. Patient noncompliance within the context of seeking medical care for arthritis. J Chronic Dis 1973; 26:689-698.
20. Brand F, Smith R, Brand P. Effect of economic barriers to medical care on patients' noncompliance. Public Health Rep 1977; 92:72-78.
21. Clinite JC, Kabat HF. Prescribed drugs, errors during self-administration. J Am Pharm Assoc 1969; NS9:450-452.
22. Glick BS. Dropout in an outpatient, double-blind drug study. Psychosomatics 1965; 6:44-48.
23. Gordis L, Markowitz M. Evaluation of the effectiveness of comprehensive and continuous pediatric care. Pediatrics 1971; 48:766-776.

24. Hemminki E, Heikkila J. Elderly people's compliance with prescriptions, and quality of medication. Scand J Soc Med 1975; 3:87–92.
25. Stuart RB. Behavioral control of overeating. Behav Res Ther 1967; 5:357–365.
26. Gilbert JR, Evans CE, Haynes RB, Tugwell P. Predicting compliance with a regimen of digoxin therapy in family practice. Can Med Assoc J 1980; 123:119–122.
27. Bowen RG, Rich R, Schlotfeldt RM. Effects of organized instruction for patients with the diagnosis of diabetes mellitus. Nurs Res 1961; 10:151–159.
28. Gordis L, Markowitz M, Lilienfeld AM. Studies in the epidemiology and preventability of rheumatic fever. IV. A quantitative determination of compliance in children on oral penicillin prophylaxis. Pediatrics 1969; 43:173–182.
29. Moulding TS, Halper AR, Mkutu MP, Halper S. Self-administration of isoniazid and thiacetazone studied by the medication monitor. Unpublished paper.
30. Ritson B. Involvement in treatment and its relation to outcome amongst alcoholics. Br J Addict 1969; 64:23–29.
31. Haynes RB, Taylor DW, Sackett DL, et al. Can simple clinical measurements detect patient noncompliance? Hypertension 1980; 2:757–764.
32. Stephenson BJ, Rowe BH, Macharia WM, et al. Is this patient taking their medication? JAMA 1993; 269:2779–2781.
33. Frisk PA, Cooper JW, Campbell NA. Community-hospital pharmacist detection of drug-related problems upon patient admission to small hospitals. Am J Hosp Pharm 1977; 34:738–742.
34. Hammel RW, Williams PO. Do patients receive prescribed medication? Am Pharm Assoc J 1964; 4:331–334.
35. McKenney JM, Slining JM, Henderson HR, et al. The effect of clinical pharmacy services on patients with essential hypertension. Circulation 1973; 48:1104–1111.
36. Gupta RN, Haynes RB, Logan AG, et al. Liquid-chromatographic determination of nadolol in plasma. Clin Chem 1983; 29:1085–1087.
37. Briggs WA, Lowenthal DT, Cirksena WJ, et al. Propranolol in hypertensive dialysis patients: efficacy and compliance. Clin Pharmacol Ther 1975; 18:606–612.
38. Porter AM. Drug defaulting in a general practice. Br Med J 1969; 1:218–222.
39. Maenpaa H, Manninen V, Heinonen OP. Compliance with medication in the Helsinki Heart Study. Eur J Clin Pharmacol 1992; 42:15–19.
40. Rudd P, Ahmed S, Zachary V, et al. Improved compliance measures: applications in an ambulatory hypertensive drug trial. Clin Pharmacol Ther 1990; 48: 676–685.
41. Haynes RB, Lacourciere Y, Rabkin SW, et al. Practice guidelines for the diagnosis of hypertension in adults: Report of the Canadian Hypertension Society Consensus Conference Committee on Diagnosis. Can Med Assoc J 1993; 149: 409–418.
42. Medical Research Council Working Party. MRC trial of treatment of mild hypertension: principal results. Br Med J 1985; 291:97–104.
43. Collins R, Peto R, MacMahon S, et al. Blood pressure, stroke, and coronary heart disease. Part 2. Short-term reductions in blood pressure: overview of randomised drug trials in their epidemiological context. Lancet 1990; 335:827–838.

44. National Heart, Lung and Blood Institute Working Group on Patient Compliance. Management of patient compliance in the treatment of hypertension. Hypertension 1982; 4:415–423.
45. Logan AG, Haynes RB. Determinants of physicians' competence in the management of hypertension. J Hypertens 1986; 4(suppl 5):S367–S369.
46. Haynes RB, Wang E, Da Mota Gomes M. A critical review of interventions for improved compliance with prescribed medications. Patient Educ Counsel 1987; 10:155–166.
47. Johnson AL, Taylor DW, Sackett DL, et al. Self-recording of blood pressure in the management of hypertension. Can Med Assoc J 1978; 119:1034–1039.
48. Shepard DS, Foster SB, Stason WB, et al. Cost-effectiveness of interventions to improve compliance with antihypertensive therapy. Prev Med 1979; 8:229.
49. Sackett DL, Haynes RB, Gibson ES, et al. Randomized clinical trial of strategies for improving medication compliance in primary hypertension. Lancet 1975; 1:1205–1207.
50. Levine DM, Green LW, Deeds SG, et al. Health education for hypertensive patients. JAMA 1979; 241:1700–1703.
51. Becker LA, Glanz K, Sobel E, et al. A randomized trial of special packaging for antihypertensive medications. J Fam Pract 1986; 22:357–361.
52. Haynes RB, Sackett DL, Gibson ES, et al. Improvement of medication compliance in uncontrolled hypertension. Lancet 1976; 2:1265–1268.
53. Logan AS, Milne BJ, Achber C, et al. Treatment of hypertensive patients at the worksite by specially-trained nurses: a controlled trial. Lancet 1979; 2:1175–1178.
54. Logan AS, Milne BJ, Achber C, et al. Cost-effectiveness of a worksite hypertension treatment program. Hypertension 1981; 3:211–218.
55. Bass MJ, McWhinney IR, Donner A. Do family physicians need medical assistants to detect and manage hypertension? Can Med Assoc J 1986; 134:1247–1255.
56. Nessman DG, Carnahan JE, Nugent CA. Increasing compliance: patient operated hypertension groups. Arch Intern Med 1980; 140:1427–1431.
57. Swain MA, Steckel SB. Influencing adherence among hypertensives. Res Nurs Health 1981; 4:213–218.
58. Morisky D. Five-year blood pressure control and mortality following health education for hypertensive patients. Am J Public Health 1983; 73:153–162.
59. Takala J, Niemela N, Rosti J, Sivers K. Improving compliance with therapeutic regimens in hypertensive patients in a community health center. Circulation 1979; 59:540–543.
60. Leventhal H, Cameron L. Behavioral theories and the problem of compliance. Patient Educ Counsel 1987; 10:117–138.
61. Tinkelman DG, Vanderpool GE, Carroell MS. Compliance differences following administration of theophylline at six and twelve hour intervals. Ann Allergy 1980; 44:283–286.
62. Baird MG, Bentley-Taylor MM, Carruthers SG, et al. A study of the efficacy tolerance and compliance of once-daily versus twice-daily metoprolol (Betaloc^{R}) in hypertension. Clin Invest Med 1984; 7:95–102.

63. Taggart AJ, Johnston GD, McDevitt DG. Does the frequency of daily dosage influence compliance with digoxin therapy? Br J Clin Pharmacol 1981; 1:31–34.
64. Takala J, Niemela N, Rosti J, Sivers K. Improving compliance with therapeutic regimens in hypertensive patients in a community health center. Circulation 1979; 59:540–543.
65. Macharia WM, Leon G, Rowe BH, et al. An overview of interventions to improve appointment keeping for medical services. JAMA 1992; 267:1813–1817.
66. Haynes RB, Sackett DL, Gibson ES, et al. Improvement of medication compliance in uncontrolled hypertension. Lancet 1976; 1:1265–1268.
67. Haynes RB, Dantes R. Patient compliance and the design and interpretation of clinical trials. Controlled Clin Trials 1987; 8:12–19.
68. Haynes RB. Patient compliance then and now (editorial). Patient Educ Counsel 1987; 10:103–105.

Index

About the Editors

NORMAN M. KAPLAN is Professor of Internal Medicine at the University of Texas Southwestern Medical Center at Dallas. A Fellow of the American College of Physicians' Council for High Blood Pressure Research and Council for Cardiovascular Epidemiology, he is the author or coauthor of over 300 professional papers that reflect his research interests in the clinical aspects of hypertension. A recipient of the National Institutes of Health Academic Award for the teaching of preventive cardiology, Dr. Kaplan received the M.D. degree (1954) from the University of Texas Southwestern Medical School, Dallas.

C. VENKATA S. RAM is Professor of Internal Medicine at the University of Texas Southwestern Medical Center at Dallas, Director of the Hypertension Clinic at Parkland Memorial Hospital and of the Hypertension Unit at St. Paul Medical Center, Dallas, Texas. The author or coauthor of more than 150 professional papers, he is a Fellow of the American College of Cardiology, the American College of Chest Phyusicians, the Council of High Blood Pressure Research of the American Heart Association, the American College of Clinical Pharmacology, and the American College of Physicians, and a member of many other organizations. Dr. Ram received the M.D. degree (1972) from Osmania University, Hyderabad, India. He undertook his residency and fellowship training at the Rhode Island Hospital, Providence, and at the Hospital of the University of Pennsylvania, Philadelphia. He is a Diplomate of the American Board of Internal Medicine.